Interventional Spine and Joint

A Fluoroscopic Atlas and...
Business Primer For The Pain Proceduralist

TERMS/ABBREVIATIONS

ACDF anterior cervical discectomy and fusion

AP articular pillar

A/P x-ray beam passes from anterior to posterior

CAUDAL TILT image intensifier toward patient's feet

CEPHALAD TILT image intensifier toward patient's head

CESI cervical interlaminar epidural steroid injection

CLO contralateral oblique

CSF cerebrospinal fluid

DRG dorsal root ganglion

ESI epidural steroid injection

GTB greater trochanteric bursa

IAP inferior articular process

IEP inferior endplate

IVF intervertebral foramen

LESI lumbar interlaminar epidural steroid injection

LF ligamentum flavum

LOR loss of resistance

MBB medial branch block

P/A x-ray beam passes from posterior to anterior

PILL posterior interlaminar line

PLIF posterior lumbar interbody fusion

RFNA radiofrequency nerve ablation

SAP superior articular process

SCS spinal cord stimulation

SEP superior endplate

SI sacroiliac

SNRB selective nerve root block

SP spinous process

TESI thoracic interlaminar epidural steroid injection

TFESI transforaminal epidural steroid injection

TON third occipital nerve

TP transverse process

VILL ventral interlaminar line

Cervical Levels
C1
C2
C3
C4
C5
C6
C7

Thoracic Levels
T1
T2
T3
T4
T5
T6
T7
T8
T9
T10
T11
T12

Lumbar Levels
L1
L2
L3
L4
L5

Sacral Levels
S1
S2
S3
S4
S5

Interventional Spine and Joint

A Fluoroscopic Atlas and...
Business Primer For The Pain Proceduralist

Albert G. Singh, M.D.
Director Interventional Spine & Pain
Suri Medical, LLC
www.surimedical.com

SURI

MEDICAL

SURI
MEDICAL

INTERVENTIONAL SPINE AND JOINT, A FLUOROSCOPIC ATLAS AND
BUSINESS PRIMER FOR THE PAIN PROCEDURALIST

NOTICES

Medicine is an ever-changing science and further research and clinical experience may necessitate the change in professional practices. The author and publisher have made every effort to ensure that all information and advice in this book is true and accurate at the date of publication. Nevertheless, neither the publisher nor author gives a warranty, express or implied, with respect to the material contained herein or for any errors or omissions that may have been made. Every reader should examine carefully the package inserts accompanying each drug and should carefully check whether the dosage schedules mentioned therein or the contraindications stated by the manufacturer differ from the statements made in this book. It is the responsibility of practitioners, relying on their own experience and knowledge of their patients, to make diagnoses, to determine dosages and the best treatment for each individual patient, and to take all appropriate safety precautions.

Practitioners and researchers must always rely on their own experience and knowledge in evaluating and using any information, methods, compounds, or experiments described herein. In using such information or methods, they should be mindful of their own safety and the safety of others, including parties for whom they have a professional responsibility.

To the fullest extent of the law, neither the publisher nor the author, assume any liability for any injury and/or damage to persons or property as a matter of products liability, negligence or otherwise, or from any use or operation of any methods, products, instructions, or ideas contained in the material herein.

To Rassmita for her love and companionship.
To Livya for her enthusiasm.
To Jenica for her support.
To Mom and Dad, who taught me to aim high.

To all of my previous educators – Without your guidance and instruction, this project would not have been possible.

To all of the fellows I have had the pleasure of teaching – Continue to learn, prepare, and care!

To all of the patients that I have had the honor of caring for, either directly or indirectly – Thank you!

Preface

"The conditions necessary for the Surgeon [the Proceduralist] are four; First, he should be learned; Second, he should be expert; Third, he must be ingenious; and Fourth, he should be able to adapt himself."
–Guy de Chauliac, *Ars Chirurgica*

Now, more than ever, the field of Interventional Pain requires "The Proceduralist" to satisfy all of the aforementioned conditions. With the increasing concerns surrounding effective and safe management of pain conditions, it is the proceduralist's moral responsibility to be learned, knowledgeable, expert, and at times ingenious, on ways to effectively perform interventional pain techniques, allowing for excellent patient outcomes with less reliance on medications possessing potentially harmful long-term effects.

This textbook is not meant to serve as a substitute for proper training in the field of Interventional Pain Medicine, but rather as a supplemental guide for those who have properly been trained in the specialty. By no means should any of the procedures discussed in this book be performed by inexperienced physicians or those who have not had formal training or do not have an understanding of anatomy, indications, and contraindications to each procedure discussed.

My primary goal when starting this textbook was to provide **multiple "real world" examples each** of several of the more commonly performed procedures in the field of Interventional Pain. The impetus for this endeavor came from the realization that, to date, there has been no comprehensive reference that presents multiple examples each for a given procedure while also providing **specific fluoroscopic angles** needed to obtain an ideal view. Over the years, my patients have given me the privilege of learning from them, and honing my procedural skills as I encountered varying and unexpected anatomical presentations. With this textbook, the reader can now reference precise fluoroscopic angle adjustments, with an accompanying explanation, to obtain the ideal view for a wide collection of varying anatomy.

In the atlas part of this book, each chapter begins by presenting a step-by-step guide on how to perform the procedure discussed. This is followed by multiple "real world" patient examples, taken from my practice over the years, which fluoroscopically walk the reader through each mentioned procedural step – providing exact angles of obliquity and cephalocaudal tilting along the way. The reasoning behind each fluoroscopic angular adjustment is presented in detail such that the proceduralist may gain a better understanding of how to obtain an ideal radiologic view – *which very often is more than half the battle.* For many chapters, a concluding "additional discussion" section is also provided to further examine **key concepts** and offer **procedural pearls**.

The second part of this textbook focuses on the business side of medicine. Having solely been in private practice, over time I have come to appreciate the intricacies of the business side of medicine, which is often omitted in formal medical training. Thus, in this section, I have strived to once again present **"real world" pricing, reimbursement, and profit analysis** – based upon actual data from my private practice – for each procedure discussed in part one of this textbook. Moreover, the reader will note that each unique procedure from part 1 of this textbook is cross-referenced to part 2 by a green box indicating the connecting page number. It is my hope that the proceduralist may use this information to gain a practical understanding of the business of an Interventional Pain practice.

My passion for teaching and improving patient outcomes fueled the creation of this textbook. It is my hope that you, as my colleague, will find procedural concepts that can be applied to your practice – thereby allowing this book to serve patients on a macro level. I encourage you to send me comments at textbook@surimedical.com.

Albert G. Singh, M.D.

Author Biography

Albert G. Singh, M.D. received his Bachelors in Science in Electrical Engineering from Purdue University, with a special focus on biomedical engineering. He completed his internship, residency training in Physical Medicine & Rehabilitation, and Interventional Pain fellowship training from the Indiana University School of Medicine. He has been in private practice since 2012.

Dr. Singh is board certified in Physical Medicine and Rehabilitation and Pain Medicine. He is the founder, CEO, and medical director of Suri Medical LLC, and provides care in both Indiana and Illinois. He has been involved in the education and training of fellows and established physicians in interventional pain techniques, and serves as a consultant on the product advisory board of one of the largest biotechnology companies in the world. Dr. Singh's area of interest includes the diagnosis and treatment of musculoskeletal and spinal disorders, with a key focus on the use of neuromodulation to treat complex pain patterns. He has lectured extensively at the local, national, and international level on using advanced interventional pain therapies to treat complex spinal pain.

In addition to clinical practice, Dr. Singh's interests also lie in research. He has served as a principal investigator on prospective clinical outcomes studies pertaining to radiofrequency nerve ablation. He has also been published in numerous research articles and textbooks, including "Sports Medicine & Rehabilitation: A Sport-Specific Approach" and "Musculoskeletal, Sports, and Occupational Medicine."

Dr. Singh enjoys teaching on interventional spine and peripheral joint treatment, procedural risk mitigation strategies, and billing/coding. In addition, having been in a private practice setting for nearly a decade, Dr. Singh has a passion for educating on the business side of medicine. He has been a national recipient of the "Outstanding 50 Asian Americans in Business" award and was selected as a "Top 40 under 40" in Indianapolis.

Albert G. Singh, M.D.

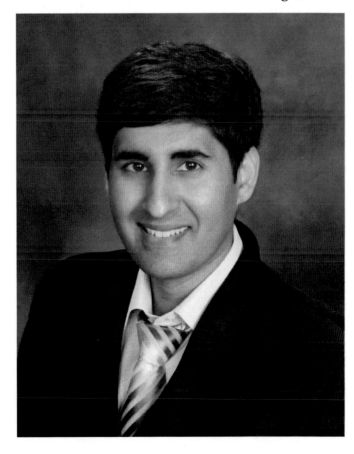

Contents

Fluoroscopic Atlas

Chapter 1
Lumbar Transforaminal Epidural Steroid Injection

- Obtain an A/P view and, if needed, oblique such that the spinous process at the targeted level is midline and equally spaced between the left and right pedicles – "True A/P" view.

- Apply cephalocaudal tilting as needed to square off the endplates at the targeted vertebral level – if both the SEP & IEP cannot be squared simultaneously, preference should be given to squaring the SEP. This step allows the needle to be parallel to the endplates and the pedicles – providing the best opportunity for the needle tip to enter the superior aspect of the foramen, and away from the exiting nerve root (see page 39 for further discussion). *Of note, cephalocaudal tilting of the C-arm can also be done in the next step (i.e., the oblique view) – see below.*

- Oblique the C-arm ipsilaterally until the SAP below the targeted foramen is at, or just medial to, the 6 o'clock position of the pedicle above. *As a rule of thumb, begin with an ipsilateral oblique of 20° from the "True A/P" view, as this angle of obliquity works well in many instances – but NOT always (see page 42 for further discussion).* Place the needle in a coaxial view (i.e., parallel to the fluoroscopic beam – see Figure 1-3D) just inferior to the 6 o'clock position of the pedicle above the targeted foramen, which will ultimately allow the needle tip to enter the superior foramen. The needle is advanced until it approaches the foramen – at this depth one may often feel a subtle increase in resistance. *If there is any question regarding needle depth during advancement in this view, intermittent A/P fluoroscopy may be used to assess needle positioning (see below).*

- Once the needle approaches the foramen in the prior oblique view, obtain an A/P view and ensure that the needle is not advanced any further than the lateral border of the vertebral body. *If the needle is not seen to be at this position, use intermittent oblique fluoroscopy to advance the needle to this desired position.* Further needle advancement is performed in the lateral view where needle depth can be better assessed (see below).

- In the lateral view, further advance the needle carefully into the superior and posterior half of the foramen – away from the exiting nerve root.

- Finally, obtain an A/P view to confirm needle positioning. As a rule of thumb, in this view the needle should be typically seen no further medial than the 6 o'clock position of the pedicle, to prevent puncturing the dura. *At times, the needle tip may be slightly medial to this position depending upon patient positioning, varying spinal anatomy, foraminal stenosis, a "non-true" A/P, etc.*

- After negative aspiration, administer contrast under live fluoroscopy and ensure that there is no vascular uptake with a proper neurogram and epidurogram – *see Page 44.*

Right L4-L5

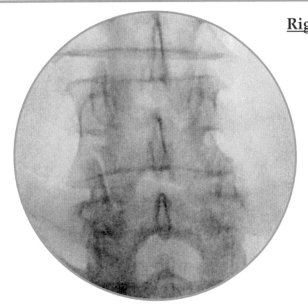

Figure 1-1A
Tilt: 0°
Oblique: 0°

A/P View. The spinous process looks fairly midline, and the L4 SEP fairly squared. Squaring the SEP above the targeted foramen allows for an open view of the neural foramen, and sets up the needle trajectory for placement in the superior foramen.

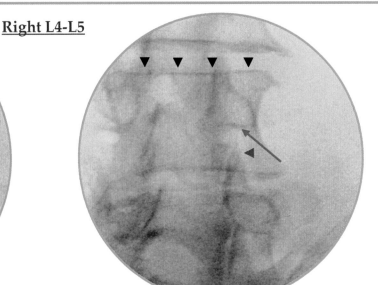

Figure 1-1B
Tilt: 0°
Oblique: 20° Right

Oblique View. Oblique ipsilaterally until the tip of the SAP below the foramen (red arrowhead) is at, or just medial to, the 6 o'clock position of the pedicle above (blue arrow). Additionally, reconfirm that the L4 SEP is squared (black arrowheads).

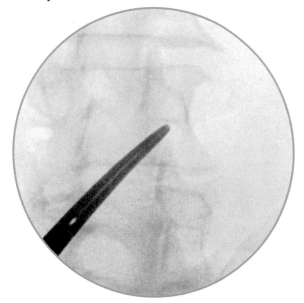

Figure 1-1C
Tilt: 0°
Oblique: 20° Right

Oblique View. Pointer showing location of ideal needle placement – just inferior to the 6 o'clock position of the pedicle at the targeted neural foramen.

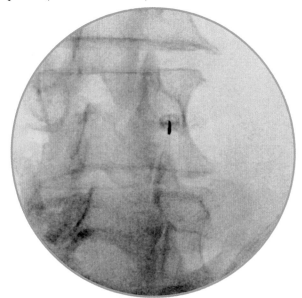

Figure 1-1D
Tilt: 0°
Oblique: 20° Right

Oblique View. Needle placed just inferior to the 6 o'clock position of the pedicle, which allows for the needle tip to remain in the superior foramen and away from the exiting spinal nerve. As the needle approaches the foramen, a subtle increase in resistance may be felt.

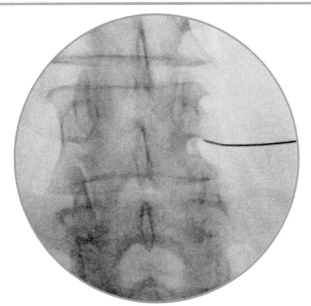

Figure 1-1E
Tilt: 0°
Oblique: 0°

A/P View. After noting a subtle increase in resistance with needle advancement in the prior oblique view, the needle tip is typically seen just lateral to the lateral border of the vertebral body in the A/P view – at this needle position, a lateral view is obtained.

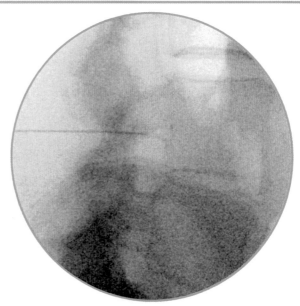

Figure 1-1F
Tilt: 0°
Oblique: 90° Right

Lateral View. The needle is advanced towards the superior aspect of the neural foramen (away from the exiting nerve root), and typically in the posterior half of the foramen.

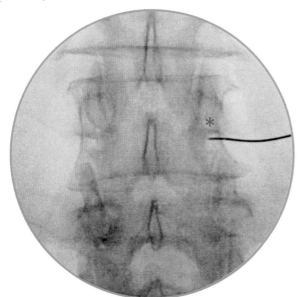

Figure 1-1G
Tilt: 0°
Oblique: 0°

A/P View. Once the needle has entered the neural foramen, the needle tip typically should be seen no further medial than approximately the 6 o'clock position of the pedicle above (blue star) to avoid dural puncture – *exceptions include stenosis and/or lack of a "true" A/P image.*

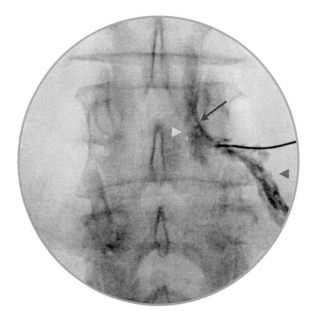

Figure 1-1H
Tilt: 0°
Oblique: 0°

A/P View. After negative aspiration, contrast is administered and shows an appropriate right L4 neurogram *(blue arrowhead)* and epidurogram *(yellow arrowhead)*. Contrast spread can be seen wrapping around the pedicle *(red arrow)* and entering the epidural space.

See Page 268

Right L4-L5
"Squaring the SEP"

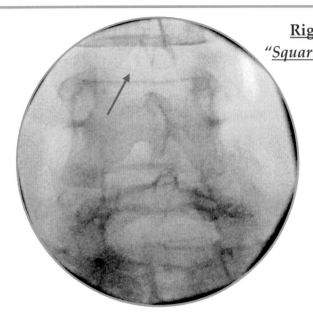

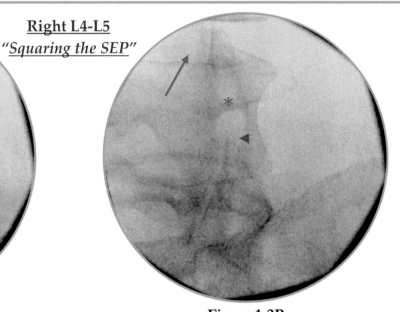

Figure 1-2A
Tilt: 0°
Oblique: 0°

Figure 1-2B
Tilt: 0°
Oblique: 30° Right

A/P View. Note that the L4 spinous process is slightly obliqued towards the right. Therefore, when obliquing for a right L4-L5 TFESI, one will likely need to oblique more than 20° to get the ideal view. Also, note that the L4 SEP is elliptical and not squared (blue arrow).

Oblique View. The SAP (red arrowhead) below the targeted neural foramen is seen to be at approximately the 6 o'clock position of the pedicle above (blue star) – ideal position. However, note the elliptical shape of the L4 SEP – indicating it is NOT squared (blue arrow).

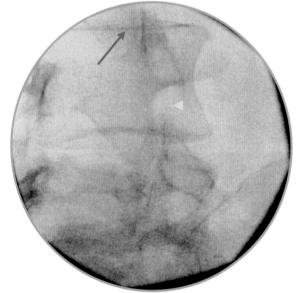

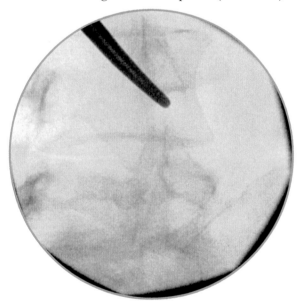

Figure 1-2C
Tilt: 10° Cephalad
Oblique: 30° Right

Figure 1-2D
Tilt: 10° Cephalad
Oblique: 30° Right

Oblique View. A cephalad tilt (image intensifier tilted towards patient's head) provides a more crisply squared SEP (blue arrow), and allows for a clearer view of the targeted neural foramen (yellow arrowhead). *Compare this SEP and view of the targeted neural foramen to Figure 1-2B.*

Oblique View. Pointer showing location of ideal needle placement – just inferior to the 6 o'clock position of the pedicle.

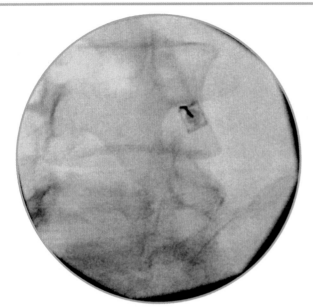

Figure 1-2E
Tilt: 10° Cephalad
Oblique: 30° Right

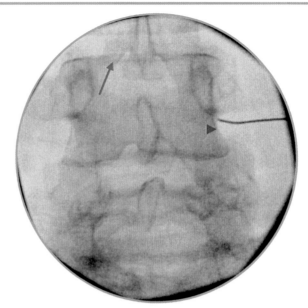

Figure 1-2F
Tilt: 10° Cephalad
Oblique: 5° Right

Oblique View. The needle is placed just inferior to the 6 o'clock position of the pedicle, allowing the needle tip to remain in the superior foramen. Once the needle approaches the foramen, one may feel some increased resistance, at which time an A/P view is obtained.

A/P View. The SEP is squared (blue arrow) and SP more midline for a "true" A/P view - *compare to Figure 1-2A*. Do not advance the needle beyond the lateral border of the vertebral body. Further advancement is carried out in the lateral view to assess needle depth.

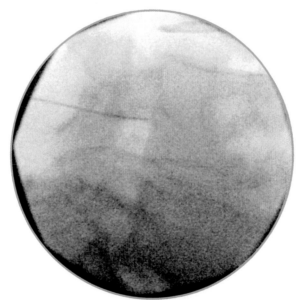

Figure 1-2G
Tilt: 0°
Oblique: 90° Right

Lateral View. One may feel a distinct "pop" as the needle tip enters its final position. By initially squaring the SEP, the needle trajectory remains parallel to the SEP and provides the best chance of placing the needle in the superior aspect of the foramen. Additionally, note that the needle tip is seen in the anterior aspect of the foramen in this case – *this may occur if the needle bevel is rotated more laterally during advancement, with varying patient anatomy/positioning, and/ or varying degrees of foraminal stenosis.*

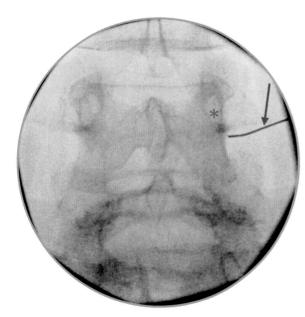

Figure 1-2H
Tilt: 0°
Oblique: 5° Right

A/P View. Note the needle's cephalocaudad trajectory (red arrow) without a fluoroscopic tilt to square the L4 SEP – *compare to Figure 1-2F*. If the needle is directed more laterally during advancement, the final position of the needle tip may be seen in the anterior foramen in the lateral view & lateral to the pedicle's 6 o'clock position (blue star) in the A/P view.

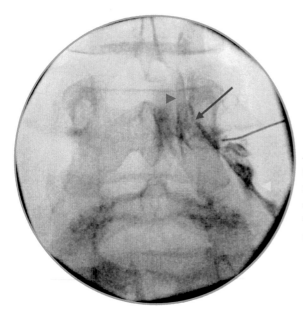

Figure 1-2I
Tilt: 0°
Oblique: 5° Right

A/P View. After negative aspiration, contrast is administered and shows an appropriate right L4 neurogram *(yellow arrowhead)* and epidurogram *(blue arrowhead)*. Appropriate contrast spread can be seen wrapping around the pedicle *(red arrow)* and entering the epidural space.

Left L4-L5 & L5-S1

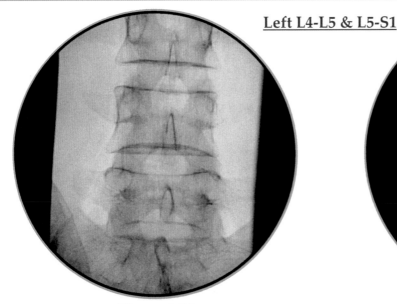

Figure 1-3A
Tilt: 0°
Oblique: 0°

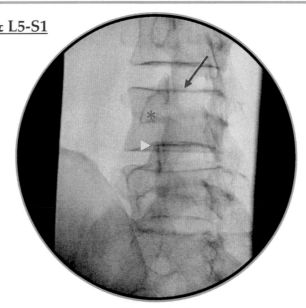

Figure 1-3B
Tilt: 0°
Oblique: 20° Left

A/P View. The spinous processes at L4 and L5 are approximately midline. Additionally, the L4 SEP looks fairly squared, but comparatively the L5 SEP does not. Thus, for the L4 vertebral level, no tilt is needed to obtain the proper view for optimal needle trajectory.

Oblique View. For the L4-L5 foramen, note that the SEP of L4 (red arrow) is confirmed to be fairly squared in this view. The SAP (yellow arrowhead) below the targeted neural foramen is just medial to the 6 o'clock position of the pedicle above (blue star) – ideal position.

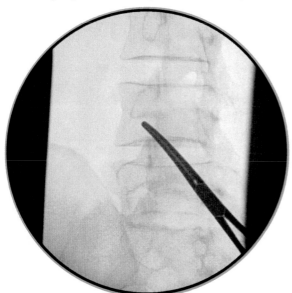

Figure 1-3C
Tilt: 0°
Oblique: 20° Left

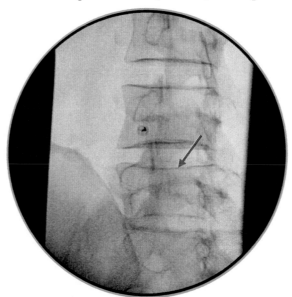

Figure 1-3D
Tilt: 0°
Oblique: 20° Left

Oblique View. Pointer showing the location of ideal needle placement just inferior to the 6 o'clock position of the left L4 pedicle.

Oblique View. Needle placed coaxially just inferior to the left L4 pedicle until a subtle increase in resistance is felt – *if not felt, use intermittent A/P fluoroscopy to keep the needle just lateral to the vertebral body.* For the left L5-S1 level, note that the L5 SEP is not squared (red arrow).

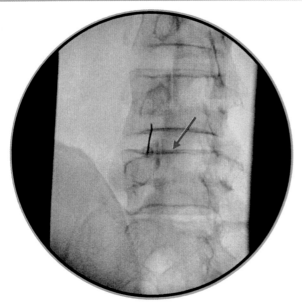

Figure 1-3E
Tilt: 10° Cephalad
Oblique: 20° Left

Oblique View. Tilting the C-arm cephalad (image intensifier towards patient's head) squares the L5 SEP (red arrow) – *compare to Figure 1-3D*. Additionally, note how the L5-S1 neural foramen is more clearly visualized with this tilt *(compare to Figure 1-3D).*

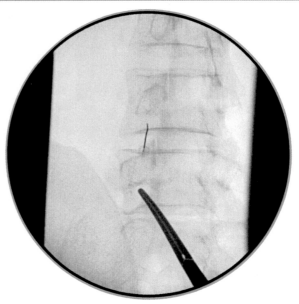

Figure 1-3F
Tilt: 10° Cephalad
Oblique: 20° Left

Oblique View. Pointer showing the location of ideal needle placement just inferior to the 6 o'clock position of the left L5 pedicle.

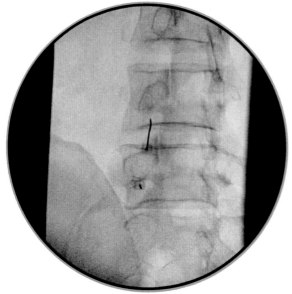

Figure 1-3G
Tilt: 10° Cephalad
Oblique: 20° Left

Oblique View. The needle is placed just inferior to the left L5 pedicle until a subtle increase in resistance is felt. *Of note, if an increase in resistance is not felt at the expected depth, one should check an A/P view as needed to ensure that the needle is not advanced beyond the lateral vertebral border.*

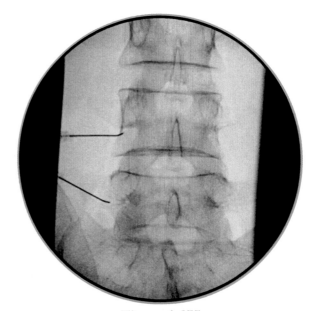

Figure 1-3H
Tilt: 0°
Oblique: 0°

A/P View. Note that this view is without a tilt, showing a non-squared L5 SEP. The needle tips are typically seen at approximately the lateral vertebral border. *If needed, the needle may be advanced deeper in the prior oblique view until this needle position is seen.* Next, a lateral view is obtained.

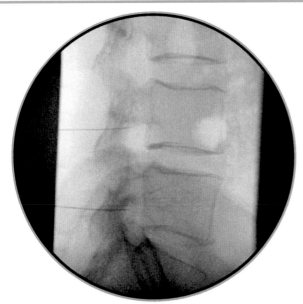

Figure 1-3I
Tilt: 0°
Oblique: 90° Right

Lateral View. Needle tips are advanced into the superior and posterior half of the L4-L5 and L5-S1 neural foramen.

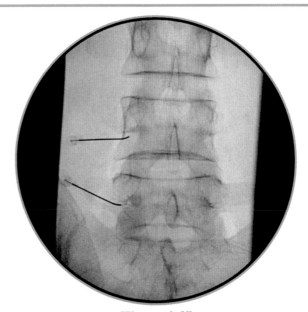

Figure 1-3J
Tilt: 0°
Oblique: 0°

A/P View. Needle position in the A/P view after the needles have been placed in the neural foramen in the prior lateral view (Figure 1-3I). Note the relation of the needle tips to the 6 o'clock position of their respective pedicles.

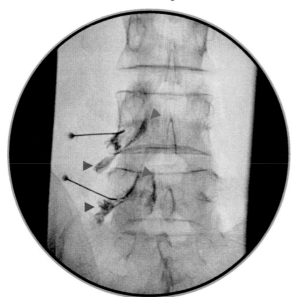

Figure 1-3K
Tilt: 0°
Oblique: 0°

A/P View. After negative aspiration, contrast is administered showing a proper left L4 and L5 neurogram (red arrowheads) and epidurogram (blue arrowheads), with contrast wrapping around the pedicles and into the epidural space.

See Page 269

Left L3-L4 & L4-L5

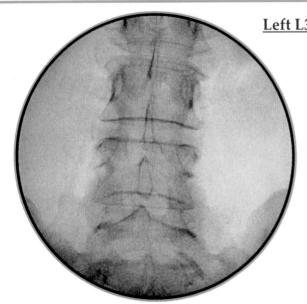

Figure 1-4A
Tilt: 0°
Oblique: 0°

A/P View. Note that the spinous processes of L3 and L4 appear to be midline – "true" A/P. However, the endplates of L3 and L4 are not ideally squared.

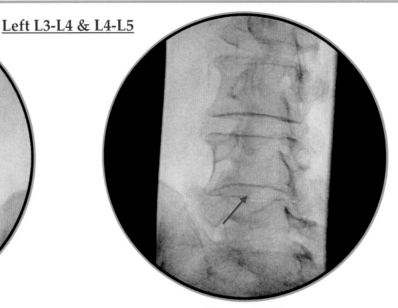

Figure 1-4B
Tilt: 0°
Oblique: 20° Left

Oblique View. When targeting the left L4-L5 foramen, note that the L4 SEP & IEP (red arrow) is not squared.

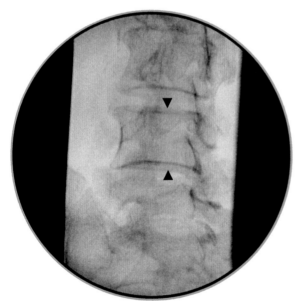

Figure 1-4C
Tilt: 5° Cephalad
Oblique: 20° Left

Oblique View. With a slight cephalad tilt, note that the L4 SEP and IEP becomes more optimally squared (black arrowheads). Squaring the endplates provides the best chance of creating a needle trajectory that places the tip in the superior foramen.

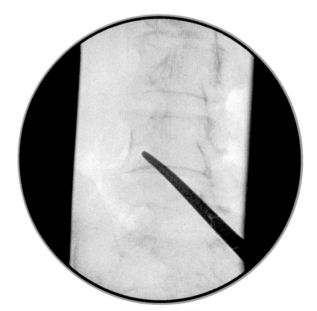

Figure 1-4D
Tilt: 5° Cephalad
Oblique: 20° Left

Oblique View. Pointer showing the location of ideal needle placement just inferior to the 6 o'clock position of the left L4 pedicle.

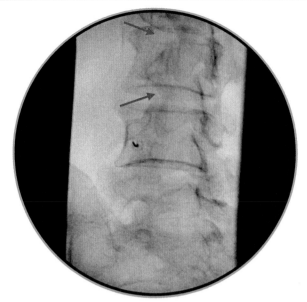

Figure 1-4E
Tilt: 5° Cephalad
Oblique: 20° Left

Oblique View. Coaxial needle placement just inferior to the left L4 pedicle.

Next, for targeting the left L3-L4 neural foramen, note that the endplates of L3 are not squared (red arrows).

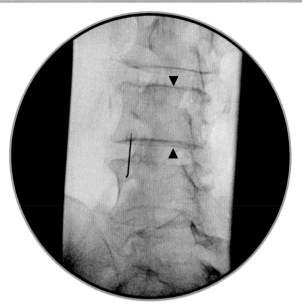

Figure 1-4F
Tilt: 5° Caudal
Oblique: 20° Left

Oblique View. Note that with a caudal tilt, the endplates of L3 become more optimally squared (black arrowheads) – *compare to Figure 1-4B*.

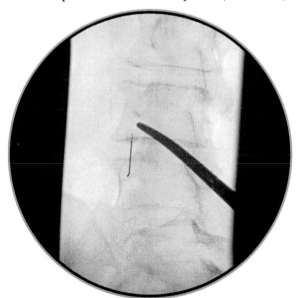

Figure 1-4G
Tilt: 5° Caudal
Oblique: 20° Left

Oblique View. Pointer showing the location of ideal needle placement just inferior to the left L3 pedicle.

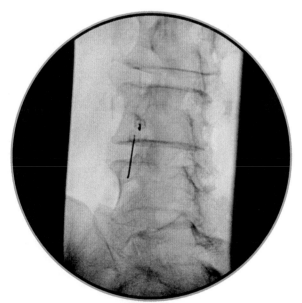

Figure 1-4H
Tilt: 5° Caudal
Oblique: 20° Left

Oblique View. Coaxial needle placement just inferior to the 6 o'clock position of the left L3 pedicle.

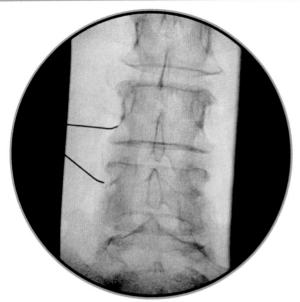

Figure 1-4I
Tilt: 5° Caudal
Oblique: 0°

A/P View. Note that with a caudal tilt, the L3 endplates are squared *(compare to Figure 1-4A)*. As the needle approaches the neural foramen, ensure that the needle is not advanced beyond the lateral border of the vertebral bodies in the A/P view. Next, obtain a lateral view.

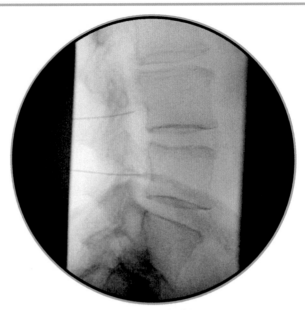

Figure 1-4J
Tilt: 0°
Oblique: 90° Right

Lateral View. The needles are advanced into the superior aspect of each neural foramen. Initially squaring the endplates for each vertebral level prior to needle placement allows for the needles to be parallel to their respective endplates and land superiorly in the foramen.

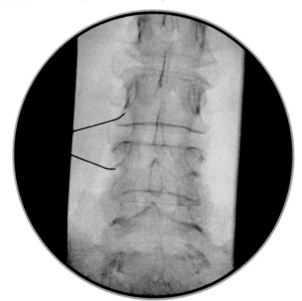

Figure 1-4K
Tilt: 0°
Oblique: 0°

A/P View. Needle position in the A/P view after the needles have been placed in the neural foramen in the prior lateral view. For each needle, note the needle tip position relative to the 6 o'clock position of its respective pedicle.

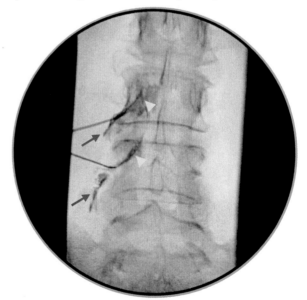

Figure 1-4L
Tilt: 0°
Oblique: 0°

A/P View. After negative aspiration, contrast is administered and shows a proper left L3 and L4 neurogram (red arrows) and epidurogram, with contrast seen to be wrapping around the pedicles and into the epidural space (yellow arrowheads).

Bilateral L5-S1

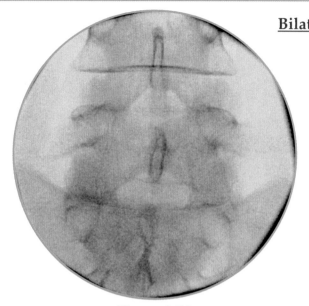

Figure 1-5A
Tilt: 0°
Oblique: 0°

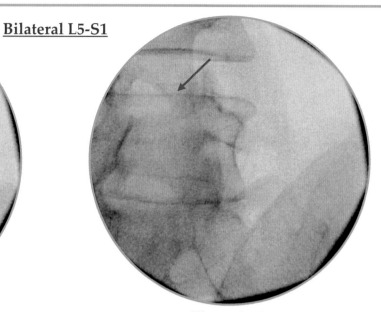

Figure 1-5B
Tilt: 5° Cephalad
Oblique: 20° Right

A/P View. The spinous process of L5 appears to be midline ("true" A/P), but the L5 SEP does not appear ideally squared.

Oblique View. Note that even with a slight cephalad tilt of 5°, the L5 SEP still does NOT appear to be squared (red arrow). Further cephalad tilting will result in a more optimally squared L5 SEP – *see Figure 1-5C.*

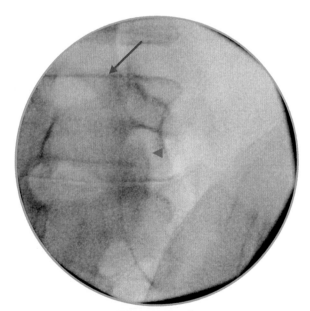

Figure 1-5C
Tilt: 10° Cephalad
Oblique: 20° Right

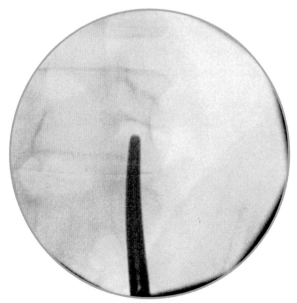

Figure 1-5D
Tilt: 10° Cephalad
Oblique: 20° Right

Oblique View. With further cephalad tilting, note that the L5 SEP is now better squared and seen as a crisp line (red arrow). Additionally, note that the right S1 SAP (blue arrowhead) is just medial to the 6 o'clock position of the right L5 pedicle – ideal view.

Oblique View. Pointer showing the location of ideal needle placement just inferior to the right L5 pedicle.

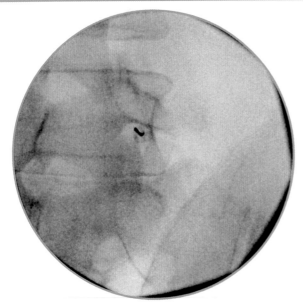

Figure 1-5E
Tilt: 10° Cephalad
Oblique: 20° Right

Oblique View. Coaxial needle placement just inferior to the right L5 pedicle, until a subtle increase in resistance is felt – *if not felt, use intermittent A/P fluoroscopy as needed to confirm needle positioning.* Next, a similar approach is carried out on the contralateral side.

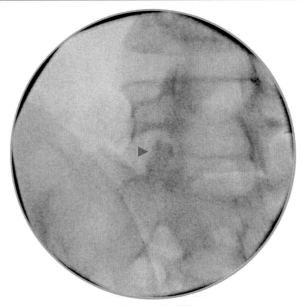

Figure 1-5F
Tilt: 10° Cephalad
Oblique: 20° Left

Oblique View. Note that the L5 SEP remains nicely squared. The left S1 SAP (blue arrowhead) is seen to be just medial to the 6 o'clock position of the left L5 pedicle, which is the ideal position.

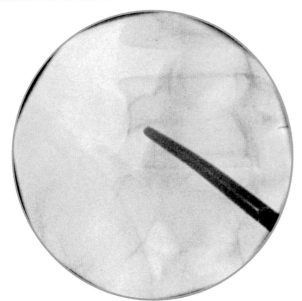

Figure 1-5G
Tilt: 10° Cephalad
Oblique: 20° Left

Oblique View. Pointer showing the location of needle placement just inferior to the left L5 pedicle.

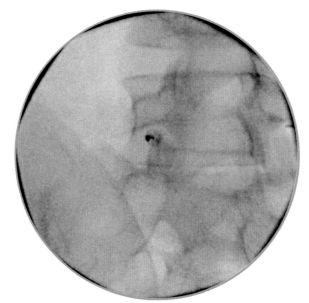

Figure 1-5H
Tilt: 10° Cephalad
Oblique: 20° Left

Oblique View. Coaxial needle placement just inferior to the left L5 pedicle. Once the needle approaches the neural foramen, one can often feel a subtle increase in resistance. Next, an A/P view is obtained.

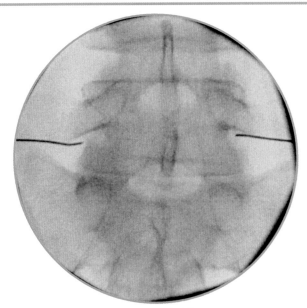

Figure 1-5I
Tilt: 10° Cephalad
Oblique: 0°

A/P View. Note that the needles are not seen to be beyond the lateral vertebral border. Next, with this needle positioning confirmed, a lateral view is obtained.

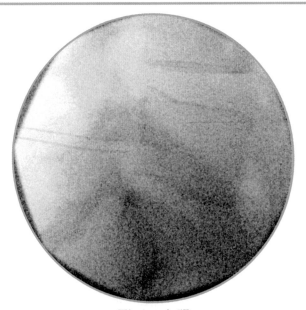

Figure 1-5J
Tilt: 0°
Oblique: 90° Right

Lateral View. The needles are advanced into the superior aspect of the L5-S1 neural foramen. Note that squaring the SEP prior to needle placement allows for the needle trajectory to be parallel to the SEP and the needle tip to land in the superior foramen, away from the nerve root.

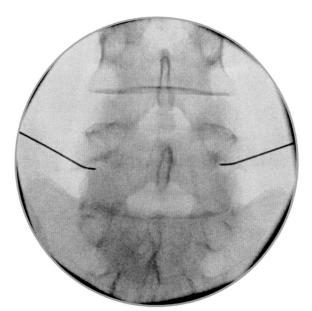

Figure 1-5K
Tilt: 0°
Oblique: 0°

A/P View. After the needle has been placed in the neural foramen in the prior view, note the needle positions in the A/P view. Compare the cephalocaudal needle trajectory in this view to the A/P view with a cephalad tilt *(Figure 1-5I)*.

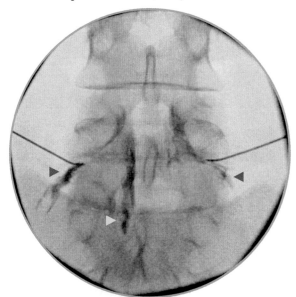

Figure 1-5L
Tilt: 0°
Oblique: 0°

A/P View. After negative aspiration, contrast is administered and shows a proper bilateral L5 neurogram (red arrowheads) and epdiurogram, with contrast wrapping around the pedicles. Note the epidural spread towards the left sacral nerve roots (yellow arrowhead).

See Page 270

<u>Bilateral L3-L4</u>

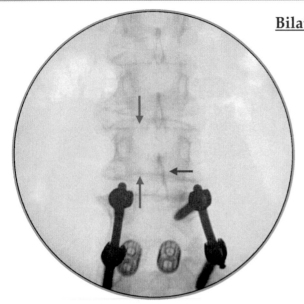

Figure 1-6A
Tilt: 0°
Oblique: 0°

A/P View. Note that the L3 spinous process (red arrow) is not in the midline. Additionally, the L3 endplates are not squared (blue arrows).

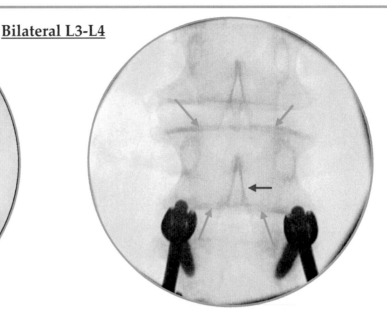

Figure 1-6B
Tilt: 10° Caudal
Oblique: 5° Right

A/P View. With the correct amount of oblique and caudal tilt, the L3 spinous process is now in the midline (red arrow - "True A/P" view) and the L3 endplates squared (green arrows) – *compare to Figure 1-6A.*

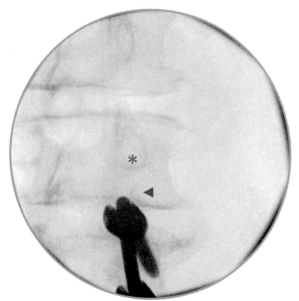

Figure 1-6C
Tilt: 10° Caudal
Oblique: 25° Right

Oblique View. Note that this is an appropriate amount of oblique, as the right L4 SAP (red arrowhead) is seen to be at approximately the 6 o'clock position of the right L3 pedicle (blue star).

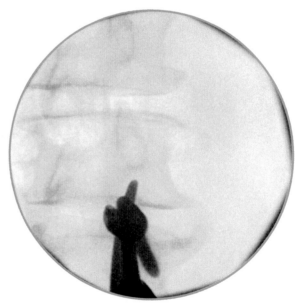

Figure 1-6D
Tilt: 10° Caudal
Oblique: 25° Right

Oblique View. Pointer showing the location of ideal needle placement just inferior to the right L3 pedicle.

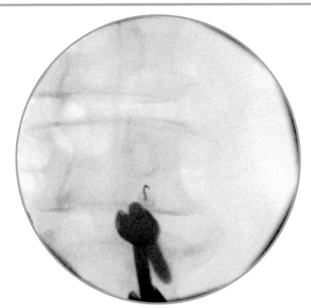

Figure 1-6E
Tilt: 10° Caudal
Oblique: 25° Right

Oblique View. Coaxial needle placement just inferior to the right L3 pedicle. Advance until a subtle increase in resistance is felt – *if not felt, use intermittent A/P fluoroscopy as needed to confirm needle positioning.* Next, plan for a similar approach on the contralateral side.

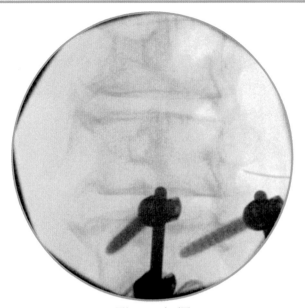

Figure 1-6F
Tilt: 10° Caudal
Oblique: 20° Left

Oblique View. Note that since the "non-true" A/P view showed the spinous process to be right of midline *(see Figure 1-6A)*, less oblique is needed to visualize the left L3-L4 foramen compared to the right (i.e., 20° left vs 25° right – *compare to Figure 1-6C*).

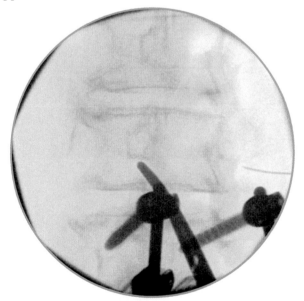

Figure 1-6G
Tilt: 10° Caudal
Oblique: 20° Left

Oblique View. Pointer showing the location of ideal needle placement just inferior to the left L3 pedicle.

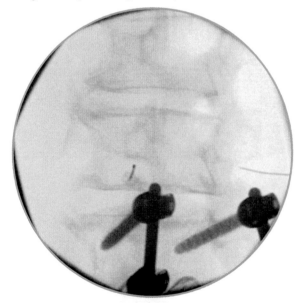

Figure 1-6H
Tilt: 10° Caudal
Oblique: 20° Left

Oblique View. Coaxial needle placement just inferior to the left L3 pedicle. Once the needle approaches the neural foramen, one can often feel a subtle increase in resistance. Next, obtain an A/P view.

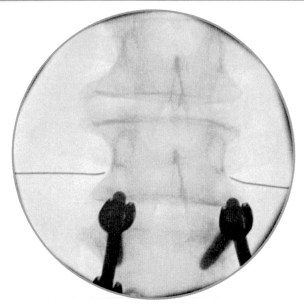

Figure 1-6I
Tilt: 10° Caudal
Oblique: 0°

A/P View. Ensure that the needles are at, and NOT beyond, approximately the lateral border of the vertebral body. Next, a lateral view can be obtained.

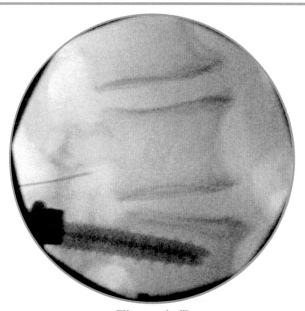

Figure 1-6J
Tilt: 0°
Oblique: 90° Right

Lateral View. The needles are advanced into the superior aspect of the L3-L4 neural foramen. Note that initially squaring the SEP prior to needle placement allows for the final needle position to be parallel to the L3 SEP – leading to easier placement in the superior foramen.

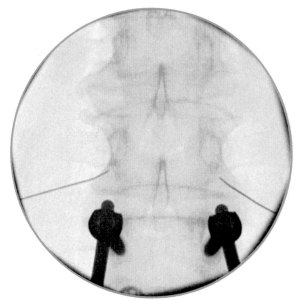

Figure 1-6K
Tilt: 0°
Oblique: 5° Right

A/P View. Needle positioning in the "true A/P" view (spinous process midline) after the needles have been advanced in the neural foramen in the lateral view. Note the cephalocaudal needle trajectory in the A/P view without squaring the endplates – *Compare to Figure 1-6I.*

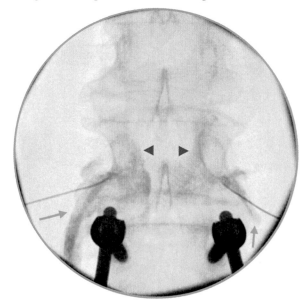

Figure 1-6L
Tilt: 0°
Oblique: 5° Right

A/P View. After negative aspiration, contrast is administered and shows a proper bilateral L3 neurogram (green arrows) and epidurogram, with contrast wrapping around the pedicles (red arrowheads) and into the epidural space.

Right L2-L3, L3-L4, L4-L5

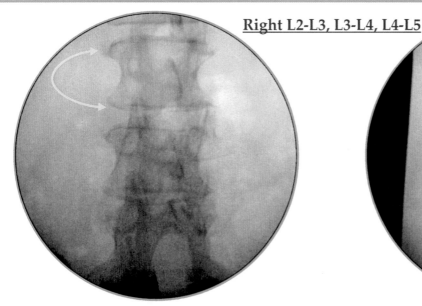

Figure 1-7A
Tilt: 0°
Oblique: 0°

A/P View. Note that the spinous processes are not midline, but obliqued towards the right. The endplates of L2 are fairly squared (curved yellow arrow), but the endplates of L3 and L4 are not.

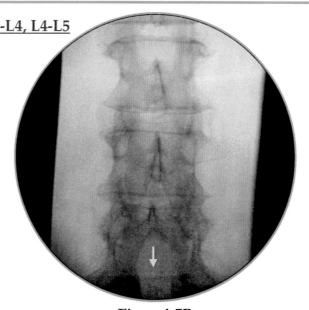

Figure 1-7B
Tilt: 0°
Oblique: 5° Right

A/P View. With this small amount of oblique, the spinous processes now appear to be more evenly spaced between the pedicles – "True A/P" view (compare to Figure 1-7A). *Note the laminectomy towards the bottom of the image* (yellow arrow).

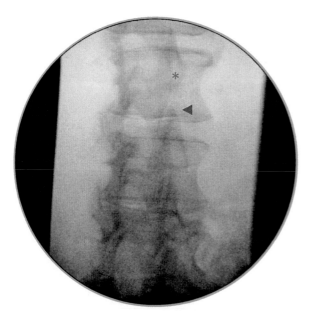

Figure 1-7C
Tilt: 0°
Oblique: 25° Right

Oblique View. The right L3 SAP (red arrowhead) is seen to be at approximately the 6 o'clock position of the right L2 pedicle (blue star) – ideal amount of rotation. The endplates of L2 are confirmed to be fairly squared.

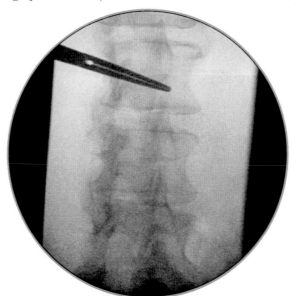

Figure 1-7D
Tilt: 0°
Oblique: 25° Right

Oblique View. Pointer showing the location of needle placement just inferior to the right L2 pedicle.

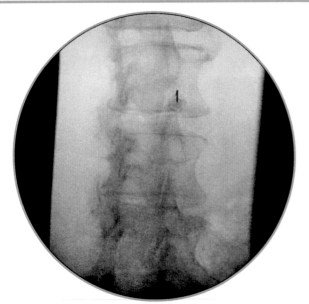

Figure 1-7E
Tilt: 0° Cephalad
Oblique: 25° Right

Oblique View. Coaxial needle placement just inferior to the right L2 pedicle until a subtle increase in resistance is felt – if *not felt, use intermittent A/P fluoroscopy to confirm needle positioning.* Next, for targeting the right L3-L4 foramen, note that the L3 endplates are not squared.

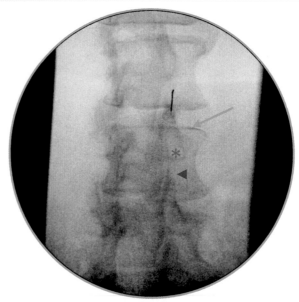

Figure 1-7F
Tilt: 5° Cephalad
Oblique: 25° Right

Oblique View. With a slight amount of cephalad tilt, the L3 SEP now appears better squared (green arrow) – *compare to Figure 1-7E.* The right L4 SAP (red arrowhead) is seen to be just medial to the 6 o'clock position of the right L3 pedicle (blue star) – ideal amount of rotation.

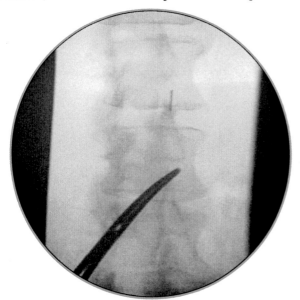

Figure 1-7G
Tilt: 5° Cephalad
Oblique: 25° Right

Oblique View. Pointer showing the location of ideal needle placement just inferior to the right L3 pedicle.

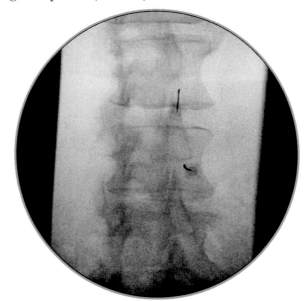

Figure 1-7H
Tilt: 5° Cephalad
Oblique: 25° Right

Oblique View. Coaxial needle placement just inferior to the right L3 pedicle until a subtle increase in resistance is felt – *if not felt, use intermittent A/P views as needed to confirm needle positioning.* Next, for targeting the right L4-L5 foramen, note that the L4 endplates are not squared.

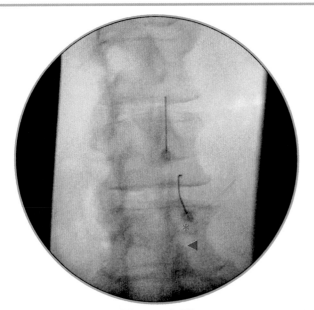

Figure 1-7I
Tilt: 10° Cephalad
Oblique: 25° Right

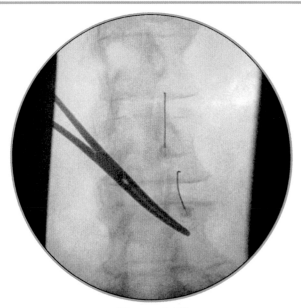

Figure 1-7J
Tilt: 10° Cephalad
Oblique: 25° Right

Oblique View. With further cephalad tilting, the L4 SEP becomes more squared (green arrow) – *compare to Figure 1-7H*. The right L5 SAP (red arrowhead) is seen to be just medial to the 6 o'clock position of the right L4 pedicle (blue star) – ideal amount of rotation.

Oblique View. Pointer showing the location of ideal needle placement just inferior to the right L4 pedicle.

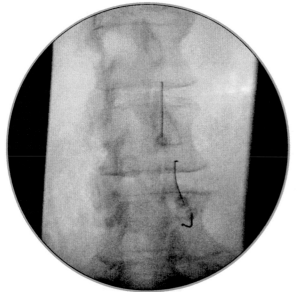

Figure 1-7K
Tilt: 10° Cephalad
Oblique: 25° Right

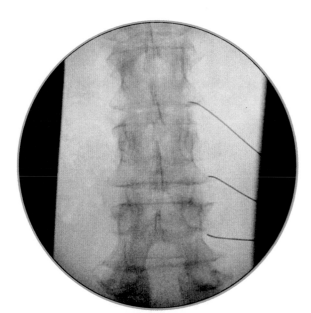

Figure 1-7L
Tilt: 10° Cephalad
Oblique: 5° Right

Oblique View. Coaxial needle placement just inferior to the right L4 pedicle until a subtle increase in resistance is felt – *if not felt, use intermittent A/P views as needed to confirm needle positioning*. Next, obtain an A/P view.

A/P View. Ensure that the needles are approximately at, and NOT beyond, the lateral border of the vertebral bodies.

Next, a lateral view is obtained.

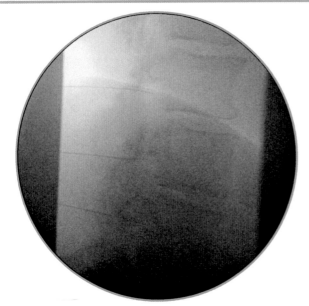

Figure 1-7M
Tilt: 0°
Oblique: 90° Right

Lateral View. The needles are advanced into the superior aspect of the L2-L3, L3-L4, and L4-L5 neural foramen. Note that initially squaring the SEP prior to needle placement allows for the needle trajectories to be parallel to their respective SEP and land in the superior foramen.

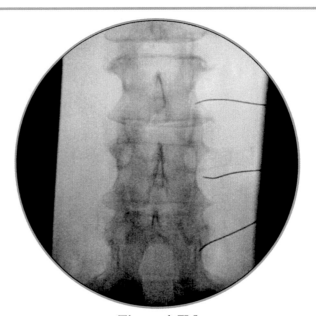

Figure 1-7N
Tilt: 0°
Oblique: 5° Right

A/P View. Needle positioning after each needle has been advanced into its neural foramen in the lateral view. Note the angles of the needles in this view without tilting, compared to the A/P view with a cephalad tilt *(compare to Figure 1-7L)*.

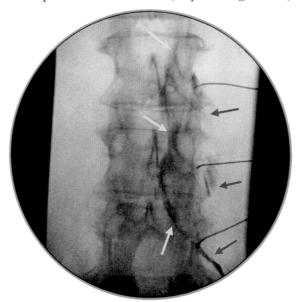

Figure 1-7O
Tilt: 0°
Oblique: 5° Right

A/P View. After negative aspiration, contrast is administered and shows a poper right L2, L3, and L4 neurogram (red arrows) and epidurogram, with contrast wrapping around the pedicles (yellow arrows) and into the epidural space.

See Page 271

Left L3-L4, L4-L5, L5-S1

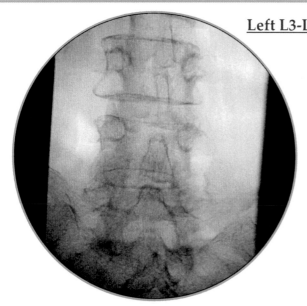

Figure 1-8A
Tilt: 0°
Oblique: 0°

A/P View. Note that the spinous processes are not midline, but rather obliqued towards the right. The endplates of L3 appear fairly squared, but those of L4 and L5 are not.

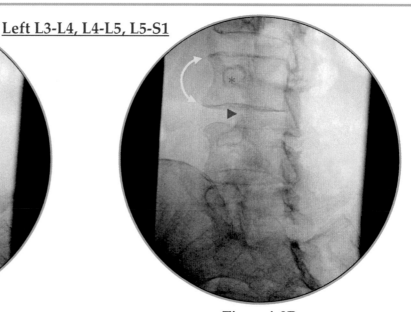

Figure 1-8B
Tilt: 0°
Oblique: 20° Left

Oblique View. The left L4 SAP (red arrowhead) is seen to be just medial to the 6 o'clock position of the left L3 pedicle (blue star) – ideal amount of rotation. Note that the endplates of L3 are confirmed to be fairly squared (curved yellow arrow)

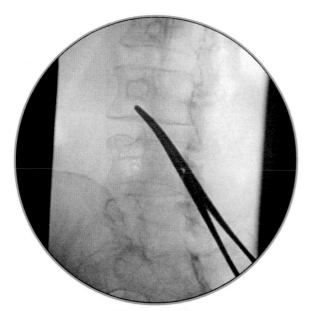

Figure 1-8C
Tilt: 0°
Oblique: 20° Left

Oblique View. Pointer showing the location of ideal needle placement just inferior to the left L3 pedicle.

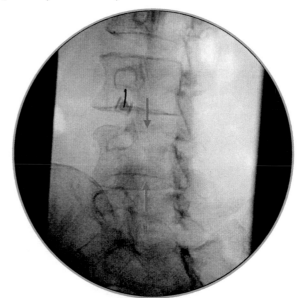

Figure 1-8D
Tilt: 0°
Oblique: 20° Left

Oblique View. Coaxial needle placement just inferior to the left L3 pedicle, until a subtle increase in resistance is felt – *if not felt, use intermittent A/P views to assess needle positioning.* Next, for targeting the left L4-L5 foramen, note that the L4 endplates (blue arrows) are not squared.

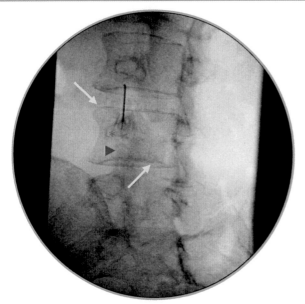

Figure 1-8E
Tilt: 10° Cephalad
Oblique: 20° Left

Oblique View. A cephalad tilt more optimally squares the L4 endplates (yellow arrows). Note that the left L5 SAP (red arrowhead) is seen to be just medial to the 6 o'clock position of the left L4 pedicle (blue star) – ideal amount of rotation.

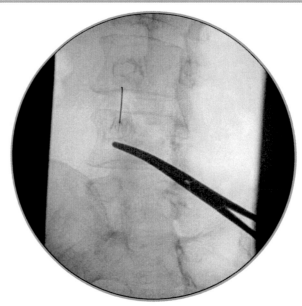

Figure 1-8F
Tilt: 10° Cephalad
Oblique: 20° Left

Oblique View. Pointer showing the location of ideal needle placement just inferior to the left L4 pedicle.

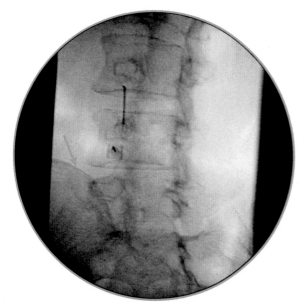

Figure 1-8G
Tilt: 10° Cephalad
Oblique: 20° Left

Oblique View. Coaxial needle placement just inferior to the left L4 pedicle until a subtle increase in resistance is felt – *if not felt, use intermittent A/P views to assess needle positioning*. Note that the left iliac crest (green arrow) is obstructing the left L5-S1 foramen.

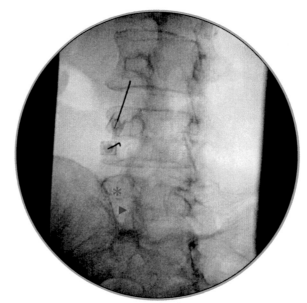

Figure 1-8H
Tilt: 10° Cephalad
Oblique: 15° Left

Oblique View. A lesser oblique creates a better view of the left L5-S1 foramen. The left S1 SAP (red arrowhead) is seen to be just medial to the 6 o'clock position of the left L5 pedicle (blue star) – ideal view. *Note that a more cephalad tilt could have even better squared the L5 SEP.*

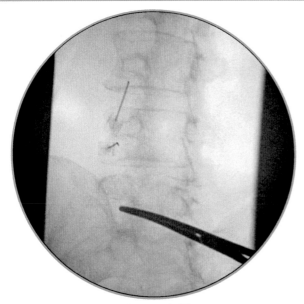

Figure 1-8I
Tilt: 10° Cephalad
Oblique: 15° Left

Oblique View. Pointer showing the location of ideal needle placement just inferior to the left L5 pedicle.

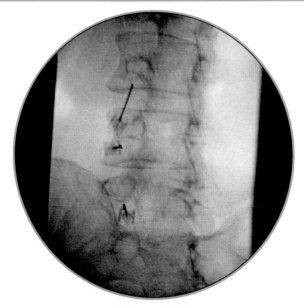

Figure 1-8J
Tilt: 10° Cephalad
Oblique: 15° Left

Oblique View. Coaxial needle placement just inferior to the left L5 pedicle, until a subtle increase in resistance is felt – *if not felt, use intermittent A/P fluoroscopy as needed to assess needle positioning.* Next, obtain an A/P view.

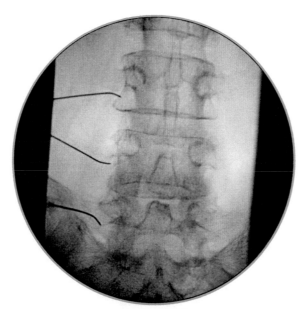

Figure 1-8K
Tilt: 0°
Oblique: 5° Right

A/P View. This is a more "true A/P" view – compare to Figure 1-8A. Ensure that the needle tips are approximately at, and NOT beyond, the lateral border of the vertebral bodies. Next, obtain a lateral view.

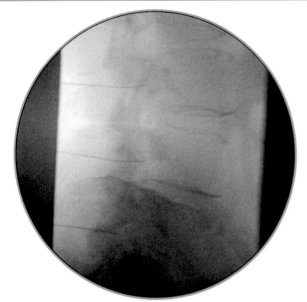

Figure 1-8L
Tilt: 0°
Oblique: 90° Right

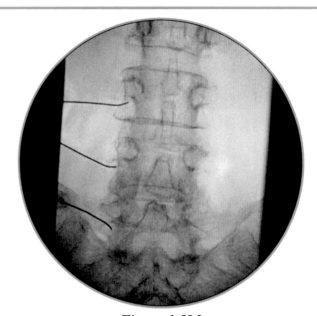

Figure 1-8M
Tilt: 0°
Oblique: 5° Right

Lateral View. The two superior needles are advanced into the superior aspect of their respective foramen. Note how the inferior needle is not parallel to the L5 SEP, which was initially not optimally squared – making it more challenging to enter the superior L5-S1 foramen.

A/P View. Needle positioning after each needle has been placed in its respective neural foramen in the prior lateral view.

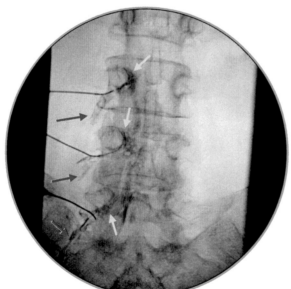

Figure 1-8N
Tilt: 0°
Oblique: 5° Right

A/P View. In this "True A/P view," after negative aspoiration, contrast is administered and shows a proper left L3, L4, and L5 neurogram (red arrows) and epidurogram, with contrast seen wrapping around the pedicles (yellow arrows) and into the epidural space.

See Page 271

Right L3-L4
Bilateral L4-L5

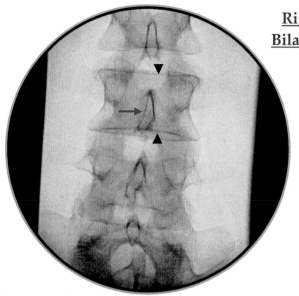

Figure 1-9A
Tilt: 0°
Oblique: 0°

A/P View. Note that the L3 spinous process is close to midline (red arrow) – "true" A/P view. Additionally, the endplates of L3 are also fairly squared (black arrowheads) – so no tilting of the C-arm will be needed for targeting the L3-L4 foramen.

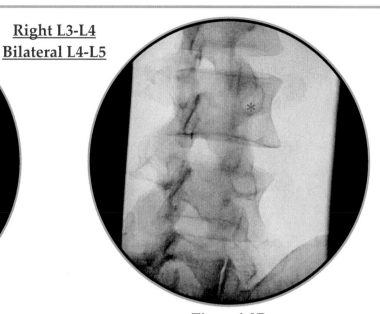

Figure 1-9B
Tilt: 0°
Oblique: 20° Right

Oblique View. With this amount of oblique, the right L4 SAP (green arrowhead) is seen to be just medial to the 6 o'clock position of the right L3 pedicle (blue star) – ideal amount of rotation.

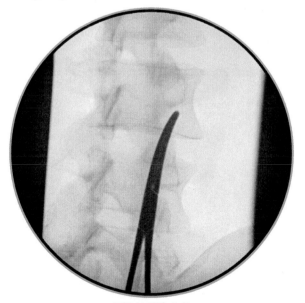

Figure 1-9C
Tilt: 0°
Oblique: 20° Right

Oblique View. Pointer showing the location of ideal needle placement just inferior to the right L3 pedicle.

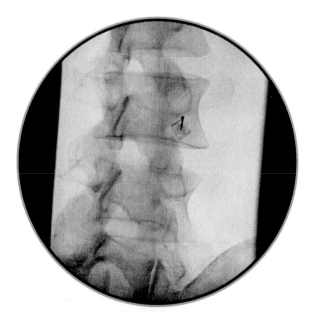

Figure 1-9D
Tilt: 0°
Oblique: 20° Right

Oblique View. Coaxial needle placement just inferior to the right L3 pedicle, until a subtle increase in resistance is felt – *if not felt, use intermittent A/P views as needed to assess needle positioning*. Next, for targeting the right L4-L5 foramen, note that the endplates of L4 are not squared.

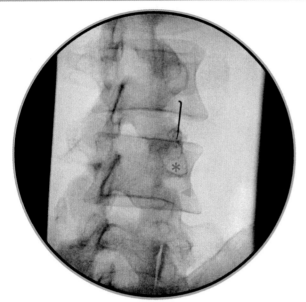

Figure 1-9E
Tilt: 10° Cephalad
Oblique: 20° Right

Oblique View. With this amount of oblique, the right L5 SAP (green arrowhead) is seen to be at the 6 o'clock position of the right L4 pedicle (blue star) – ideal amount of rotation. Note that a cephalad tilt more optimally squares the L4 SEP *(compare to Figure 1-9D)*.

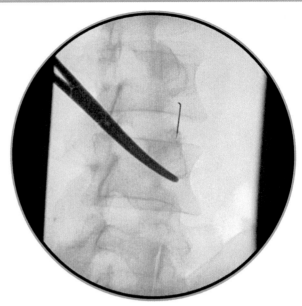

Figure 1-9F
Tilt: 10° Cephalad
Oblique: 20° Right

Oblique View. Pointer showing the location of ideal needle placement just inferior to the right L4 pedicle.

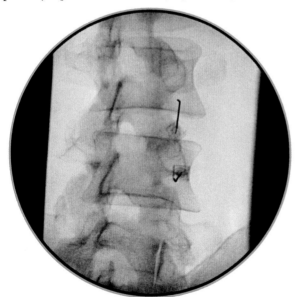

Figure 1-9G
Tilt: 10° Cephalad
Oblique: 20° Right

Oblique View. Coaxial needle placement just inferior to the right L4 pedicle, until a subtle increase in resistance is felt – *if not felt, use intermittent A/P views as needed to assess needle positioning.* Next, for targeting the left L4-L5 foramen, oblique to the contralateral side.

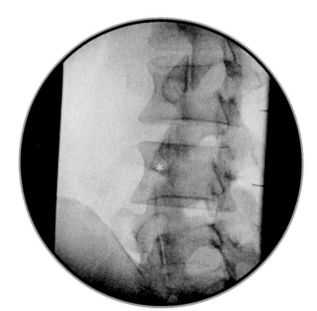

Figure 1-9H
Tilt: 10° Cephalad
Oblique: 20° Left

Oblique View. With this amount of oblique, the left L5 SAP (green arrowhead) is NOT at – or slightly medial to – the 6 o'clock position of the left L4 pedicle (yellow star). Further oblique will be needed to obtain a more ideal view prior to needle placement *(see Figure 1-9I)*.

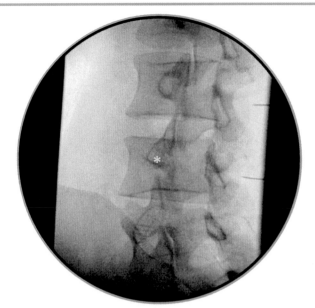

Figure 1-9I
Tilt: 10° Cephalad
Oblique: 30° Left

Oblique View. With this amount of oblique, the left L5 SAP (green arrowhead) is now seen to be at the 6 o'clock position of the left L4 pedicle (yellow star) – ideal amount of rotation. *Compare to Figure 1-9H.*

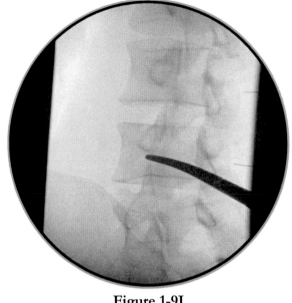

Figure 1-9J
Tilt: 10° Cephalad
Oblique: 30° Left

Oblique View. Pointer showing the location of ideal needle placement just inferior to the left L4 pedicle.

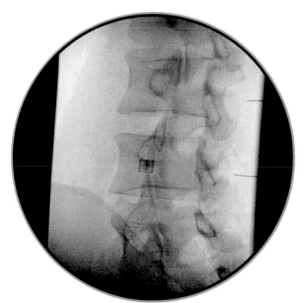

Figure 1-9K
Tilt: 10° Cephalad
Oblique: 30° Left

Oblique View. Coaxial needle placement just inferior to the left L4 pedicle, until a subtle increase in resistance is felt – *if not felt, use intermittent A/P views as needed to assess needle positioning.* Next, obtain an A/P view.

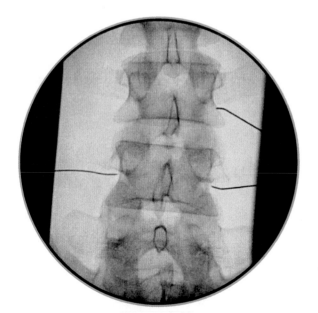

Figure 1-9L
Tilt: 10° Cephalad
Oblique: 0°

A/P View. The needles tips should be at approximately the lateral border of the vertebral bodies – *if this is not seen, advance further in the prior oblique view using intermittent fluoroscopy as needed.* Once the needle tips are in this position, a lateral view is obtained.

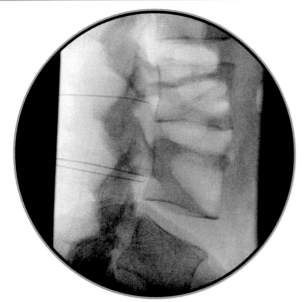

Figure 1-9M
Tilt: 0°
Oblique: 90° Right

Lateral View. The needles are advanced into the superior aspect of the L3-L4 & L4-L5 neural foramen. Note that squaring the SEP prior to needle placement allows for the final needle trajectories to be parallel to each SEP, with each needle tip placed in the superior foramen.

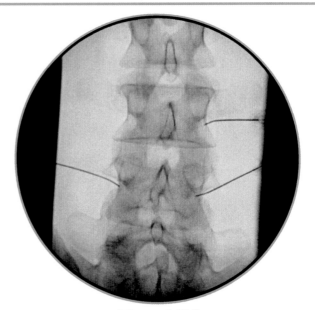

Figure 1-9N
Tilt: 0°
Oblique: 0°

A/P View. Needle positioning after each needle has been placed in its respective neural foramen in the prior lateral view. Note the cephalocaudal needle angles in this view without tilting, compared to the A/P view with a cephalad tilt *(compare to Figure 1-9L)*.

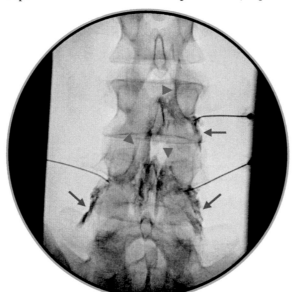

Figure 1-9O
Tilt: 0°
Oblique: 0°

A/P View. After negative aspiration, contrast is administered and shows a proper right L3 and bilateral L4 neurogram (red arrows) and epidurogram, with contrast seen to be wrapping around the pedicles (blue arrowheads) and into the epidural space.

See Page 272

<u>**Right L3-L4 & Bilateral L4-5**</u>
<u>*"Challenging Scoliotic Spine"*</u>

The principles of needle placement do not change...

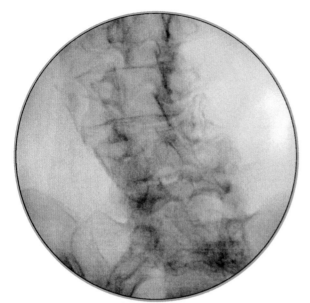

Figure 1-10A
Tilt: 0°
Oblique: 0°

A/P View. In this scoliotic spine, note that the spinous processes appear to be obliqued right and the endplates are not squared.

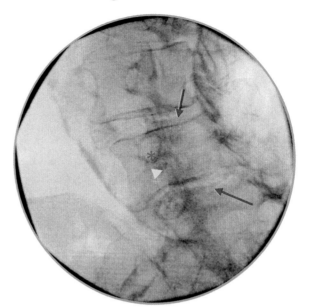

Figure 1-10B
Tilt: 0°
Oblique: 20° Left

Oblique View. With this amount of oblique, the left L5 SAP (yellow arrowhead) is seen to be just medial to the 6 o'clock position of the left L4 pedicle (blue star) – ideal amount of rotation. However, the L4 endplates are not optimally squared (red arrows).

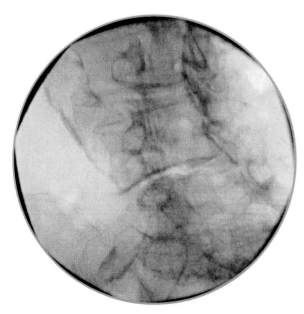

Figure 1-10C
Tilt: 10° Cephalad
Oblique: 20° Left

Oblique View. Note that the L4 endplates now appear to be a bit better squared (*compare to Figure 1-10B*). *It will be challenging to get crisp SEP and IEP lines in this case given the significant amount of scoliosis.*

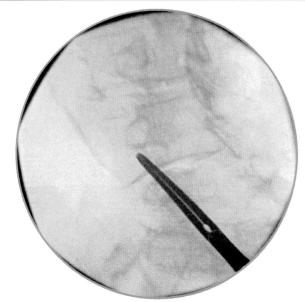

Figure 1-10D
Tilt: 10° Cephalad
Oblique: 20° Left

Oblique View. Pointer showing the location of ideal needle placement just inferior to the left L4 pedicle.

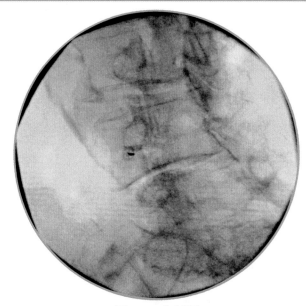

Figure 1-10E
Tilt: 10° Cephalad
Oblique: 20° Left

Oblique View. Coaxial needle placement just inferior to the left L4 pedicle, until a subtle increase in resistance is felt – *if not felt, use intermittent A/P views as needed to assess needle positioning.* Next, plan to target the right L4-L5 foramen.

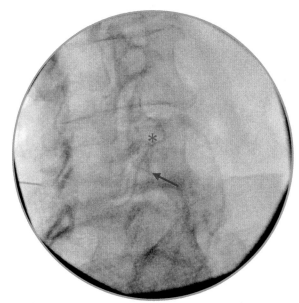

Figure 1-10F
Tilt: 10° Cephalad
Oblique: 50° Right

Oblique View. Note the significant amount of ipsilateral oblique needed to get the right L5 SAP (red arrow) just medial to the 6 o'clock position of the right L4 pedicle (blue star).

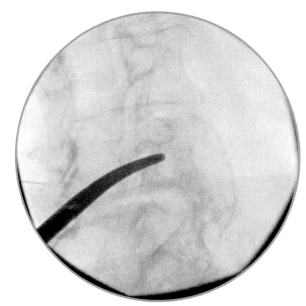

Figure 1-10G
Tilt: 10° Cephalad
Oblique: 50° Right

Oblique View. Pointer showing the location of ideal needle placement just inferior to the right L4 pedicle.

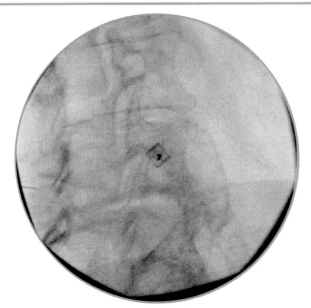

Figure 1-10H
Tilt: 10° Cephalad
Oblique: 50° Right

Oblique View. Coaxial needle placement just inferior to the right L4 pedicle, until a subtle increase in resistance is felt – *if not felt, use intermittent A/P views as needed to assess needle positioning.* Next, plan to target the right L3-L4 foramen.

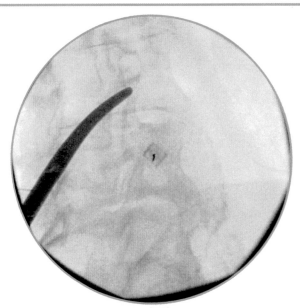

Figure 1-10I
Tilt: 10° Cephalad
Oblique: 50° Right

Oblique View. Pointer showing the location of needle placement just inferior to the right L3 pedicle. Note that the right L4 SAP is at approximately the 6 o'clock position of the right L3 pedicle. However, note that the L3 endplates are NOT ideally squared.

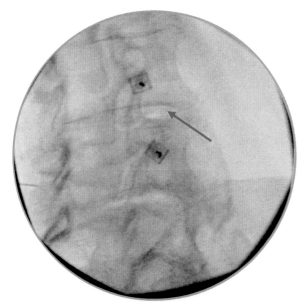

Figure 1-10J
Tilt: 10° Cephalad
Oblique: 50° Right

Oblique View. Needle placed just inferior to the right L3 pedicle. Note that a more caudal tilt could have been used to better square the L3 endplates (blue arrow at the non-squared L3 IEP) – *see how this eventually affects needle positioning in the lateral view (Figure 1-10L).*

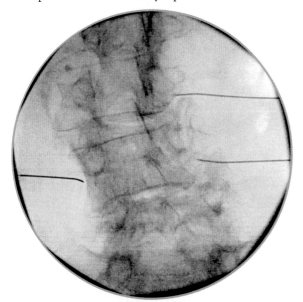

Figure 1-10K
Tilt: 10° Cephalad
Oblique: 0°

A/P View. Once the needle approaches the neural foramen (often a subtle increase in resistance can be felt when this occurs), obtain an A/P view and ensure that the needles are at approximately the lateral border of the vertebral bodies. Next, obtain a lateral view.

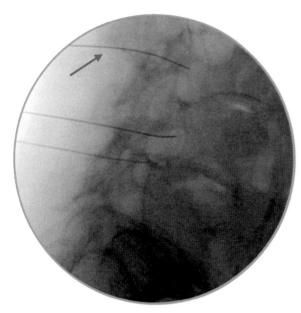

Figure 1-10L
Tilt: 0°
Oblique: 90° Right

Lateral View. Note that the individual foramen are much more difficult to assess due to scoliosis and varying angles of spinal curvature. Therefore, extra care is taken to slowly advance the needles into the superior aspect of each foramen. If any paresthesias are reported during needle advancement, withdraw the needle slightly and adjust accordingly.

Note how NOT squaring the L3 endplates in the A/P view prior to needle placement created a non-parallel needle to the L3 endplates (blue arrow) – making it much more challenging to place the needle tip in the superior aspect of the L3-L4 foramen.

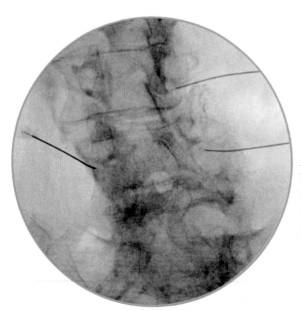

Figure 1-10M
Tilt: 0°
Oblique: 0°

A/P View. Note the needle positioning after the needles have been placed in their respective neural foramen in the prior lateral view. This is NOT a "true" A/P view since the spinous processes are not midline and equally spaced between their respective pedicles.

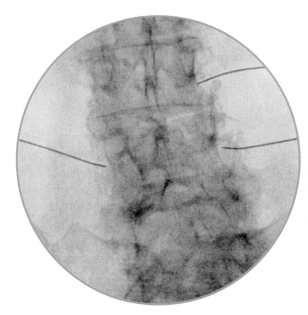

Figure 1-10N
Tilt: 0°
Oblique: 15° Right

A/P View. Note that by applying a 15° oblique towards the right, a more "true" A/P view is seen with the spinous processes midline and equidistant between their respective left and right pedicles.

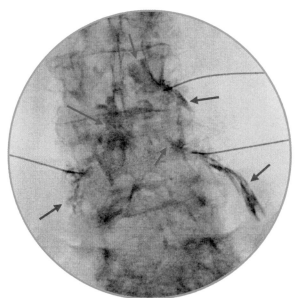

Figure 1-10O
Tilt: 0°
Oblique: 15° Right

A/P View. After negative aspiration, contrast is administered and shows a proper right L3 and bilateral L4 neurogram (red arrows) and epidurogram, with contrast seen to be wrapping around the pedicles and into the epidural space (blue arrows).

Additional Discussion:
"Visualizing the L5-S1 Foramen"

When targeting the L5-S1 foramen in the oblique view, often times the iliac crest can present a challenge in getting an adequate view of the foramen. In these instances, adjusting the ipsilateral oblique and cephalad tilt will be needed. The below examples present such scenarios and the specific fluoroscopic oblique and tilt angles used to adequately "open up" and clearly visualize the L5-S1 foramen prior to needle placement.

Example 1

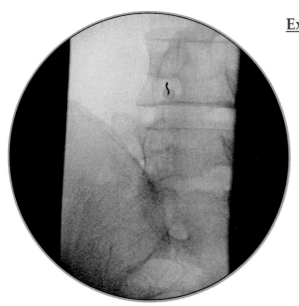

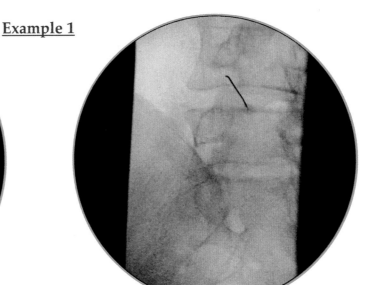

Figure 1-11A
Tilt: 0°
Oblique: 20° Left

Figure 1-11B
Tilt: 5° Cephalad
Oblique: 25° Left

Oblique View. The above view shows an adequate view of the L4-L5 foramen with needle placement just inferior to the left L4 pedicle.

However, when planning for needle placement at L5-S1, note that a further oblique will be needed since the left S1 SAP is not at the 6 o'clock position of the left L5 pedicle. However, doing so will cause the iliac crest to obstruct the foramen and make needle placement at the L5-S1 foramen impossible. Thus, in addition to a further ipsilateral oblique, a cephalad tilt will also be required to remove the iliac crest from obstructing the view of the L5-S1 foramen. This will provide a clear needle path towards the neural foramen — *see Figure 1-11B*.

Oblique View. Note how the additional oblique, and application of a cephalad tilt, provides a clear view of the left L5-S1 foramen. *Compare to Figure 1-11A.*

Example 2

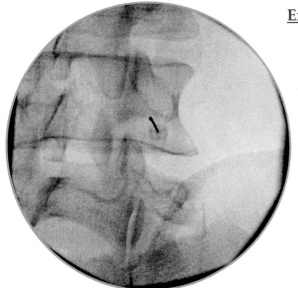

Figure 1-12A
Tilt: 0°
Oblique: 20° Right

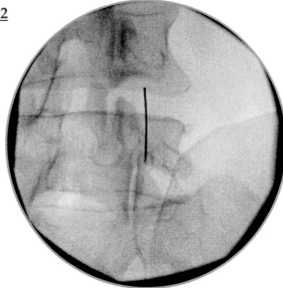

Figure 1-12B
Tilt: 10° Cephalad
Oblique: 20° Right

Oblique View. Ideal view for needle placement at the right L4-L5 foramen. However, a cephalad tilt will be needed to square the L5 SEP and get a more adequate view of the L5-S1 foramen. *Note the position of the S1 SAP relative to the L5 pedicle – further oblique will NOT be needed.*

Oblique View. Note how applying a cephalad fluoroscopic tilt creates a clear view of the right L5-S1 foramen. *Compare to Figure 1-12A.*

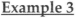

Example 3

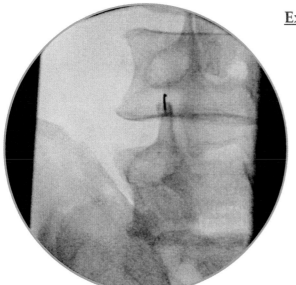

Figure 1-13A
Tilt: 5° Cephalad
Oblique: 20° Left

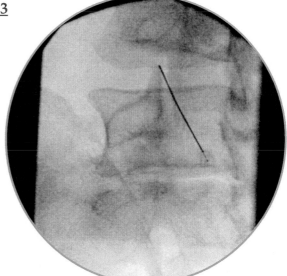

Figure 1-13B
Tilt: 20° Cephalad
Oblique: 30° Left

Oblique View. Ideal view for needle placement at the left L4-L5 foramen. However, a cephalad tilt and further oblique will be needed to get a more adequate view of the left L5-S1 foramen. *Note the position of the left S1 SAP relative to the left L5 pedicle – further oblique will be necessary.*

Oblique View. Note how the above fluoroscopic adjustments provide for a more adequate view of the left L5-S1 foramen. *Compare to Figure 1-13A.*

Even in more challenging scoliotic spines, with varying degrees of spinal curvature in multiple planes, the fluoroscopic principles still remain the same...

Example 4

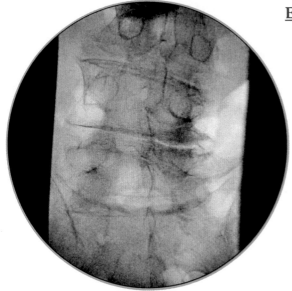

Figure 1-14A
Tilt: 0°
Oblique: 0°

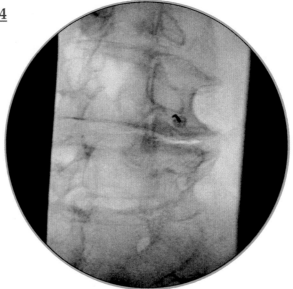

Figure 1-14B
Tilt: 0°
Oblique: 30° Right

A/P View. Note the scoliotic spine in this view. Spinal curvature can provide a significant challenge in accessing the targeted neural foramen. However, the fluoroscopic principles discussed should still be followed to provide the best chance of successful needle placement.

Oblique View. Ideal view for needle placement at the right L4-L5 foramen. However, a cephalad tilt will be needed to square the L5 SEP and get a more adequate view of the L5-S1 foramen. *Note the position of the right S1 SAP relative to the L5 pedicle – further oblique will be needed.*

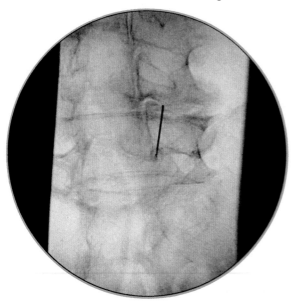

Figure 1-14C
Tilt: 15° Right
Oblique: 35° Right

Oblique View. Note how the above fluoroscopic adjustments create a clear view of the right L5-S1 foramen. *Compare to Figure 1-14B.*

Additional Discussion:
"Squaring Endplates"

Squaring the endplates (SEP and IEP) is a key part of fluoroscopic planning prior to needle placement. When the endplates are squared, the final needle trajectory will be parallel to the endplates – and the corresponding pedicle – providing the best opportunity for needle tip entry into the superior foramen (away from the exiting nerve root). *Note that if only one endplate can be squared, preference should be given to squaring the SEP.*

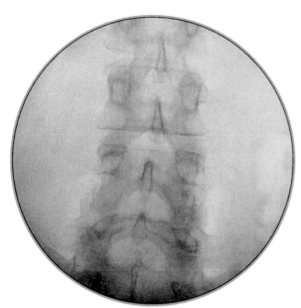

Figure 1-15A
Tilt: 0°
Oblique: 0°

A/P View. Note the elliptical shape of the SEPs in this example (i.e., non-squared endplates). In order to help determine whether a cephalad or caudal tilt will be needed to square the endplates, one should note the position of the pedicles relative to its respective SEP. For example, if the SEP appears to be elliptical, with its respective pedicles within or superior to this ellipse, then a cephalad tilt will be needed to square the SEP. In contrast, if the pedicles are seen to be inferior to the elliptically shaped SEP, then a caudal tilt will be needed to square the SEP.

Applying the principles described above, in this example a caudal tilt will be needed to square the L3 SEP, and a cephalad tilt will be needed to square the L5 SEP.

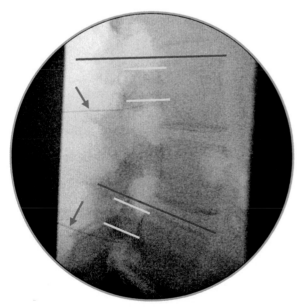

Figure 1-15B
Tilt: 0°
Oblique: 90° Right

Lateral View. Squaring the endplates prior to needle placement allows for the needles (blue arrows) to be fairly parallel to their corresponding SEPs (red lines) – and resultantly their corresponding pedicles (yellow lines). This allows for each needle to stay in the superior aspect of the foramen *(away from the exiting spinal nerve).*

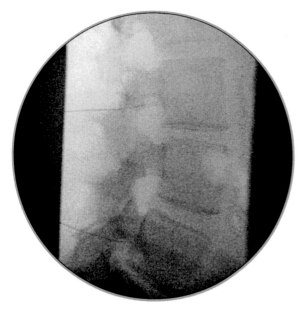

Figure 1-15C
Tilt: 0°
Oblique: 90° Right

Lateral View. *Figure 1-15B reproduced without maker lines.* The typical natural lordosis of the lumbar spine is seen in this lateral view. Note the differing angles of the L3 and L5 vertebral bodies, and the final needle tip position in the superior aspect of the L3-L4 and L5-S1 foramen.

Each needle trajectory corresponds to the angle required to square its respective SEP – slight caudal tilt for the L3 SEP and a cephalad tilt for the L5 SEP.

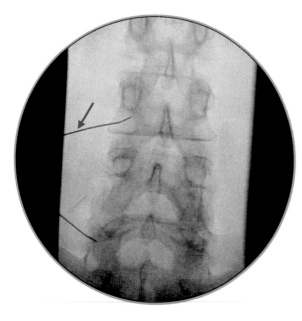

Figure 1-15D
Tilt: 0°
Oblique: 0°

A/P View. Note the final needle position in the A/P view after the needles have been placed in their respective neural foramen in the prior lateral view.

The L3-L4 needle (red arrow) has a caudad-to-cephalad angle – representing a caudal tilt used to square the L3 SEP prior to needle placement.

The L5-S1 needle (green arrow) has a cephalad-to-caudad angle – representing a cephalad tilt used to square the L5 SEP prior to needle placement.

An example of NOT squaring the endplates prior to needle placement…

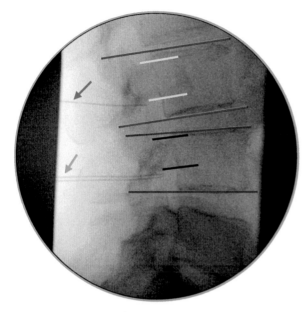

Figure 1-16A
Tilt: 0°
Oblique: 90° Right

Lateral View. Final needle position in the lateral view.

For the superior needle (blue arrow), note how it is NOT parallel to the L3 endplates (red lines) or the corresponding L3 pedicles (yellow lines). Optimal squaring of the L3 SEP was NOT performed prior to needle placement. Consequently, if further needle advancement is needed to deliver medication in the epidural space, it will be challenging to keep this needle tip in the superior foramen – *posing an increased risk of the needle contacting the exiting nerve root.*

In contrast, the L4 endplates were properly squared prior to needle placement. As a result, the inferior needles at L4-L5 (green arrow) are seen to be fairly parallel to the L4 endplates (purple lines) and pedicles (black lines) – allowing the needle tips to be easily placed in the desired superior aspect of the foramen.

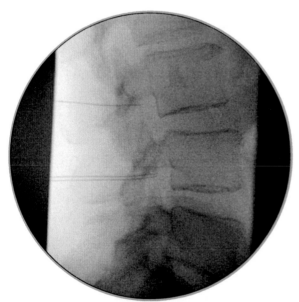

Figure 1-16B
Tilt: 0°
Oblique: 90° Right

Lateral View. *Figure 1-16A reproduced without marker lines.* One can clearly see in this image the effect of not squaring (superior needle) vs. squaring (inferior needles) the endplates prior to needle placement – note the needle trajectories as they enter their foramen.

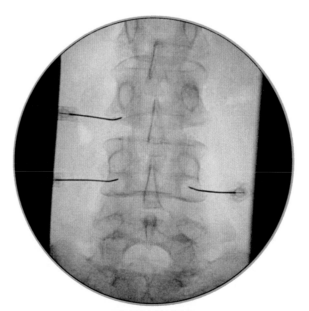

Figure 1-16C
Tilt: 0°
Oblique: 0°

A/P View. Final needle position after placement in the prior lateral view (Figure 1-16B). *Note how the left superior and inferior needles are fairly parallel even though the L3 and L4 SEPs are not parallel – this is NOT ideal.*

Additional Discussion:
The 20° Ipsilateral Oblique is only meant to be a "Rule of Thumb"...

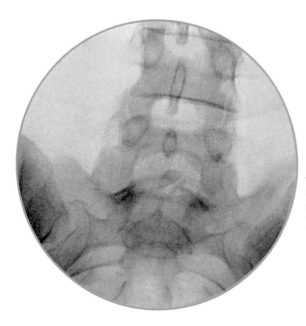

Figure 1-17A
Tilt: 0°
Oblique: 0°

A/P View. Note that the L5 spinous process is fairly midline. Thus, given this "true" A/P view, as a rule of thumb, a 20° ipsilateral oblique may be used to target the L5-S1 foramen.

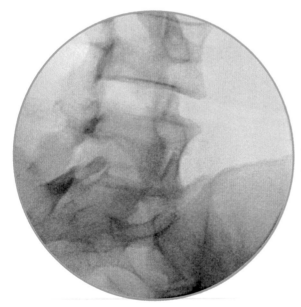

Figure 1-17B
Tilt: 0°
Oblique: 20° Right

Oblique View. Using the "Rule of Thumb" of 20° ipsilateral oblique to view the targeted foramen, in this example the right S1 SAP is still NOT seen to be at (or slightly medial to) the 6 o'clock position of the right L5 pedicle, which would have been the ideal amount of rotation. Therefore, further oblique will be needed.

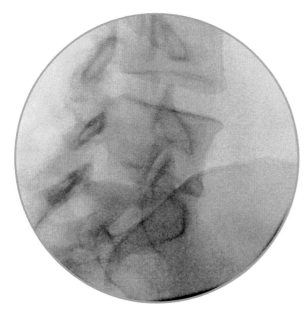

Figure 1-17C
Tilt: 5° Cephalad
Oblique: 40° Right

Oblique View. An ipsilateral oblique angle of double the "Rule of Thumb" was required to get an adequate view of this targeted foramen. Note that the position of the right S1 SAP is now at approximately the 6 o'clock position of the right L5 pedicle, which is the ideal amount of rotation *(Compare to Figure 1-17B)*.

Also, note how a slight cephalad tilt better squares the L5 SEP *(Compare to Figure 1-17B)*.

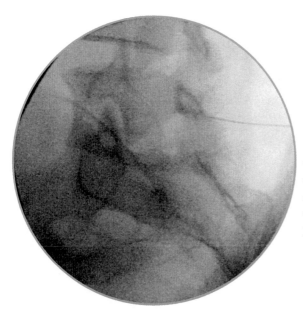

Figure 1-17D
Tilt: 5° Cephalad
Oblique: 50° Left

Oblique View. In this same patient, an even greater oblique is required to the get an ideal view of the left L5-S1 foramen. Note the position of the left S1 SAP at approximately the 6 o'clock position of the left L5 pedicle – ideal amount of rotation.

Additional Discussion:
Transforaminal Epidural vs. Selective Nerve Root Block

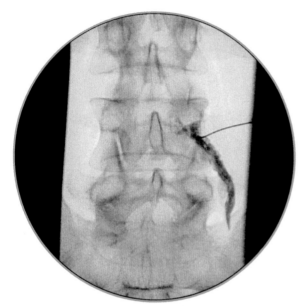

Figure 1-18
Tilt: 0°
Oblique: 0°

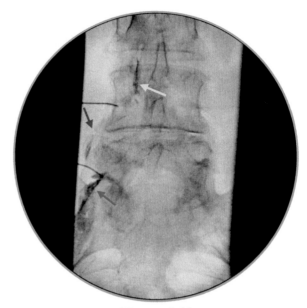

Figure 1-19
Tilt: 0°
Oblique: 0°

A/P View. Note that contrast spread is seen to be outlining the right L4 nerve root. However, there is no significant contrast spread seen wrapping around the L4 pedicle and into the epidural space. This represents a SNRB and NOT a TFESI.

A/P View.

Superior Needle – Note that contrast spread is seen to be outlining the left L4 nerve root (red arrow), and wrapping around the L4 pedicle into the epidural space (yellow arrow) – this represents a TFESI.

Inferior Needle – Note that contrast spread is seen to be outlining the left L5 nerve root (blue arrow), but NOT wrapping around the L5 pedicle and into the epidural space – this represents a SNRB.

With a Selective Nerve Root Block, contrast spread is seen around the nerve root (neurogram), but NOT wrapping around the pedicle and into the epidural space.

In order to obtain transforaminal epidural spread, the needle will need to be adjusted. This may be accomplished by simply advancing the needle a bit further in its current oblique trajectory. If this does not produce the desired epidurogram, alternatively, the needle may also be withdrawn slightly and advanced in a more medial trajectory towards the targeted foramen – the proceduralist must carefully monitor for any reported paresthesias throughout needle manipulation.

Additional Discussion:
Varying Transforaminal Epidural Contrast Spread Patterns
Because no two patients are exactly alike...

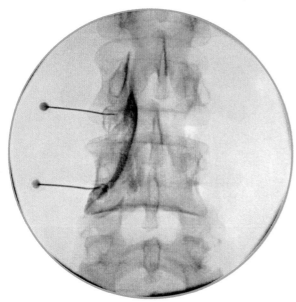

Figure 1-20

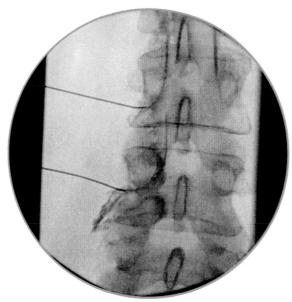

Figure 1-21

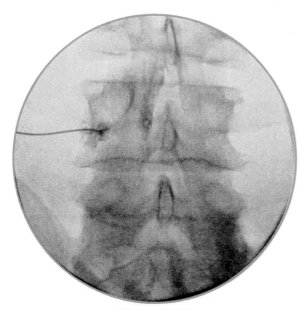

Figure 1-22

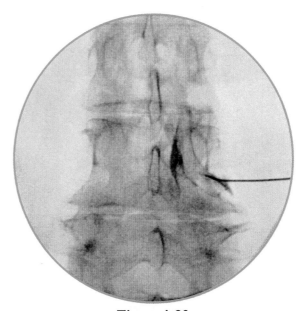

Figure 1-23

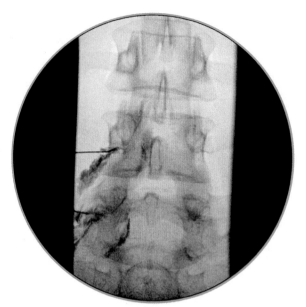

Figure 1-24

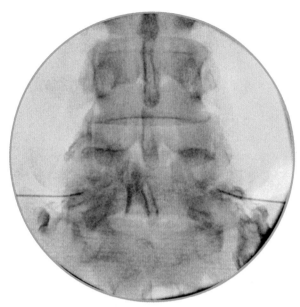

Figure 1-25

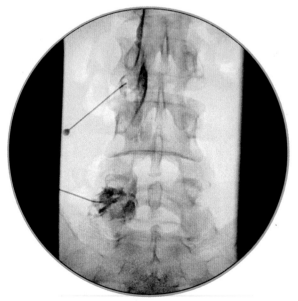

Figure 1-26

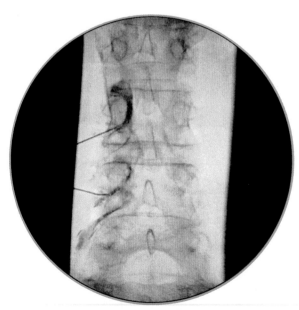

Figure 1-27

Chapter 2
S1 Transforaminal Epidural Steroid Injection

- Obtain an A/P view to identify the sacral endplate and S1 pedicle on the targeted side. The S1 dorsal sacral foramen is located just inferior to the S1 pedicle. Often times, the S1 foramen can be easily identified with a "straight A/P" view (i.e., without a tilt). However, if the S1 foramen is not clearly visualized with this view, a cephalad tilt and/or a slight ipsilateral oblique may be applied. Although using a more pronounced cephalad tilt to line up the sacral endplate can be attempted, it is the author's experience that often times only a slight cephalad tilt is needed to clearly visualize the S1 foramen – while also being technically less challenging.

> *It is important that the proceduralist does not confuse the S1 foramen with the larger S2 dorsal sacral foramen, which is more inferior to the expected location of the S1 foramen. See page 54 for an "Additional Discussion" on the use of anatomical landmarks to accurately estimate the location of the S1 nerve in the S1 dorsal sacral foramen.*

- Once the S1 foramen has been clearly visualized, place the needle coaxially towards the superomedial aspect of the foramen, as this helps to avoid the needle tip contacting the S1 nerve which typically runs inferolateral. Once the needle approaches the foramen, one may feel a subtle increase in resistance. However, the proceduralist should not solely rely on this increased resistance, and should implement the use of intermittent lateral fluoroscopy as needed to assess needle depth. Alternatively, one may also consider walking the needle off the sacral periosteum in order to estimate needle depth.

- After the needle tip approaches the foramen, a lateral view is obtained so that needle depth can be clearly assessed while further advancement is carried out. The needle tip should be advanced to a depth just anterior to the ventral epidural space, and should not be advanced to the floor of the sacral canal.

- Next, obtain an A/P view to confirm needle positioning. After negative aspiration, administer contrast under live fluoroscopy to ensure that there is no vascular uptake with a noted proper S1 neurogram and epidurogram.

Left S1 Dorsal Foramen

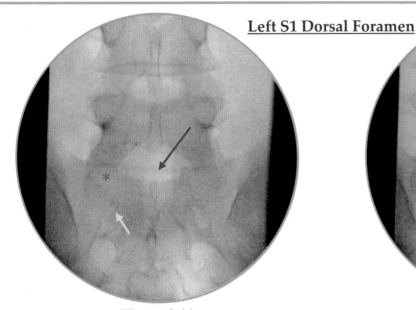

Figure 2-1A
Tilt: 0°
Oblique: 0°

A/P View. Note the sacral endplate (red arrow) and left S1 pedicle (blue star). The left S1 dorsal sacral foramen is not clearly visualized in this view (yellow arrow) – further fluoroscopic adjustment may be used for better visualization.

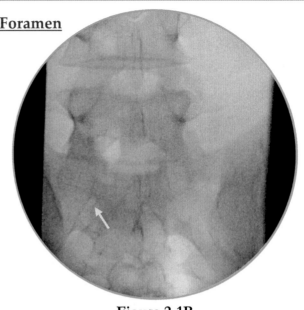

Figure 2-1B
Tilt: 0°
Oblique: 5° Left

Oblique View. Note how a slight ipsilateral oblique allows for better visualization of the left S1 dorsal sacral foramen (yellow arrow) – *Compare to Figure 2-1A.*

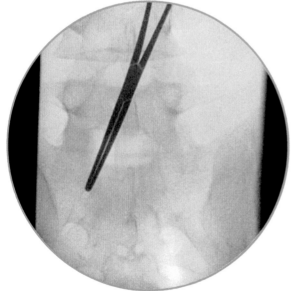

Figure 2-1C
Tilt: 0°
Oblique: 5° Left

Oblique View. Pointer showing location of ideal needle placement at the left S1 dorsal sacral foramen. One should aim to be towards the superomedial aspect of the foramen, to avoid the spinal nerve which typically runs in the inferolateral aspect of the foramen.

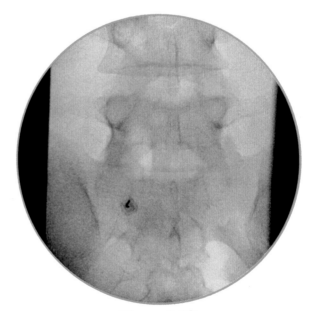

Figure 2-1D
Tilt: 0°
Oblique: 5° Left

Oblique View. Needle placed coaxially at the superomedial aspect of the left S1 foramen. Once the needle approaches the foramen, often a subtle increase in resistance can be felt. *If not felt, use intermittent lateral fluoroscopy or consider slightly walking off the sacral periosteum.*

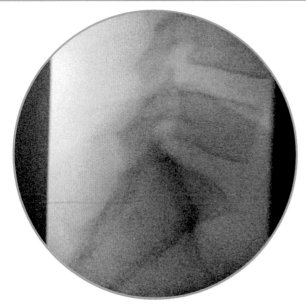

Figure 2-1E
Tilt: 0°
Oblique: 90° Right

Lateral View. After the needle approaches the foramen in the prior view, the lateral view is used to perform further advancement just anterior to the ventral epidural space. Do NOT advance the needle tip to the floor of the sacral canal.

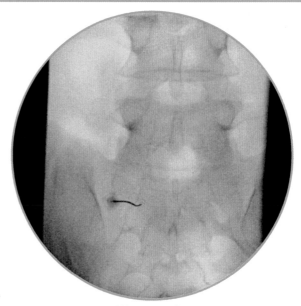

Figure 2-1F
Tilt: 0°
Oblique: 0°

A/P View. Needle placement within the left S1 dorsal sacral foramen after it has been advanced to its final position in the prior lateral view.

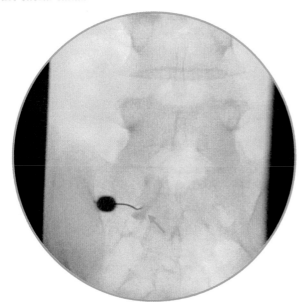

Figure 2-1G
Tilt: 0°
Oblique: 0°

A/P View. After negative aspiration, a small amount of contrast is administered and begins to show spread outlining the left S1 nerve root (green arrow).

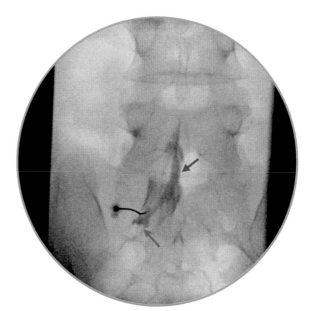

Figure 2-1H
Tilt: 0°
Oblique: 0°

A/P View. With administration of additional contrast, a proper epidurogram (red arrow) and left S1 neurogram (blue arrow) is now seen.

See Page 268

Left S1 Dorsal Foramen

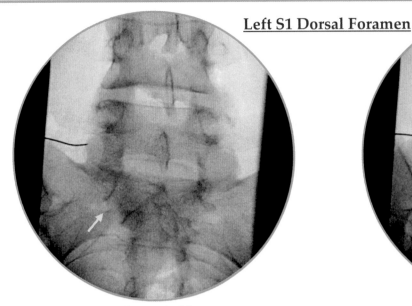

Figure 2-2A
Tilt: 0°
Oblique: 0°

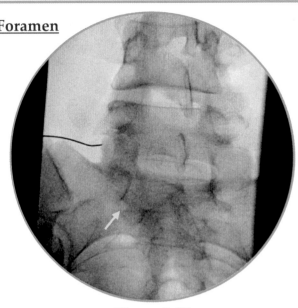

Figure 2-2B
Tilt: 0°
Oblique: 5° Left

A/P View. In this view, one can somewhat see the left S1 dorsal sacral foramen (yellow arrow). However, a further ipsilateral oblique may be considered for better visualization of the foramen – see Figure 2-2B. *Note the additional needle placed towards the left L5-S1 foramen.*

Oblique View. Note how a slight ipsilateral oblique provides better visualization of the left S1 dorsal sacral foramen (yellow arrow).

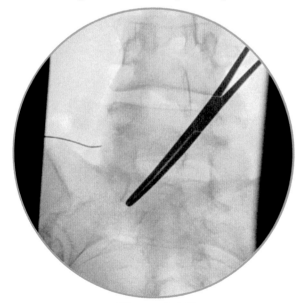

Figure 2-2C
Tilt: 0°
Oblique: 5° Left

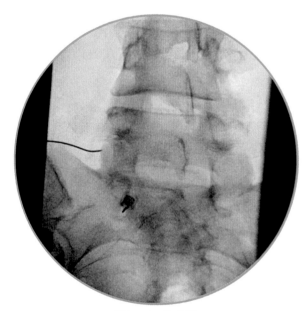

Figure 2-2D
Tilt: 0°
Oblique: 5° Left

Oblique View. Pointer showing location of ideal needle placement at the left S1 dorsal sacral foramen. One should aim to be towards the superomedial aspect of the foramen, to avoid the spinal nerve which typically runs in the inferolateral aspect of the foramen.

Oblique View. Needle placed coaxially at the superomedial aspect of the left S1 foramen. Once the needle approaches the foramen, often a subtle increase in resistance can be felt. *If not felt, use intermittent lateral fluoroscopy or consider slightly walking off the sacral periosteum.*

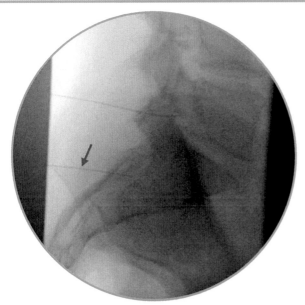

Figure 2-2E
Tilt: 0°
Oblique: 90° Right

Lateral View. After the needle approaches the foramen in the prior view, a lateral view is used to perform further advancement until the needle is just anterior to the ventral epidural space. Do NOT advance the needle tip to the floor of the sacral canal.

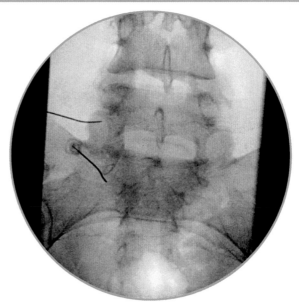

Figure 2-2F
Tilt: 0°
Oblique: 0°

A/P View. Needle placement within the left S1 dorsal sacral foramen after it has been advanced to its final position in the prior lateral view.

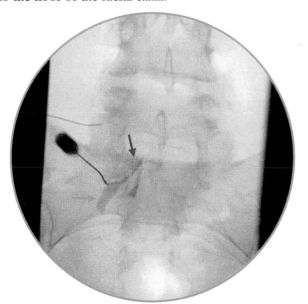

Figure 2-2G
Tilt: 0°
Oblique: 0°

A/P View. After negative aspiration, a small amount of contrast is administered and begins to show a proper epidurogram (red arrow) and left S1 neurogram (green arrow).

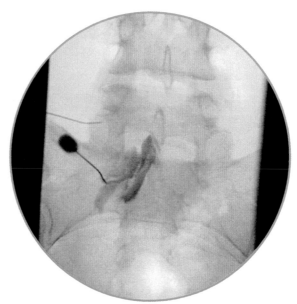

Figure 2-2H
Tilt: 0°
Oblique: 0°

A/P View. After further administration of contrast, note the epidural spread towards the L5-S1 disc space. *Of note, contrast agent has not been administered at the needle placed at the left L5-S1 foramen.*

Left S1 Dorsal Foramen

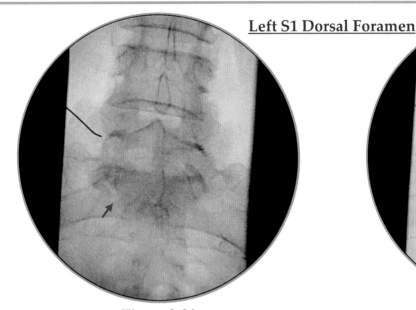

Figure 2-3A
Tilt: 0°
Oblique: 5° Left

Oblique View. Left S1 dorsal sacral foramen (red arrow). *Note the additional needle placed towards the left L5-S1 foramen.*

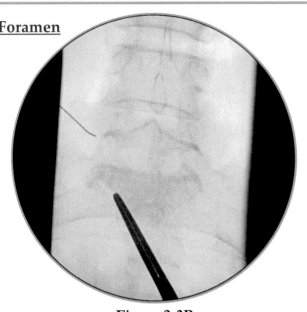

Figure 2-3B
Tilt: 0°
Oblique: 5° Left

Oblique View. Pointer showing location of needle placement at the left S1 dorsal sacral foramen. One should aim to be towards the superomedial aspect of the foramen, to avoid the spinal nerve which typically runs in the inferolateral aspect of the foramen.

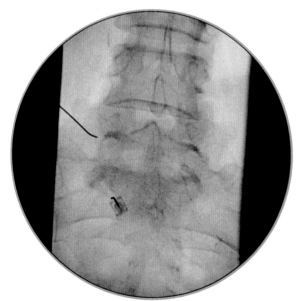

Figure 2-3C
Tilt: 0°
Oblique: 5° Left

Oblique View. Needle placed coaxially at the superomedial aspect of the left S1 foramen. Once the needle approaches the foramen, often a subtle increase in resistance can be felt. *If not felt, use intermittent lateral fluoroscopy or consider slightly walking off the sacral periosteum.*

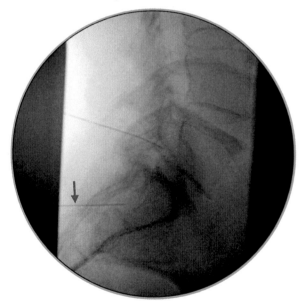

Figure 2-3D
Tilt: 0°
Oblique: 90° Right

Lateral View. After the needle approaches the foramen in the prior view, the needle (red arrow) is further advanced in the lateral view until it is just anterior to the ventral epidural space. Do NOT advance the needle tip to the floor of the sacral canal.

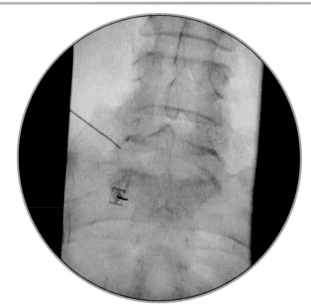

Figure 2-3E
Tilt: 0°
Oblique: 0°

A/P View. Needle placement within the left S1 dorsal sacral foramen after it has been advanced to its final position in the prior lateral view.

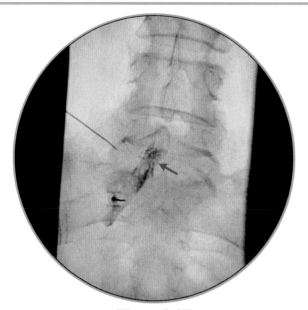

Figure 2-3F
Tilt: 0°
Oblique: 0°

A/P View. After negative aspiration, contrast is administered and shows a proper epidurogram (red arrow) and left S1 neurogram (green arrow).

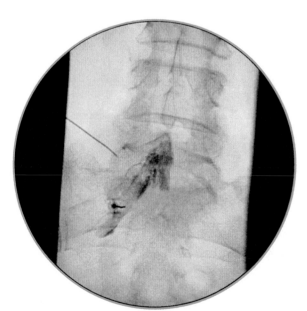

Figure 2-3G
Tilt: 0°
Oblique: 0°

A/P View. After further administration of contrast, note the epidural spread towards the L5 vertebral level. *Of note, contrast has not been administered at the needle placed at the left L5-S1 foramen.*

Additional Discussion:
Using Anatomical Landmarks to Locate the S1 Foramen

In certain instances, it may be difficult to visualize the S1 dorsal sacral foramen due to patient anatomy, advanced degenerative changes, poor image quality related to patient body habitus, or inadequate C-arm contrast/brightness adjustments. In these scenarios, it is helpful to have a sound understanding of anatomical landmarks which can be used to properly estimate the "typical location" of the foramen. This can allow the proceduralist to focus on a specific area of the image without getting distracted by various hyperlucencies which may mimic the foramen.

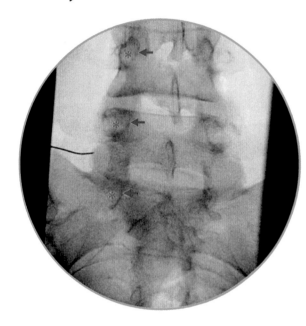

Figure 2-4A
Tilt: 0°
Oblique: 0°

A/P View. *Figure 2-2A reproduced.* Note the left L4, L5, and S1 pedicles (blue stars), as well as the medial border of each pedicle (red arrows). These anatomical landmarks can be used to help focus on identifying the left S1 dorsal sacral foramen – *see Figure 2-4B.*

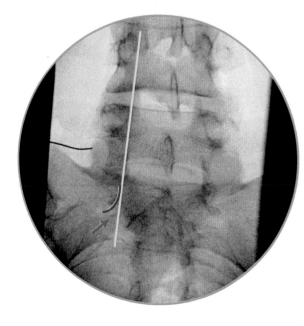

Figure 2-4B
Tilt: 0°
Oblique: 0°

A/P View. *Figure 2-2A reproduced.* In order to accurately estimate the location of the left S1 dorsal sacral foramen, draw an imaginary line connecting the medial borders of the left L4, L5, and S1 pedicles (yellow straight line). Additionally, identify the medial outline of the left S1 pedicle (red curved line).

The S1 dorsal sacral foramen (blue arrow) can be estimated to be just inferomedial to the medial outline of the S1 pedicle and just lateral to the imaginary line connecting the medial borders of the L4-S1 pedicles.

Chapter 3
Caudal Epidural Steroid Injection

☐ Obtain a lateral view to clearly visualize the sacrococcygeal junction. In this view, the location of the sacral hiatus can typically be easily and accurately identified (see Figure 3-1A).

☐ Needle entry should be inferior to the hiatus. Given the fairly close proximity of the sacrum and cocccyx to the skin at this level, often only a slight inferior needle placement is needed. However, it is imperative that a shallow needle angle into the hiatus is used in order to facilitate an inferior-to-superior needle trajectory through the hiatus. A shallow angle also allows the needle to be passed superiorly without encountering resistance from the sacrococcygeal periosteum. Of note, too shallow an angle will increase the probability of the needle lying posterior to the sacrum, whereas too steep an angle may not allow entry through the hiatus and potentially cause the needle to pass anteriorly through the sacrum. With the correct trajectory, the needle is advanced gently through the sacral hiatus. *Once the needle has entered through the sacral hiatus, do not perform further advancement since mediolateral needle positioning cannot be assessed in this view.*

☐ After the needle tip has been confirmed to be through and just beyond the sacral hiatus, and after negative aspiration, contrast is administered under live fluoroscopy to ensure that there is no vascular uptake with proper epidural spread – *spread should be seen within the sacral canal and not posterior or anterior to the sacrum.*

☐ Next, an A/P view is obtained. In this view, the needle is advanced further and adjusted mediolaterally as needed to target a specific side (or midline for both sides if needed). The proceduralist should aim to advance the needle tip no further cephalad than the S3 level to avoid potential dural puncture – as the dural sac typically ends at S2 in adults. After final needle advancement and positioning has been completed, further contrast may be administered in a similar fashion as previously discussed to ensure spread cephalad and on the desired side(s).

Example 1

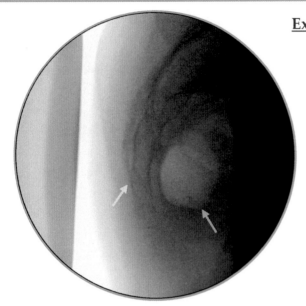

Figure 3-1A
Tilt: 0°
Oblique: 90° Right

Lateral View. Use of collimation reduces radiation exposure and also allows for a clearer view of the sacrum and sacral hiatus (yellow arrow). Note the bowel gas pattern just anterior to the sacrum (green arrow).

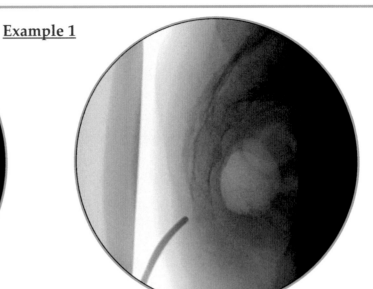

Figure 3-1B
Tilt: 0°
Oblique: 90° Right

Lateral View. Pointer showing the location of needle entry, inferior to the sacral hiatus. A shallow needle angle facilitates needle advancement through the hiatus and futher superiorly, without encountering resistance from the sacrococcygeal periosteum.

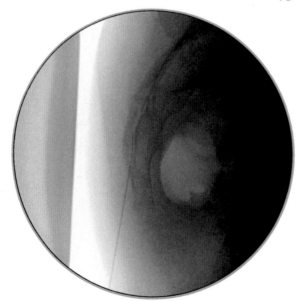

Figure 3-1C
Tilt: 0°
Oblique: 90° Right

Lateral View. Needle placement through the sacral hiatus. Note that the needle is seen to be within the sacral canal. *Needle angle entry is important - too steep an angle may potentially lead to a needle anterior to the sacrum, whereas too shallow an angle may cause the needle to be posterior to the sacrum.*

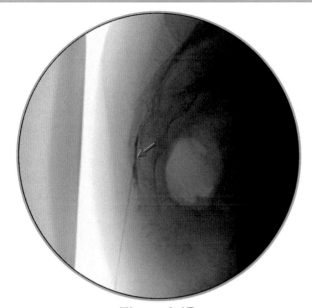

Figure 3-1D
Tilt: 0°
Oblique: 90° Right

Lateral View. After negative aspiration, contrast is administered and shows proper epidural spread within the sacral canal (red arrow).

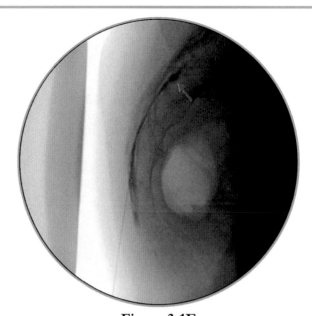

Figure 3-1E
Tilt: 0°
Oblique: 90° Right

Lateral View. After further administration of contrast, note the superior spread maintained within the sacral canal (red arrow).

Next, an A/P view is obtained (see Figure 3-1F).

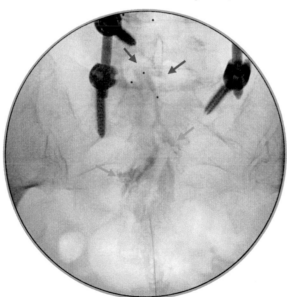

Figure 3-1F
Tilt: 0°
Oblique: 0°

A/P View. Note the epidural spread of contrast traveling superiorly towards the L5-S1 disc space (red arrows), and outlining the sacral nerve roots (green arrows). If needed, the needle tip can be further advanced and adjusted mediolaterally in this view. Aim to keep the needle tip no higher than the S3 level to avoid dural puncture, as the dura mater typically ends at S2 in adults.

See Page 274

Example 2

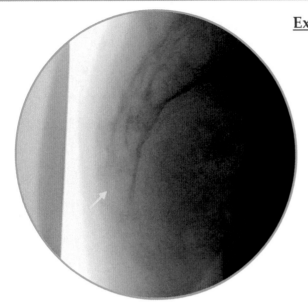

Figure 3-2A
Tilt: 0°
Oblique: 90° Right

Lateral View. Use of collimation reduces radiation exposure and also allows for a clearer view of the sacrum and sacral hiatus (yellow arrow).

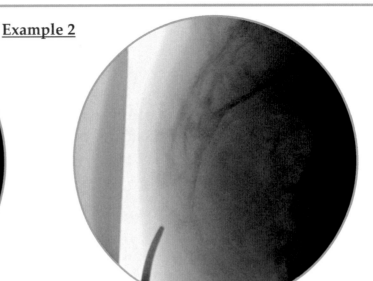

Figure 3-2B
Tilt: 0°
Oblique: 90° Right

Lateral View. Pointer showing the location of needle entry, inferior to the sacral hiatus. A shallow needle angle facilitates needle advancement through the hiatus and superiorly, without encountering resistance from the sacrococcygeal periosteum.

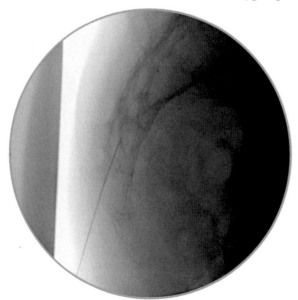

Figure 3-2C
Tilt: 0°
Oblique: 90° Right

Lateral View. Needle placement through the sacral hiatus. Note that the needle is seen to be within the sacral canal. *Needle angle entry is important - too steep an angle may potentially lead to a needle anterior to the sacrum, whereas too shallow an angle may cause the needle to be posterior to the sacrum.*

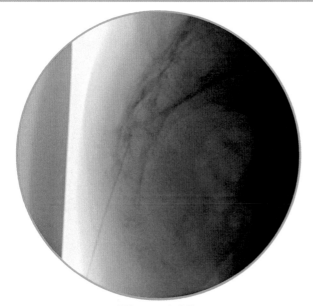

Figure 3-2D
Tilt: 0°
Oblique: 90° Right

Lateral View. After negative aspiration, contrast is administered and shows proper epidural spread within the sacral canal.

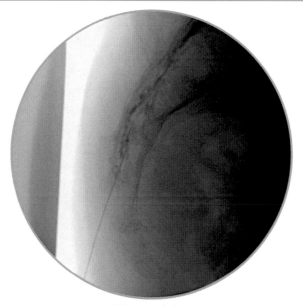

Figure 3-2E
Tilt: 0°
Oblique: 90° Right

Lateral View. After further administration of contrast, note that the spread is maintained within the sacral canal.

Next, an A/P view is obtained.

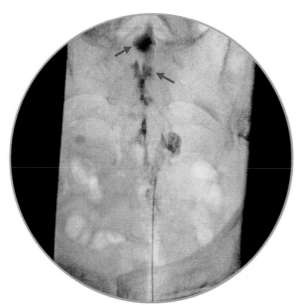

Figure 3-2F
Tilt: 0°
Oblique: 0°

A/P View. Note the epidural spread of contrast traveling superiorly (red arrows). If needed, the needle tip can be further advanced and adjusted mediolaterally in this view. Aim to keep the needle tip no higher than the S3 level to avoid dural puncture, as the dura mater typically ends at S2 in adults.

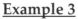
Example 3

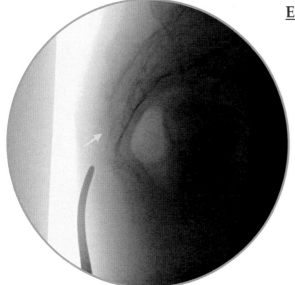

Figure 3-3A
Tilt: 0°
Oblique: 90° Right

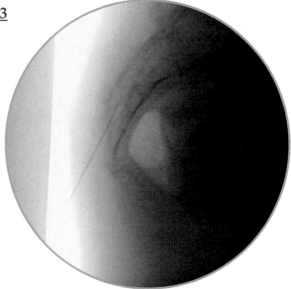

Figure 3-3B
Tilt: 0°
Oblique: 90° Right

Lateral View. Pointer showing the location of needle entry, inferior to the sacral hiatus (yellow arrow). A shallow needle angle facilitates needle advancement through the hiatus and superiorly, without encountering resistance from the sacrococcygeal periosteum.

Lateral View. Needle placement through the sacral hiatus. Note that the needle is seen to be within the sacral canal. *Needle angle entry is important - too steep an angle may potentially lead to a needle anterior to the sacrum, whereas too shallow an angle may cause the needle to be posterior to the sacrum.*

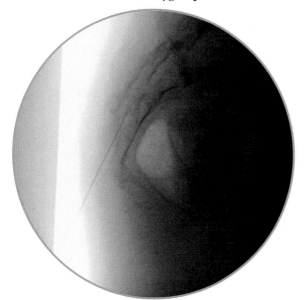

Figure 3-3C
Tilt: 0°
Oblique: 90° Right

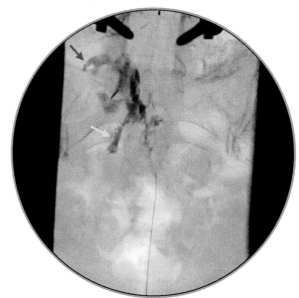

Figure 3-3D
Tilt: 0°
Oblique: 0°

Lateral View. After negative aspiration, contrast is administered and shows proper epidural spread within the sacral canal.

A/P View. Note the epidural spread of contrast traveling superiorly and outlining the left L5 (red arrow), left S1 (green arrow), and left S2 (yellow arrow) nerve roots. If needed, the needle tip can be further advanced and adjusted mediolaterally in this view.

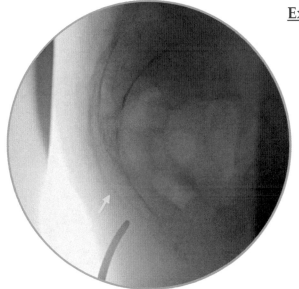

Figure 3-4A
Tilt: 0°
Oblique: 90° Right

Lateral View. Pointer showing the location of needle entry, inferior to the sacral hiatus (yellow arrow). A shallow needle angle facilitates needle advancement through the hiatus and superiorly, without encountering resistance from the sacrococcygeal periosteum.

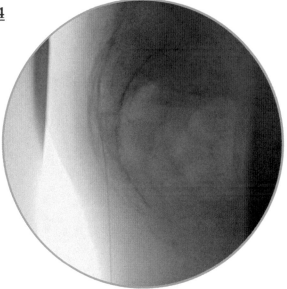

Figure 3-4B
Tilt: 0°
Oblique: 90° Right

Lateral View. Needle placement through the sacral hiatus. Note that the needle is seen to be within the sacral canal. *Needle angle entry is important - too steep an angle may potentially lead to a needle anterior to the sacrum, whereas too shallow an angle may cause the needle to be posterior to the sacrum.*

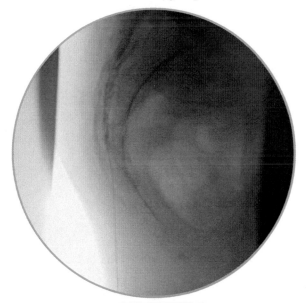

Figure 3-4C
Tilt: 0°
Oblique: 90° Right

Lateral View. After negative aspiration, contrast is administered and shows proper epidural spread within the sacral canal.

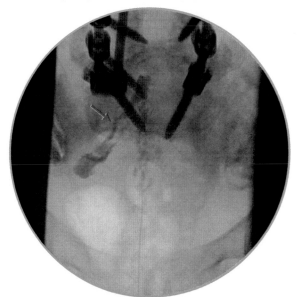

Figure 3-4D
Tilt: 0°
Oblique: 0°

A/P View. Note the epidural spread of contrast traveling superiorly and outlining the left sacral nerve root (red arrow). If needed, the needle tip can be further advanced and adjusted mediolaterally in this view.

Example 5

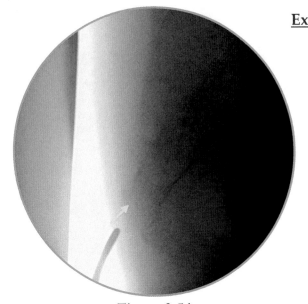

Figure 3-5A
Tilt: 0°
Oblique: 90° Right

Lateral View. Pointer showing the location of needle entry, inferior to the sacral hiatus (yellow arrow). A shallow needle angle facilitates needle advancement through the hiatus and superiorly, without encountering resistance from the sacrococcygeal periosteum.

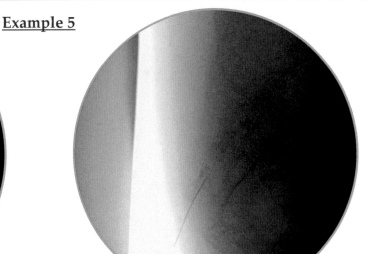

Figure 3-5B
Tilt: 0°
Oblique: 90° Right

Lateral View. Needle placement through the sacral hiatus. Note that the needle is seen to be within the sacral canal. *Needle angle entry is important - too steep an angle may potentially lead to a needle anterior to the sacrum, whereas too shallow an angle may cause the needle to be posterior to the sacrum.*

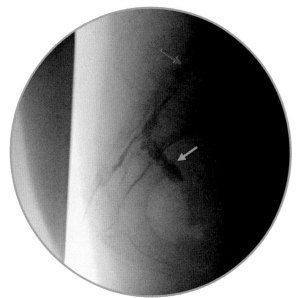

Figure 3-5C
Tilt: 0°
Oblique: 90° Right

Lateral View. After negative aspiration, contrast is administered and shows proper epidural spread (red arrow) within the sacral canal, and anteriorly through the sacral foramen (green arrow). Next, an A/P view is obtained.

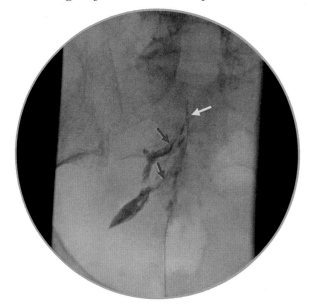

Figure 3-5D
Tilt: 0°
Oblique: 0°

A/P View. Note the epidural spread of contrast, traveling superiorly and outlining the left sacral nerve roots (red arrows). If needed, the needle tip can be further advanced and adjusted mediolaterally in this view.

Chapter 4
Lumbar Interlaminar Epidural Steroid Injection

- ☐ Obtain an A/P View to visualize the targeted interspace.

- ☐ Apply a fluoroscopic tilt as needed to open up the interlaminar space.

- ☐ Place a Tuohy epidural needle towards the targeted interspace, in either a midline or paramedian position if targeting a specific side. The needle entry can be directly overlying the targeted interspace. However, it is the author's preference to perform needle entry inferior and paramedian to the midline of the targeted interlaminar space, as this allows the laminar edge to be used as an additional safety measure for needle depth assessment in the A/P view (see Figure 4-1D). In addition, with this approach a caudad-to-cephalad needle trajectory is created, which further facilitates smooth entry into the interlaminar space. The needle is advanced towards the interspace, and once it enters the ligamentum flavum, often an increase in resistance is felt. *However, this increased resistance should not be solely relied upon and the use of intermittent lateral fluoroscopy is recommended as needed to avoid inadvertent dural puncture during needle advancement.*

- ☐ Once the needle is noted to be approaching, or at, the ligamentum flavum, a lateral view is obtained, where needle depth can be properly assessed during further advancement. The loss of resistance (LOR) syringe should also be attached at this point, and the needle is then advanced using the LOR technique, using intermittent lateral fluoroscopy as needed, until LOR is achieved. *Of note, intermittent use of biplanar imaging (i.e., A/P and lateral) throughout the procedure will help to ensure that the needle tip stays either midline or on the desired symptomatic side.*

- ☐ Next, after negative aspiration, administer contrast under live fluoroscopy and ensure that there is no vascular uptake with proper spread in the posterior epidural space.

- ☐ Finally, obtain an A/P view and administer additional contrast in a similar fashion as previously described to confirm appropriate epidural contrast spread in the desired location.

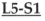

L5-S1

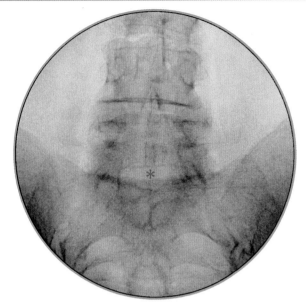

Figure 4-1A
Tilt: 0°
Oblique: 0°

A/P View. Note the L5-S1 interspace (blue star). The interspace is fairly "open," so an additional caudal tilt is not needed.

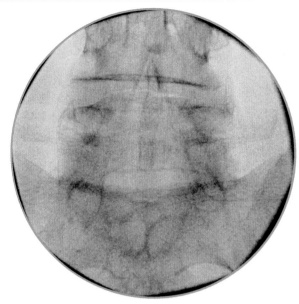

Figure 4-1B
Tilt: 0°
Oblique: 0°

A/P View. Using collimation, one may focus on the targeted interspace while also reducing radiation exposure to both the patient and proceduralist.

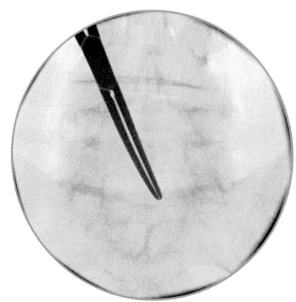

Figure 4-1C
Tilt: 0°
Oblique: 0°

A/P View. Pointer showing location of needle placement inferior and paramedian to the midline of the targeted interspace. With this type of needle trajectory, the laminar edge can be used as an additional safety measure for needle depth assessment.

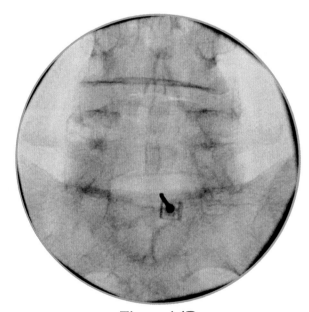

Figure 4-1D
Tilt: 0°
Oblique: 0°

A/P View. Needle placement inferior and paramedian to the interspace. Once the needle approaches the LF, often an increase in resistance is felt. *If this is not felt at the expected depth, intermittent lateral fluoroscopy should be used as needed for depth assessment.* Next, obtain a lateral view.

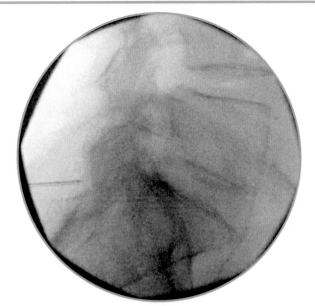

Figure 4-1E
Tilt: 0°
Oblique: 90° Right

Lateral View. Note the needle position in this view after it has approached the LF in the prior A/P view. At this needle depth, a LOR syringe is attached and the needle is advanced using intermittent fluoroscopy as needed until LOR is obtained.

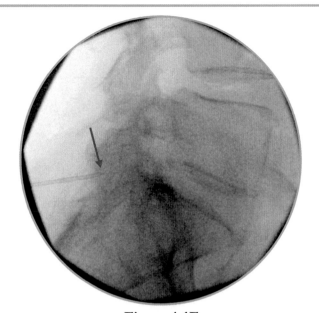

Figure 4-1F
Tilt: 0°
Oblique: 90° Right

Lateral View. Note the needle depth in this view after LOR has been achieved (red arrow) – *compare to Figure 4-1E.*

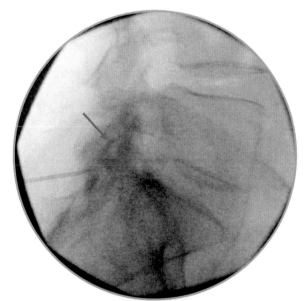

Figure 4-1G
Tilt: 0°
Oblique: 90° Right

Lateral View. After negative aspiration, contrast is administered and shows spread in the posterior epidural space (blue arrow).

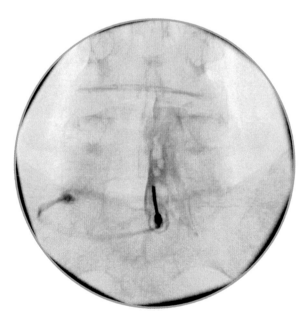

Figure 4-1H
Tilt: 0°
Oblique: 0°

A/P View. After further administration of contrast in this view, epidural contrast spread is seen traveling both cephalad and caudad to the targeted L5-S1 interspace.

See Page 275

L4-L5

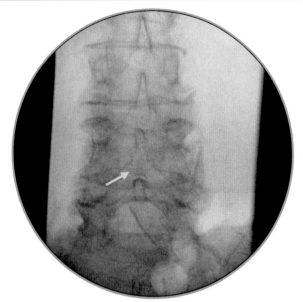

Figure 4-2A
Tilt: 0°
Oblique: 0°

A/P View. Note the L4-L5 interspace, and the large osteophyte coming off the inferior L4 spinous process (yellow arrow).

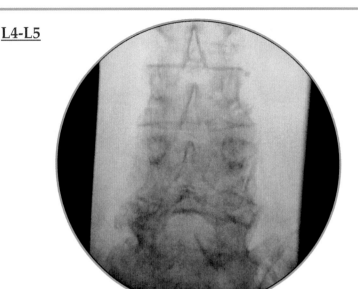

Figure 4-2B
Tilt: 0°
Oblique: 5° Right

Oblique View. Due to patient anatomy and the spinous process osteophyte, a direct midline needle placement is not possible. Therefore, fluoroscopic oblique and caudal needle entry is used to obtain a more optimal trajectory towards the interspace.

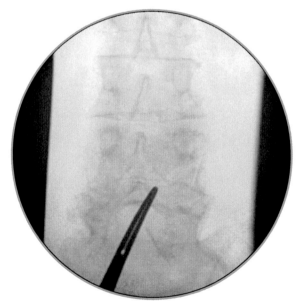

Figure 4-2C
Tilt: 0°
Oblique: 5° Right

Oblique View. Pointer showing location of needle placement inferior and paramedian to the midline of the targeted interspace. With this type of needle trajectory, the laminar edge can be used as an additional safety measure for needle depth assessment.

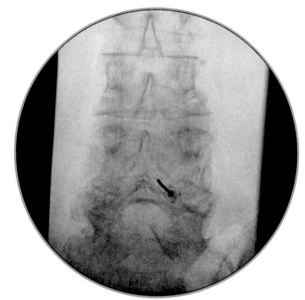

Figure 4-2D
Tilt: 0°
Oblique: 5° Right

Oblique View. Needle placement at the inferior portion of the interspace and just right of midline. The needle is advanced until it is firmly within the subcutaneous tissue and the trajectory towards midline has been established. Next, oblique back to a more "true" A/P view.

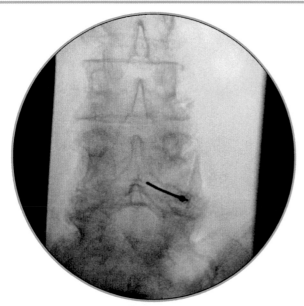

Figure 4-2E
Tilt: 0°
Oblique: 0°

A/P View. Note how the needle is advanced just lateral to the SP osteophyte. Once the needle approaches the LF, often an increase in resistance is felt. *If this is not felt at the expected depth, intermittent lateral fluoroscopy should be used as needed for depth assessment.* Next, obtain a lateral.

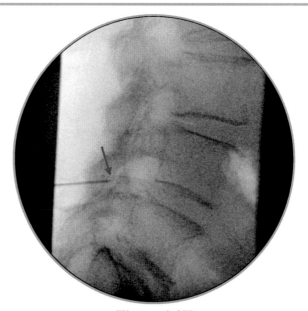

Figure 4-2F
Tilt: 0°
Oblique: 90° Right

Lateral View. The needle is advanced using the LOR technique. *Of note, during advancement in this view, continue to advance the needle towards midline.* Note the needle depth in this view after LOR has been achieved (red arrow).

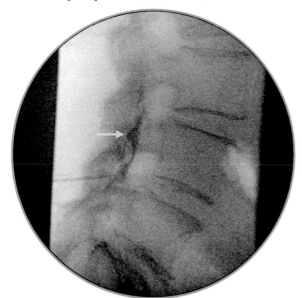

Figure 4-2G
Tilt: 0°
Oblique: 90° Right

Lateral View. After negative aspiration, contrast is administered and shows spread in the posterior epidural space (yellow arrow).

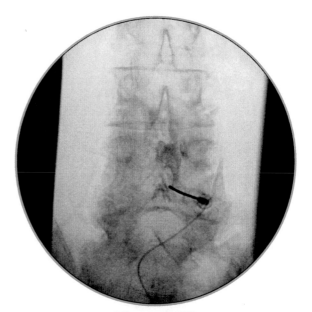

Figure 4-2H
Tilt: 0°
Oblique: 0°

A/P View. Note the epidural contrast spread traveling at and cephalad to the L4-L5 interspace.

L3-L4

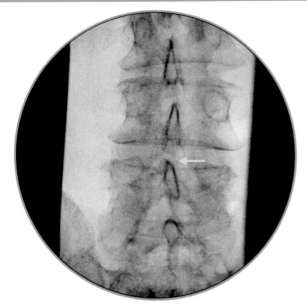

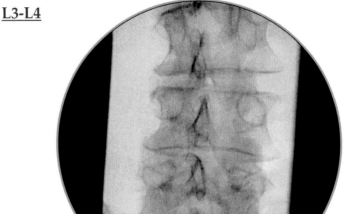

Figure 4-3A
Tilt: 0°
Oblique: 0°

Figure 4-3B
Tilt: 5° Caudad
Oblique: 5° Right

A/P View. Note the L3-L4 interspace (yellow arrow). A slight caudal tilt can be used to further "open" the interspace (see Figure 4-3B).

Oblique View. A right oblique and caudal tilt provides a more optimal view of the L3-L4 interspace – *compare to Figure 4-3A.*

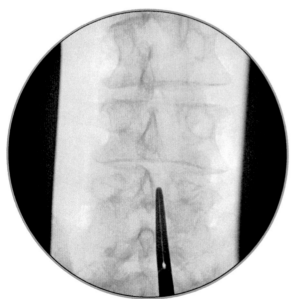

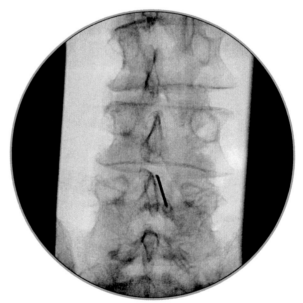

Figure 4-3C
Tilt: 5° Caudad
Oblique: 5° Right

Figure 4-3D
Tilt: 5° Caudad
Oblique: 5° Right

Oblique View. Pointer showing location of needle placement inferior and paramedian to the midline of the targeted interspace. With this type of needle trajectory, the laminar edge can be used as an additional safety measure for needle depth assessment.

Oblique View. Needle placement at the inferior portion of the interspace and just right of midline. The needle is advanced until it is firmly within the subcutaneous tissue and the trajectory towards midline has been established. Next, oblique back to a more "true" A/P view.

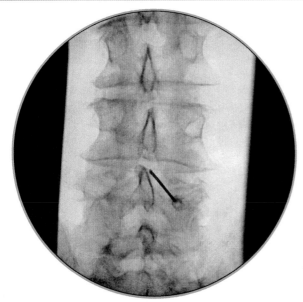

Figure 4-3E
Tilt: 5° Caudad
Oblique: 0°

A/P View. Note how the needle is advanced just lateral to the spinous process, but with a trajectory towards midline. Once the needle approaches the LF, one may often feel an increase in resistance. At this point, a lateral view is obtained.

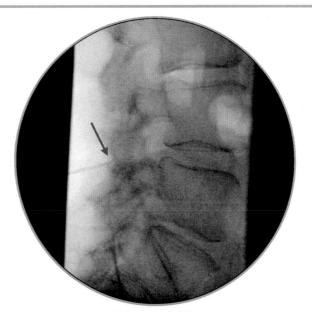

Figure 4-3F
Tilt: 0°
Oblique: 90° Right

Lateral View. Note the needle position in this view after it has approached the LF in the prior A/P view (red arrow). At this needle depth, attach a LOR syringe and advance the needle using intermittent fluoroscopy as needed, until LOR is obtained.

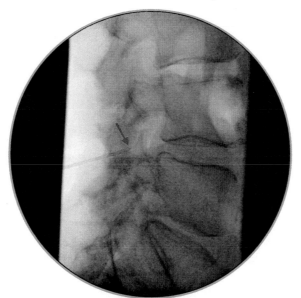

Figure 4-3G
Tilt: 0°
Oblique: 90° Right

Lateral View. Note the needle depth in this view after LOR has been achieved (red arrow).

Of note, during advancement in this view, the needle should be directed towards midline.

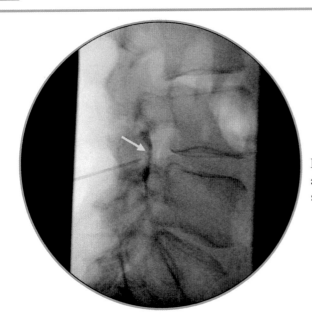

Figure 4-3H
Tilt: 0°
Oblique: 90° Right

Lateral View.   After negative aspiration, contrast is administered and shows spread in the posterior epidural space (yellow arrow).

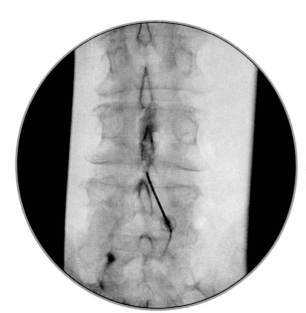

Figure 4-3I
Tilt: 0°
Oblique: 0°

A/P View. Epidural contrast spread traveling cephalad and caudad to the targeted L3-L4 interspace.

L2-L3

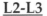

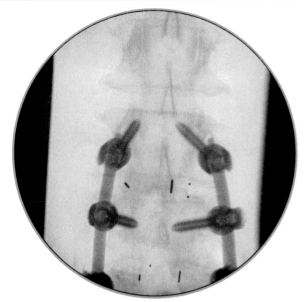

Figure 4-4A
Tilt: 0°
Oblique: 0°

A/P View. The superior pedicle screws are located at L3. Note that the L2-L3 interspace is not optimally "open" for needle placement. Thus, a fluoroscopic adjustment will be needed for optimal needle trajectory and placement.

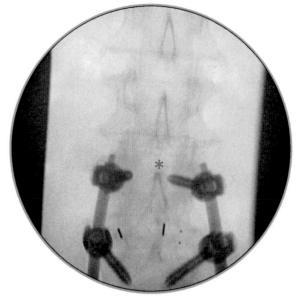

Figure 4-4B
Tilt: 15° Caudad
Oblique: 0°

A/P View. A caudal tilt provides a more optimal view of the L2-L3 interspace (blue star) – *compare to Figure 4-4A.*

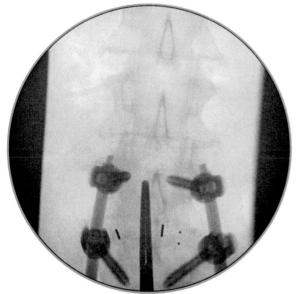

Figure 4-4C
Tilt: 15° Caudad
Oblique: 0°

A/P View. Pointer showing location of needle placement inferior and paramedian to the midline of the targeted interspace. With this type of needle trajectory, the laminar edge can be used as an additional safety measure for needle depth assessment.

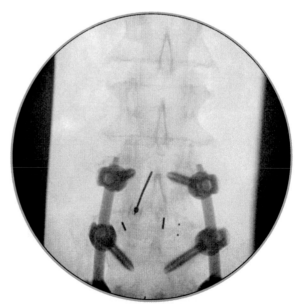

Figure 4-4D
Tilt: 15° Caudad
Oblique: 0°

A/P View. Needle placement at the inferior portion of the interspace. Once the needle approaches the LF, often an increase in resistance is felt. *If this is not felt at the expected depth, intermittent lateral fluoroscopy should be used as needed for depth assessment.* Next, obtain a lateral.

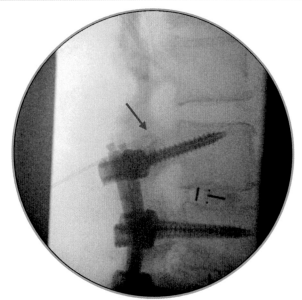

Figure 4-4E
Tilt: 0°
Oblique: 90° Right

Lateral View. Note the needle depth in this view after LOR has been achieved (red arrow).

Of note, during needle advancement in this view, continue to direct the needle towards midline.

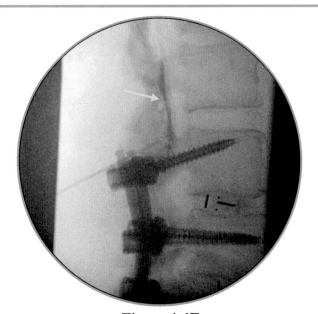

Figure 4-4F
Tilt: 0°
Oblique: 90° Right

Lateral View. After negative aspiration, contrast is administered and shows spread in the posterior epidural space (yellow arrow).

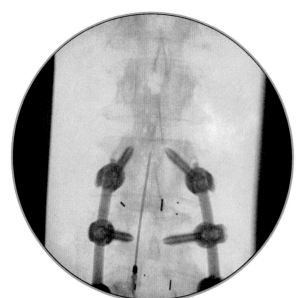

Figure 4-4G
Tilt: 0°
Oblique: 0°

A/P View. Epidural contrast spread traveling at and cephalad to the L2-L3 interspace.

L1-L2

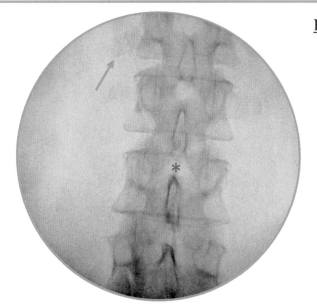

Figure 4-5A
Tilt: 10° Caudad
Oblique: 0°

A/P View. Note the 12th rib (green arrow). The L1-L2 interspace (blue star) is fairly open and visible by applying a caudal tilt.

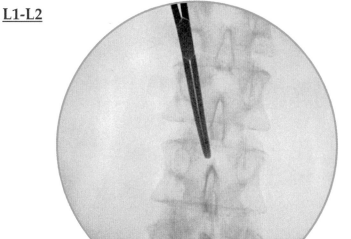

Figure 4-5B
Tilt: 10° Caudad
Oblique: 0°

A/P View. Pointer showing location of needle placement at the L1-L2 interspace.

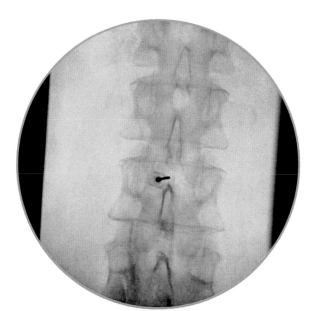

Figure 4-5C
Tilt: 10° Caudad
Oblique: 0°

A/P View. Needle placement at the L1-L2 interspace. The needle is advanced until it is firmly within the subcutaneous tissue and the trajectory towards midline has been established.

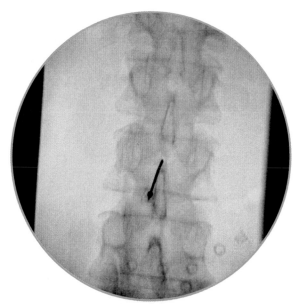

Figure 4-5D
Tilt: 0°
Oblique: 0°

A/P View. Note the needle trajectory after the caudal tilt has been removed. Once the needle approaches the LF, often an increase in resistance is felt. *If this is not felt at the expected depth, intermittent lateral fluoroscopy should be used as needed for depth assessment.* Next, obtain a lateral.

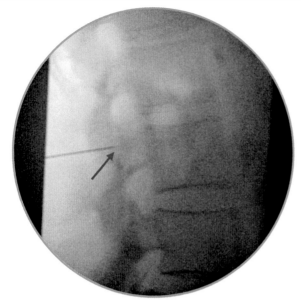

Figure 4-5E
Tilt: 0°
Oblique: 90° Right

Lateral View. Note the needle depth in this view after LOR has been obtained (red arrow).

Of note, during needle advancement in this view, continue to direct the needle towards midline.

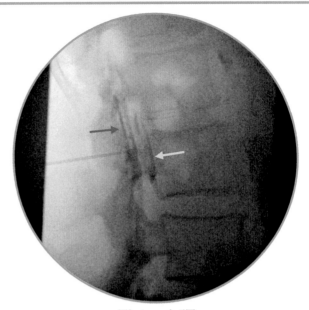

Figure 4-5F
Tilt: 0°
Oblique: 90° Right

Lateral View. After negative aspiration, contrast is administered and shows spread in the posterior (blue arrow) and anterior (yellow arrow) epidural space.

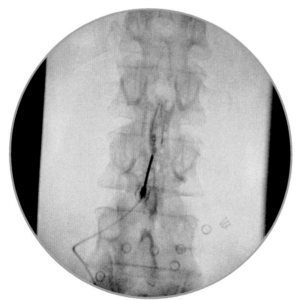

Figure 4-5G
Tilt: 0°
Oblique: 0°

A/P View. Epidural contrast spread traveling cephalad and caudad to the L1-L2 interspace.

Chapter 5
Thoracic Interlaminar Epidural Steroid Injection

The spinous process angle differs throughout the thoracic spine. The T5-T9 spinous processes have a significant downward slope, making a midline needle entry challenging, if not impossible. In contrast, typically the T1-T4 and T10-T12 spinous processes do not have such a significant slope, and a midline approach can often be successfully performed in this region.

Upper Thoracic (T1-T4) & Lower Thoracic (T10-T12) Levels:
- ☐ Obtain an A/P View to visualize the targeted interspace. If needed, apply a tilt (typically caudal) to "open" up the interlaminar space.
- ☐ Place a Tuohy epidural needle towards the targeted interspace. Due to the lack of a significant slope of the spinous processes in this region, a midline needle approach is possible *(see Figure 5-6C and 5-6D)*. However, it is the author's preference to perform needle entry inferior and paramedian to the midline interlaminar space, as this allows the laminar edge to provide an additional safety measure for assessing needle depth *(see Figure 5-1B and 5-1C)*. Once the needle enters the ligamentum flavum, often an increase in resistance is felt.
- ☐ Next, a lateral view is obtained and a LOR syringe attached. Further needle advancement is carried out in this view, where needle depth may be optimally assessed, using the LOR technique. Once LOR is achieved, and after negative aspiration, contrast is administered under live fluoroscopy to ensure that there is no vascular uptake with proper epidural spread in the posterior epidural space. *Of note, intermittent use of biplanar imaging (i.e., A/P and lateral) throughout the procedure can help to ensure that the needle tip stays midline or on the desired symptomatic side, while also preventing the risk of dural puncture. Alternatively, in place of a lateral view for needle depth assessment, one may also consider using the contralateral oblique view (see Chapter 6 for further discussion on the CLO view).*
- ☐ Next, obtain an A/P view, and administer additional contrast in a similar fashion as previously discussed to confirm appropriate epidural contrast spread in the desired location.

Mid Thoracic (T5-T9) Levels:
- ☐ Take an A/P View to visualize the targeted interspace. If needed, apply a tilt (typically caudal) to open up the interlaminar space.
- ☐ Place a Tuohy epidural needle towards the targeted interspace. Due to the significant sloping of the spinous processes in this region, a midline approach will often be impossible. Thus, a paramedian and inferolateral needle approach will likely be required. Note that this approach also allows the laminar edge to serve as an additional safety measure for assessing needle depth. Once the needle enters the ligamentum flavum, often an increase in resistance is felt.
- ☐ The remaining steps are as described above for the upper and lower thoracic spine.

Lower Thoracic
T10-T11

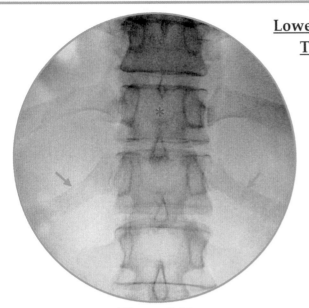

Figure 5-1A
Tilt: 0°
Oblique: 0°

A/P View. Note the targeted T10-T11 interspace (blue star) and 12th rib (green arrows). Given the lack of significant sloping of the SP in the lower thoracic spine, a midline needle placement is possible if desired.

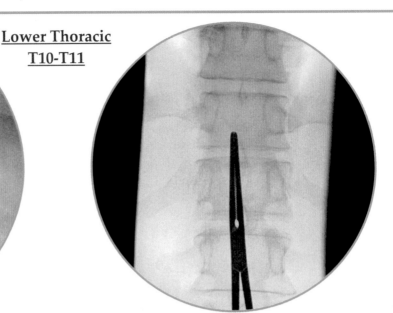

Figure 5-1B
Tilt: 0°
Oblique: 0°

A/P View. Pointer showing location of needle placement left paramedian and inferior to the T11 laminar edge. Placing the needle inferolateral to the interspace allows the lamina to provide an additional safety measure.

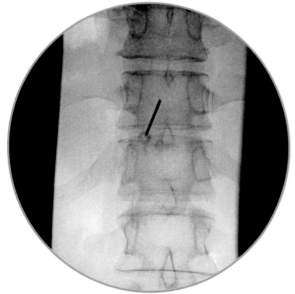

Figure 5-1C
Tilt: 0°
Oblique: 0°

A/P View. Needle advancement towards the interspace. Once the needle tip reaches the laminar edge, a lateral view is obtained. *Note that by contacting bone with the needle tip, and NOT advancing beyond the laminar edge, an additional safety measure is provided.*

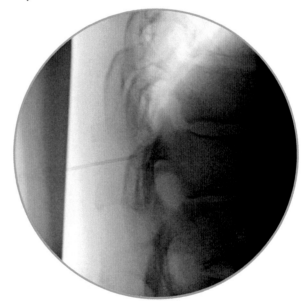

Figure 5-1D
Tilt: 0°
Oblique: 90° Right

Lateral View. Note the needle depth in this view as it approaches the laminar edge. At this point, a LOR syringe can be attached and further needle advancement carried out using the LOR technique and intermittent fluoroscopy as needed.

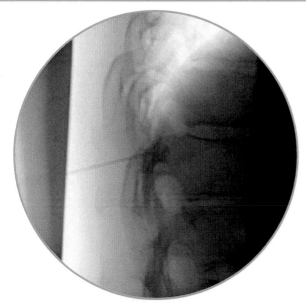

Figure 5-1E
Tilt: 0°
Oblique: 90° Right

Lateral View. Note the needle depth in this view after LOR has been achieved. While advancing the needle in this view, make sure to direct the needle towards midline or paramedian (as needed) – *intermittent A/P fluoroscopy may also be used for checking mediolateral needle positioning.*

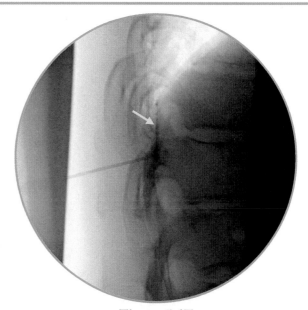

Figure 5-1F
Tilt: 0°
Oblique: 90° Right

Lateral View. After negative aspiration, contrast is administered and shows spread in the posterior epidural space (yellow arrow). Note the cephalad spread of contrast.

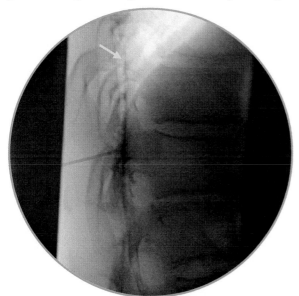

Figure 5-1G
Tilt: 0°
Oblique: 90° Right

Lateral View. After further administration of contrast, note spread cephalad towards the T9-T10 interspace (yellow arrow).

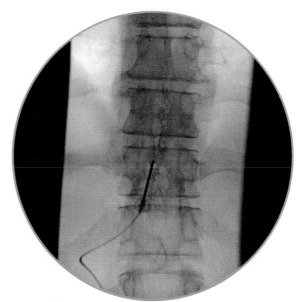

Figure 5-1H
Tilt: 0°
Oblique: 0°

A/P View. Epidural contrast spread traveling at the T10-T11 interspace, and cephalocaudad to this level.

See Page 278

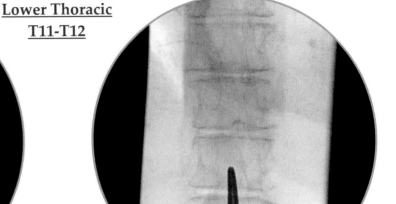

Lower Thoracic
T11-T12

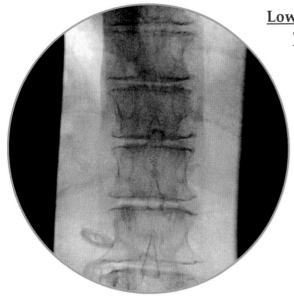

Figure 5-2A
Tilt: 0°
Oblique: 0°

A/P View. Note the T11-T12 interspace (blue star), and left 12th rib (green arrow).

Figure 5-2B
Tilt: 0°
Oblique: 5° Left

Oblique View. A slight left oblique is applied to better visualize the targeted interspace. Pointer showing location of needle placement inferior to the T12 laminar edge. With placement inferolateral to the interspace, the lamina provides an additional safety measure.

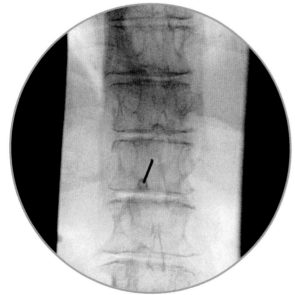

Figure 5-2C
Tilt: 0°
Oblique: 5° Left

Oblique View. Needle advancement towards the interspace. *Note that by contacting bone with the needle tip, and NOT advancing beyond the superior laminar edge, an additional safety measure is provided.*

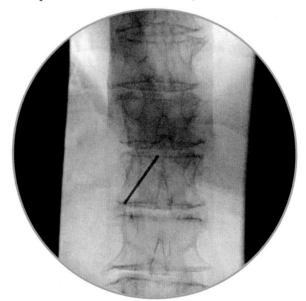

Figure 5-2D
Tilt: 0°
Oblique: 0°

A/P View. The slight oblique is removed, and the needle is slightly advanced towards midline. *Note that the proceduralist should be mindful of needle depth with any advancement beyond the laminar edge.* Next, a lateral view is obtained.

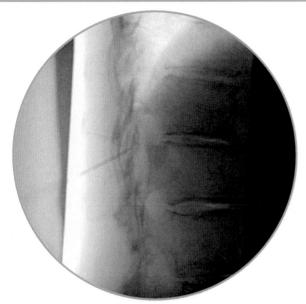

Figure 5-2E
Tilt: 0°
Oblique: 90° Right

Lateral View. Note the needle depth in this view after LOR has been achieved. While advancing the needle in this view, make sure to direct the needle towards midline or paramedian (as needed) – *intermittent A/P fluoroscopy may also be used for checking mediolateral needle positioning.*

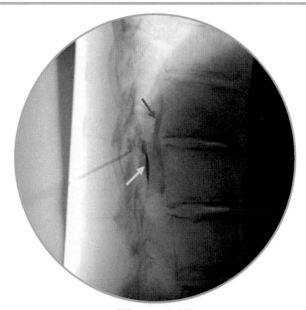

Figure 5-2F
Tilt: 0°
Oblique: 90° Right

Lateral View. After negative aspiration, contrast is administered and shows spread in the anterior (red arrow) and posterior (yellow arrow) epidural space. Note the cephalad spread of contrast.

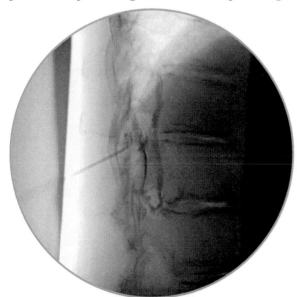

Figure 5-2G
Tilt: 0°
Oblique: 90° Right

Lateral View. Additional administration of contrast shows spread cephalad and caudad, in both the anterior and posterior epidural space.

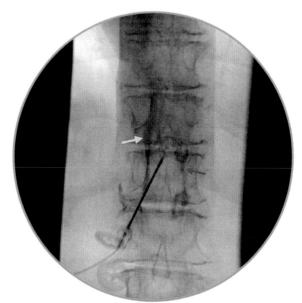

Figure 5-2H
Tilt: 0°
Oblique: 0°

A/P View. Epidural contrast spread is seen traveling at the T11-T12 interspace, cephalocaudad, and both left (yellow arrow) and right (red arrow) of midline.

Mid Thoracic
T7-T8

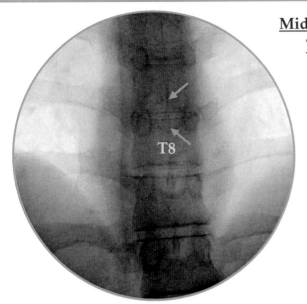

Figure 5-3A
Tilt: 0°
Oblique: 0°

A/P View. Note the T8 vertebra and corresponding superior T7-T8 interspace. Also, note the steep angle of the T7 spinous process (green arrows) overlying and obstructing the midline of the T7-T8 interspace. *Of note, this particular patient has a thin body habitus.*

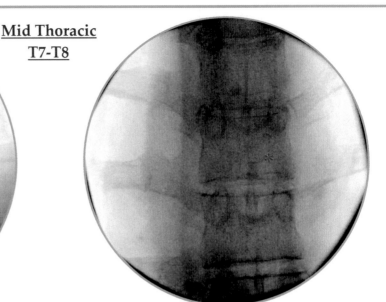

Figure 5-3B
Tilt: 0°
Oblique: 0°

A/P View. Using collimation, the proceduralist can focus on the targeted T7-T8 interspace, while reducing radiation exposure. *Due to the steep angle of the T7 spinous process, the needle entry point cannot be in the midline of the interspace and will need to be inferior and paramedian (red star).*

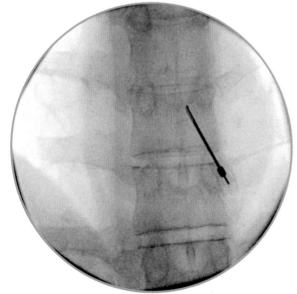

Figure 5-3C
Tilt: 0°
Oblique: 0°

A/P View. Needle placement approaching the T7-T8 interspace. *Of note, since this particular patient is of a thin body habitus, a more caudad needle entry point should not be used, as this would have created too shallow a needle trajectory to access the interspace.*

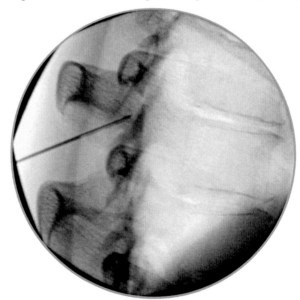

Figure 5-3D
Tilt: 0°
Oblique: 90° Right

Lateral View. Note the needle depth in this view as it approaches the epidural space. The needle is advanced using the LOR technique and intermittent fluoroscopy, while directing the needle tip midline or paramedian (as needed).

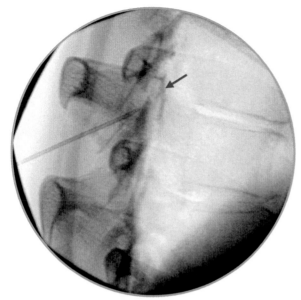

Figure 5-3E
Tilt: 0°
Oblique: 90° Right

Lateral View. After LOR has been achieved, and after negative aspiration, contrast is administered and shows spread in the posterior epidural space (red arrow).

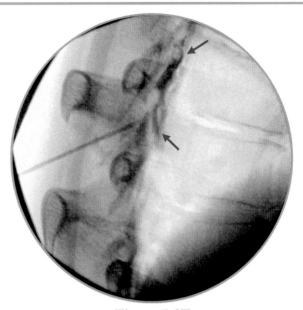

Figure 5-3F
Tilt: 0°
Oblique: 90° Right

Lateral View. Administration of additional contrast shows further spread both cephalad and caudad to the needle tip.

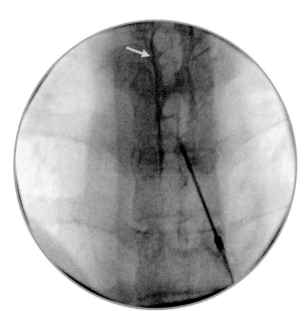

Figure 5-3G
Tilt: 0°
Oblique: 0°

A/P View. Epidural contrast spread is seen traveling at the T7-T8 interspace, cephalocaudad, and both left (yellow arrow) and right (red arrow) of midline.

Mid Thoracic
T7-T8

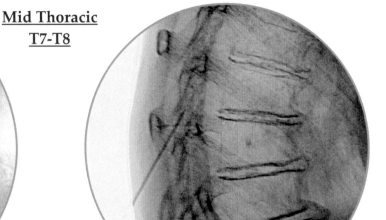

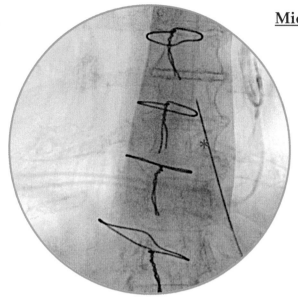

Figure 5-4A
Tilt: 0°
Oblique: 0°

Figure 5-4B
Tilt: 0°
Oblique: 90° Right

A/P View. Needle placement approaching the T7-T8 interspace, with the tip at the T8 superior laminar edge. For this particular patient's body habitus & anatomy, a more caudad needle entry point was used – *the medial border of the right T9 pedicle (red star) - compare to Figure 5-3B.*

Lateral View. Note the needle depth in this view after LOR has been achieved, and with the tip in the epidural space.

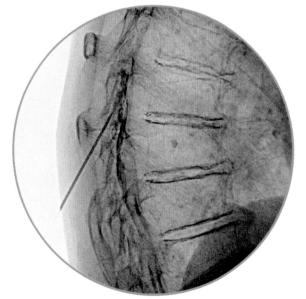

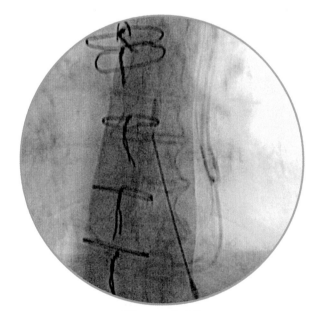

Figure 5-4C
Tilt: 0°
Oblique: 90° Right

Figure 5-4D
Tilt: 0°
Oblique: 0°

Lateral View. After negative aspiration, contrast is administered and shows spread in the posterior epidural space, and in both the cephalad and caudad direction.

A/P View. Epidural contrast spread in the A/P view.

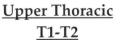

Upper Thoracic
T1-T2

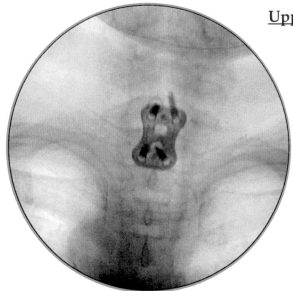

Figure 5-5A
Tilt: 0°
Oblique: 0°

A/P View. Note the ACDF hardware at C7-T1.

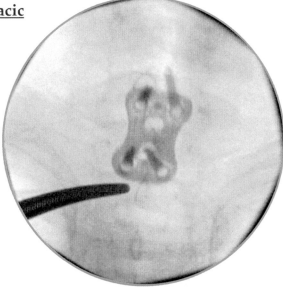

Figure 5-5B
Tilt: 0°
Oblique: 0°

A/P View. Pointer showing location of needle placement inferior and lateral to the T1-T2 interspace. Placing the needle inferolateral to the interspace allows for the lamina to provide an additional safety measure. *Do NOT advance beyond the T2 laminar edge in this view.*

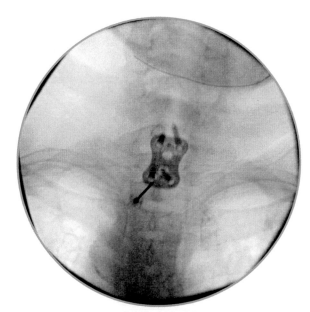

Figure 5-5C
Tilt: 0°
Oblique: 0°

A/P View. Needle advancement towards the interspace. Once the needle tip contacts the T2 superior laminar edge, a CLO view is obtained – *note that the CLO view is preferred over the lateral view due to obstruction from the shoulders (see Chapter 6 for further discussion regarding the CLO view).*

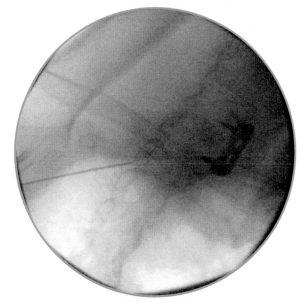

Figure 5-5D
Tilt: 0°
Oblique: 50° Right

Contralateral Oblique View. Note the needle depth as it approaches the lamina. At this point, a LOR syringe is attached and further advancement is carried out using the LOR technique and intermittent fluoroscopy – *aim to direct the needle midline or paramedian (as needed).*

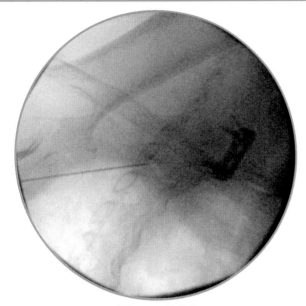

Figure 5-5E
Tilt: 0°
Oblique: 50° Right

Contralateral Oblique View. Note the needle depth in this view after LOR has been achieved. The needle tip is seen to be just beyond the VILL *(see Chapter 6 for further discussion regarding the VILL and CLO view).*

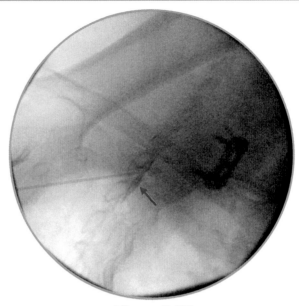

Figure 5-5F
Tilt: 0°
Oblique: 50° Right

Contralateral Oblique View. After negative aspiration, contrast is administered and shows spread in the posterior epidural space (red arrow).

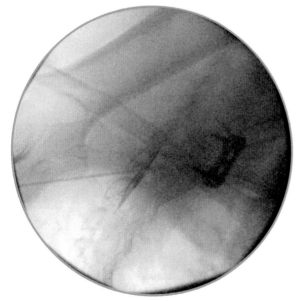

Figure 5-5G
Tilt: 0°
Oblique: 50° Right

Contralateral Oblique View. After further administration of contrast, note further spread in both the cephalad and caudad directions.

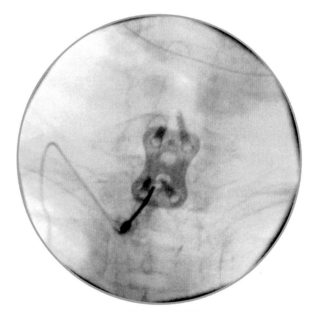

Figure 5-5H
Tilt: 0°
Oblique: 0°

A/P View. Epidural contrast spread traveling at the T1-T2 interspace, and both cephalad and caudad.

**Upper Thoracic
T4-T5**

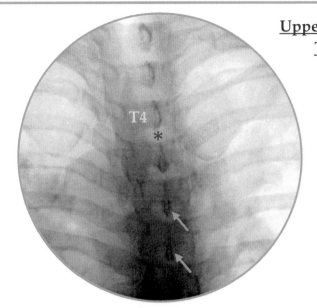

Figure 5-6A
Tilt: 0°
Oblique: 0°

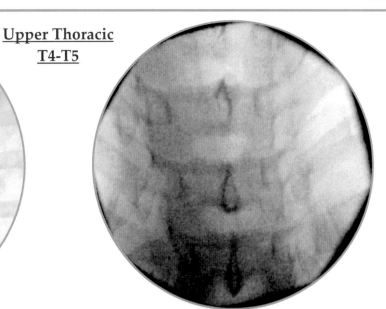

Figure 5-6B
Tilt: 0°
Oblique: 5° Right

A/P View. Note the T4 vertebra and T4-T5 interspace (red star). Given the lack of significant sloping of the SP in the upper thoracic spine, a midline needle entry is possible. *Note how the SP angle becomes steeper in the mid thoracic segments (green arrows).*

A/P View. Using collimation, the proceduralist can focus on the targeted interspace (i.e., T4-T5), while reducing radiation exposure. A slight oblique is applied to bring the spinous processes more midline and create a more "true" A/P view *(compare to Figure 5-6A).*

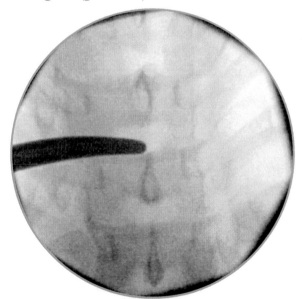

Figure 5-6C
Tilt: 0°
Oblique: 5° Right

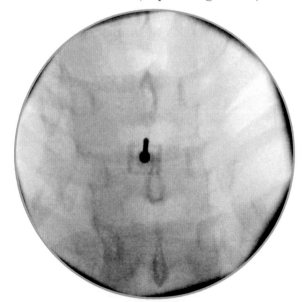

Figure 5-6D
Tilt: 0°
Oblique: 5° Right

A/P View. Pointer showing location of needle placement at the T4-T5 interspace. *Since the angle of the T4 SP is not steep in this region – in contrast to the mid thoracic segments – the needle entry point can be midline if desired.*

A/P View. Coaxial needle placement towards the interspace using a midline approach. Since the laminar edge is not being used as a safety measure, special care should be given to assessing needle depth throughout by using LOR checks and intermittent lateral fluoroscopy.

5

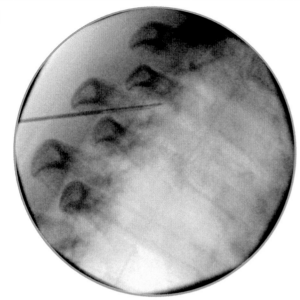

Figure 5-6E
Tilt: 0°
Oblique: 90° Right

Lateral View. Note the needle depth in this view after LOR has been obtained. During advancement in this view, direct the needle tip towards midline or paramedian (as needed). *The use of intermittent A/P fluoroscopy may also be used to assess mediolateral positioning.*

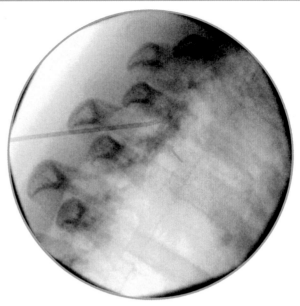

Figure 5-6F
Tilt: 0°
Oblique: 90° Right

Lateral View. After negative aspiration, contrast is administered and shows spread in the posterior epidural space (green arrow).

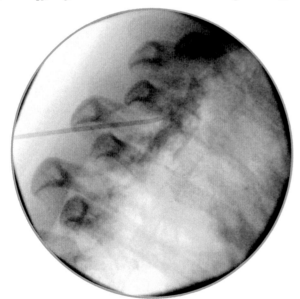

Figure 5-6G
Tilt: 0°
Oblique: 90° Right

Lateral View. After further administration of contrast, note additional spread in both the cephalad and caudad directions.

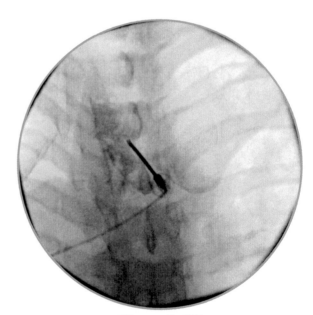

Figure 5-6H
Tilt: 0°
Oblique: 0°

A/P View. Epidural contrast spread traveling at the T4-T5 interspace, and cephalocaudad to this level, targeting the symptomatic left side. *Note the needle trajectory without the right oblique – not a "true" A/P view – compare to Figure 5-6D.*

Chapter 6
Cervical Interlaminar Epidural Steroid Injection

- [ ] Obtain an A/P view to locate the targeted interlaminar space. *Of note, if the mandible obstructs the targeted interspace, consider tilting cephalad to remove the jaw line from overlying the interspace (see Figures 6-3A & 6-3B). In addition, if targeting a specific side, a slight ipsilateral oblique towards the targeted side may also be applied (see Figure 6-2B).*

- [ ] Place a Tuohy epidural needle towards the targeted interspace. Although a midline needle approach can be performed, it is the author's preference to perform needle entry inferior and paramedian to the midline interlaminar space, as this allows the laminar edge to provide an additional safety measure for assessing needle depth *(see Figure 6-1B)*. With this approach, the needle is advanced to, but not beyond, the laminar edge *(see Figure 6-1C)*. At this point, further needle advancement is performed in either the lateral or contralateral oblique (CLO) view, where needle depth can be properly visualized and assessed. *Of note, it is the author's preference to use the CLO view in the cervical spine when assessing needle depth, since the shoulders often obstruct and prevent clear visualization of the needle tip when using the lateral view for mid to lower cervical procedures.*

- [ ] Obtain a CLO view *(see page 95 for further discussion regarding the 50° CLO angle)*. Advance the needle using the LOR technique and intermittent fluoroscopy as needed. When the needle tip enters the ligamentum flavum, often an increase in resistance is felt. *However, the proceduralist should not solely rely on this resistance, and should use intermittent CLO fluoroscopy to assess depth throughout needle advancement.* As the needle is directed towards the final target, ensure that the needle tip does not cross midline by using intermittent A/P fluoroscopy as needed *(see page 97 for further discussion regarding potential pitfalls of a needle tip in the CLO view that accesses the epidural space after crossing midline – i.e., on the same side as the image intensifier)*. The epidural space is accessed when the needle tip is seen to be just beyond the ventral interlaminar line *(see page 96 for further discussion on the VILL)*.

- [ ] Next, after negative aspiration, administer contrast under live fluoroscopy and ensure that there is no vascular uptake with proper epidural spread seen in the posterior epidural space and anterior to the VILL.

- [ ] Obtain an A/P view and administer further contrast in a similar fashion as previously described to confirm proper epidural spread in this view.

C7-T1

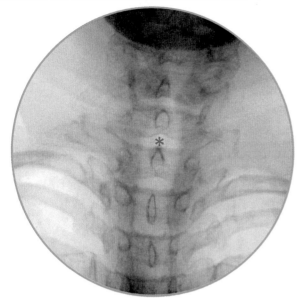

Figure 6-1A
Tilt: 0°
Oblique: 0°

A/P View. Note the targeted C7-T1 interspace (blue star).

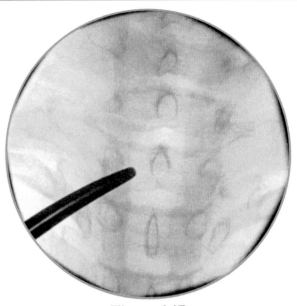

Figure 6-1B
Tilt: 0°
Oblique: 0°

A/P View. Use collimation to focus on the desired interspace, while also reducing radiation exposure to both the patient and the proceduralist. Pointer showing the location of needle placement inferior and left paramedian to the targeted C7-T1 interspace.

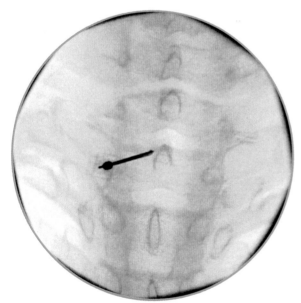

Figure 6-1C
Tilt: 0°
Oblique: 0°

A/P View. Needle placement approaching the T1 laminar edge from a left paramedian position. The lamina provides a safety measure. From this point, further needle advancement is carried out in a view where depth can be properly assessed – see next Figure.

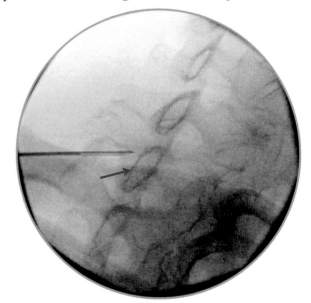

Figure 6-1D
Tilt: 0°
Oblique: 50° Right

Contralateral Oblique View. The needle is approaching the superior T1 lamina (red arrow). Next, the needle is advanced slightly cephalad towards the targeted interspace using the LOR technique. *Of note, ensure that the needle tip does not cross midline and veer toward the right side.*

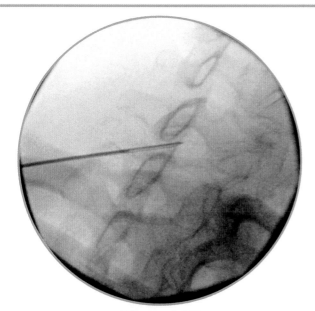

Figure 6-1E
Tilt: 0°
Oblique: 50° Right

Contralateral Oblique View. Note the depth of the needle tip after LOR has been achieved – just anterior to the VILL *(see page 96 for further discussion regarding the VILL)*.

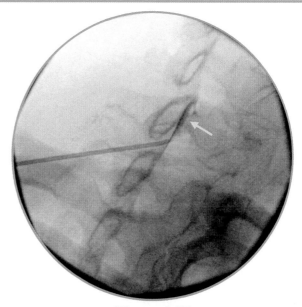

Figure 6-1F
Tilt: 0°
Oblique: 50° Right

Contralateral Oblique View. After negative aspiration, contrast is administered and shows proper spread within the posterior epidural space and just anterior to the VILL (yellow arrow).

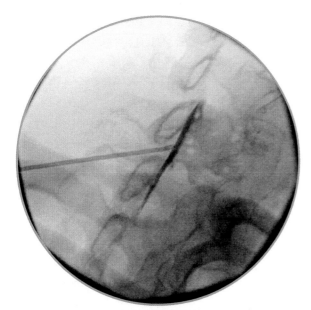

Figure 6-1G
Tilt: 0°
Oblique: 50° Right

Contralateral Oblique View. After further administration of contrast, note appropriate epidural spread in both the cephalad and caudad directions.

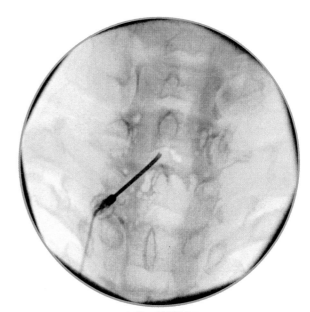

Figure 6-1H
Tilt: 0°
Oblique: 0°

A/P View. Note the spread of contrast both left and right of midline. Also note that the needle tip has not crossed midline.

See Page 278

<u>C6-C7</u>

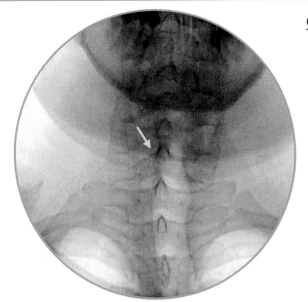

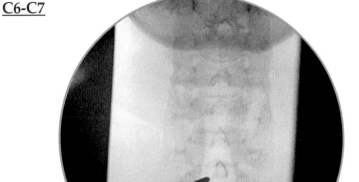

Figure 6-2A
Tilt: 0°
Oblique: 0°

Figure 6-2B
Tilt: 15° Cephalad
Oblique: 5° Left

A/P View. Note the targeted left C6-C7 interspace (yellow arrow). The interspace is not optimally visualized, with the spinous processes pointing cephalad. Further fluoroscopic adjustment will be needed – *see Figure 6-2B*.

Oblique View. Pointer showing the location of needle placement inferior and left paramedian to the targeted C6-C7 interspace. Note how the interspace is better visualized with the above fluoroscopic adjustments – *compare to Figure 6-2A.*

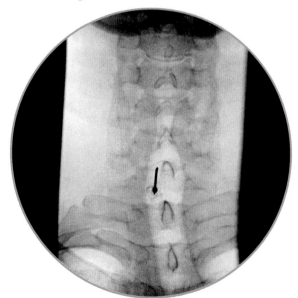

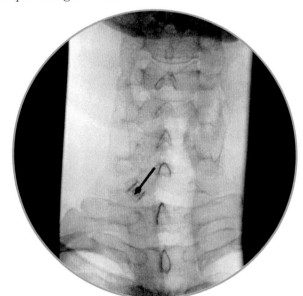

Figure 6-2C
Tilt: 15° Cephalad
Oblique: 5° Left

Figure 6-2D
Tilt: 15° Cephalad
Oblique: 0°

Oblique View. Needle placement approaching the C7 laminar edge from a left paramedian position. *Once the needle tip approaches the lamina, the slight ipsilateral oblique positioning can be removed to ensure needle positioning towards the midline of the interspace – see next Figure.*

A/P View. This is a more "true" A/P view with the spinous process midline and equidistant between the pedicles. Note that the needle tip is confirmed to be at the C7 laminar edge and approaching the interspace.

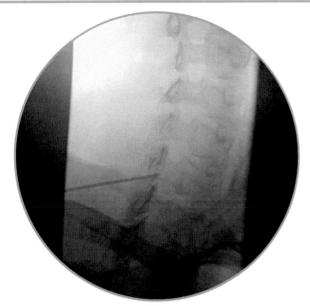

Figure 6-2E
Tilt: 15° Cephalad
Oblique: 50° Right

Contralateral Oblique View. Note the depth of the needle tip after LOR has been achieved - just anterior to the VILL.

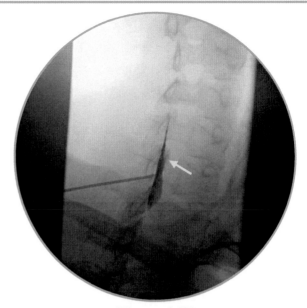

Figure 6-2F
Tilt: 15° Cephalad
Oblique: 50° Right

Contralateral Oblique View. After negative aspiration, contrast is administered and shows proper spread within the posterior epidural space and just anterior to the VILL (yellow arrow).

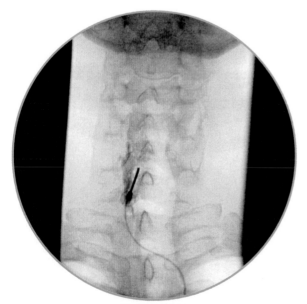

Figure 6-2G
Tilt: 15° Cephalad
Oblique: 0°

A/P View. Note the spread of contrast on the desired left side. Also note that the needle tip has not crossed midline, and remained left paramedian as desired in this particular case.

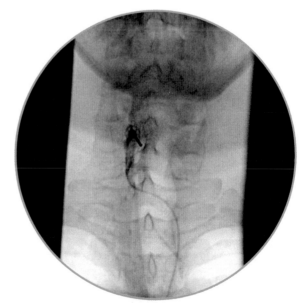

Figure 6-2H
Tilt: 0°
Oblique: 0°

A/P View. Note the needle positioning and contrast spread, after the fluoroscopic tilt has been removed.

<u>**C5-C6**</u>

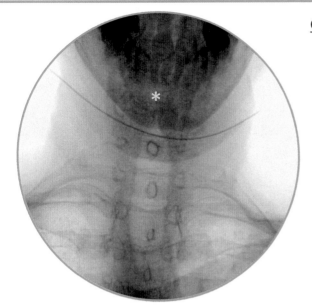

Figure 6-3A
Tilt: 0°
Oblique: 0°

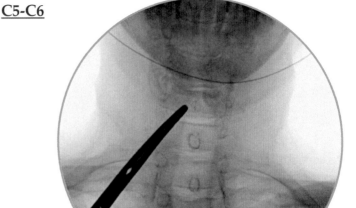

Figure 6-3B
Tilt: 10° Cephalad
Oblique: 0°

A/P View. Note the targeted C5-C6 interspace (yellow star). The interspace is not optimally viewed, due to obstruction from the patient's mandible. Further fluoroscopic adjustment will be needed – *see Figure 6-3B*.

A/P View. Note how applying a cephalad tilt removes the mandible from obstructing the targeted interspace. Pointer showing the location of needle placement inferior and left paramedian to the targeted C5-C6 interspace.

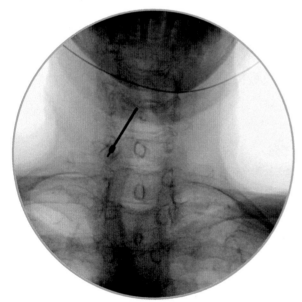

Figure 6-3C
Tilt: 10° Cephalad
Oblique: 0°

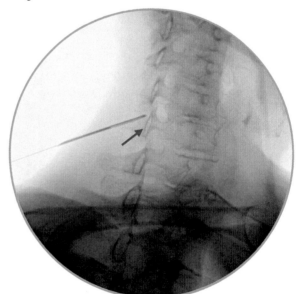

Figure 6-3D
Tilt: 10° Cephalad
Oblique: 50° Right

A/P View. Needle placement approaching the C6 laminar edge from a left paramedian position. The lamina provides a safety measure. From this point, further needle advancement is carried out in a view where depth can be properly assessed – see next Figure.

Contralateral Oblique View. The needle is approaching the superior C6 lamina (red arrow). Next, the needle is advanced slightly cephalad towards the targeted interspace using the LOR technique. *Of note, ensure that the needle tip does not cross midline and veer toward the right side.*

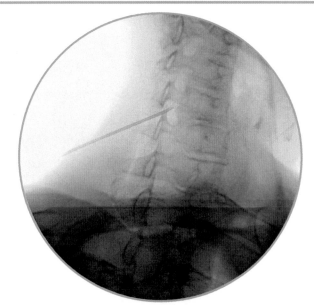

Figure 6-3E
Tilt: 10° Cephalad
Oblique: 50° Right

Contralateral Oblique View. Note the depth of the needle tip after LOR has been achieved - just anterior to the VILL.

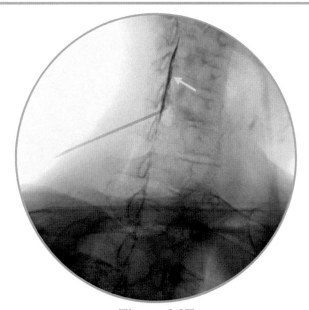

Figure 6-3F
Tilt: 10° Cephalad
Oblique: 50° Right

Contralateral Oblique View. After negative aspiration, contrast is administered and shows proper spread within the posterior epidural space and just anterior to the VILL (yellow arrow).

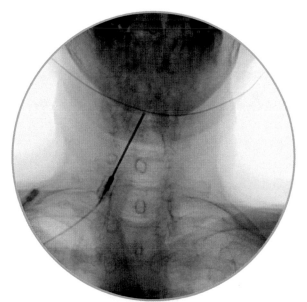

Figure 6-3G
Tilt: 10° Cephalad
Oblique: 0°

A/P View. There is spread of contrast both left and right of midline. Note how the needle tip has not crossed midline.

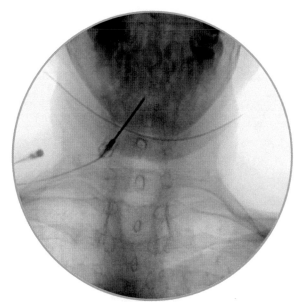

Figure 6-3H
Tilt: 0°
Oblique: 0°

A/P View. Note the change in needle positioning and contrast spread after the fluoroscopic tilt has been removed.

C7-T1
Hardware (ACDF)

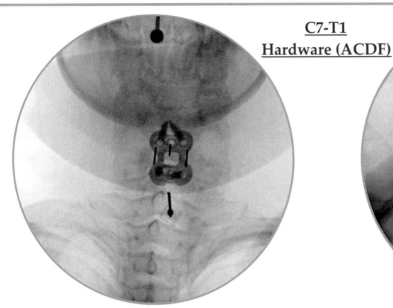

Figure 6-4A
Tilt: 0°
Oblique: 0°

A/P View. Needle placement approaching the T1 laminar edge from a right paramedian position, caudal to the ACDF hardware. From this point, further needle advancement is carried out in a view where depth can be properly assessed – see next Figure.

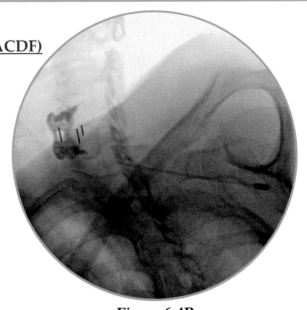

Figure 6-4B
Tilt: 0°
Oblique: 50° Left

Contralateral Oblique View. Note the depth of the needle tip after LOR has been achieved - just anterior to the VILL.

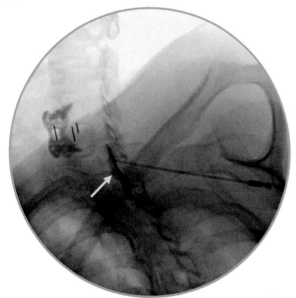

Figure 6-4C
Tilt: 0°
Oblique: 50° Left

Contralateral Oblique View. After negative aspiration, contrast is administered and shows proper spread within the posterior epidural space (yellow arrow) and just anterior to the VILL.

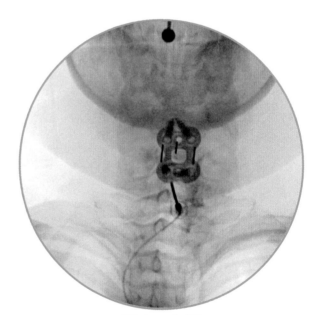

Figure 6-4D
Tilt: 0°
Oblique: 0°

A/P View. Note the spread of contrast right of midline, and traveling both cephalad (towards the location of the ACDF hardware) and caudad. Also note that the needle tip has not crossed midline.

Additional Discussion:
The Contralateral Oblique View – What's in an angle?

When performing cervical and cervicothoracic epidural access, visualization of the needle tip in a lateral view becomes very difficult, and at times impossible, in the lower cervical and upper thoracic segments. As an alternative, the CLO view is much more optimal for visualizing the needle tip and assessing depth, which is imperative to prevent inadvertent spinal cord injury. In addition, the CLO view also provides a reliable anatomical landmark to guide how far the needle can safely be advanced – i.e., the ventral interlaminar line or VILL (see page 96).

*At what angle should the C-arm be rotated to obtain the ideal CLO view? – **at an angle that is parallel to the cervical lamina located on the side of needle placement.** With this amount of contralateral obliquity, one can expect to repeatedly and reliably obtain loss of resistance when the needle tip is placed at, or within 2 mm ventral to, the VILL. Studies have shown that this angle for the lower cervical and upper thoracic segments is approximately 50° *(see Figure 6-5)*. It is the author's experience that a 50° CLO angle is consistently the most ideal angle for epidural access from C5 through T2 – **where the needle tip is consistently seen at the expected location of "at or within 2 mm ventral to" the VILL.**

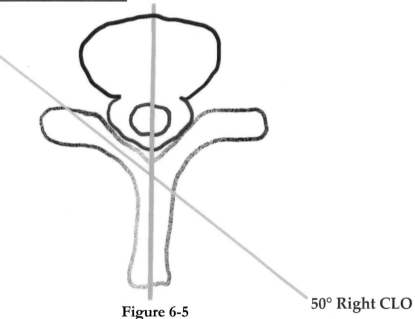

Figure 6-5   50° **Right CLO**

A CLO angle less than 50° will produce a more ventral appearing needle tip when LOR is achieved. Correspondingly, prior to epidural access, the proceduralist may experience reluctance to advance the needle due to a <u>falsely dangerous ventral appearance</u> of the needle tip with respect to the VILL – leading to superficial and incorrect needle placement.

A CLO angle greater than 50° will produce a more posterior appearing needle tip when LOR is achieved – *potentially even posterior to the VILL*. Correspondingly, despite the needle tip entering the epidural space, the proceduralist may continue to perform further dangerous needle advancement due to a <u>falsely safe superficial appearance</u> of the needle tip relative to the VILL.

Additional Discussion:
Understanding the Ventral Interlaminar Line (VILL)

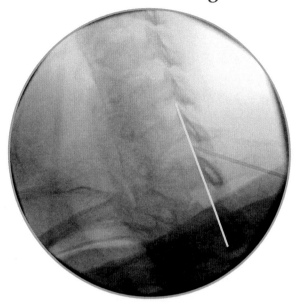

Figure 6-6A
Tilt: 0°
Oblique: 50° Left

Contralateral Oblique View. The VILL (yellow line) is a line connecting the anterior borders of the laminae. In order to acces the epidural space, the needle tip should be advanced just ventral to this line – *this is where LOR is expected to be achieved when using a CLO angle of 50°.*

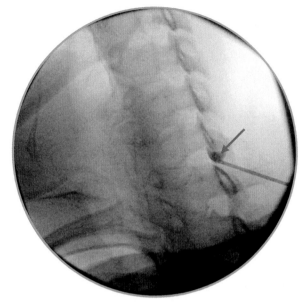

Figure 6-6B
Tilt: 0°
Oblique: 50° Left

Contralateral Oblique View. Note that if the needle tip is posterior to the VILL when contrast is administered, the spread will be outside the epidural space (blue arrow) – and not anterior to the VILL as desired for correct epidural spread.

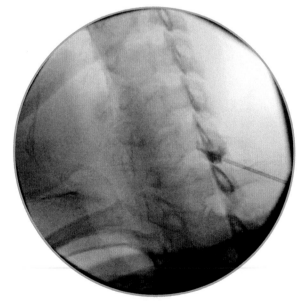

Figure 6-6C
Tilt: 0°
Oblique: 50° Left

Contralateral Oblique View. The needle tip is advanced into the epidural space just anterior to the VILL.

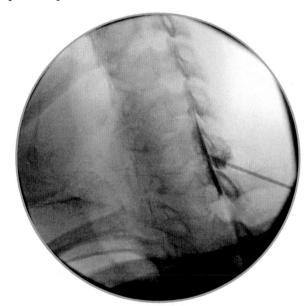

Figure 6-6D
Tilt: 0°
Oblique: 50° Left

Contralateral Oblique View. Proper epidural contrast spread anterior to the VILL – *compare to Figure 6-6B.*

Additional Discussion:
The importance of not crossing midline with the needle tip when accessing the epidural space beyond the ventral interlaminar line (VILL) in the CLO view...

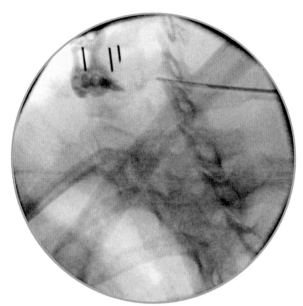

Figure 6-7A
Tilt: 0°
Oblique: 50° Left

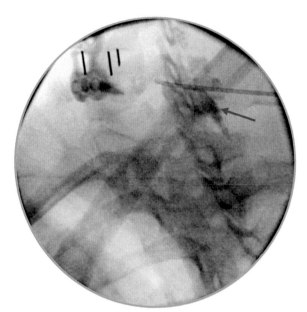

Figure 6-7B
Tilt: 0°
Oblique: 50° Left

Contralateral Oblique View. In this view, the needle has been advanced using the LOR technique. However, LOR has yet to be achieved despite the needle tip appearing dangerously ventral to the VILL. Aspiration for CSF also continues to be negative at this needle depth.

It is imperative that the proceduralist be very mindful of needle positioning in this view in order to avoid a potential dural puncture, or a more catastrophic event such as spinal cord injury. In addition to intermittent fluoroscopy, repeated checks of LOR, repeated checks for negative aspiration of CSF, and administration of contrast *(see Figure 6-7B)* should also be performed to evaluate needle depth. Further advancement of the needle should NOT be performed until the proceduralist is well aware of needle positioning and the cause of such a ventral appearing needle tip.

Contralateral Oblique View. Given the ventral appearing needle tip, contrast is administered as a safety check – but is seen to be extra-epidural (red arrow).

One such cause of a ventrally appearing needle tip with extra-epidural contrast spread is that the needle tip has crossed midline and is no longer contralateral to the image intensifier. Once this occurs, the needle tip will appear to be dangerously ventral to the VILL, despite not obtaining LOR or proper epidural contrast spread. If this is suspected, check an A/P view to confirm that the needle tip has crossed midline. In this example, this in fact is what has occurred (see Figure 6-7E).

See Figure 6-7C to understand how needle depth appearance in the CLO view changes when the image intensifier is correctly rotated to the side contralateral to the needle tip.

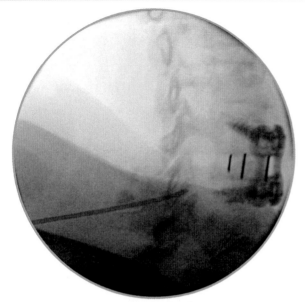

Figure 6-7C
Tilt: 0°
Oblique: 50° Right

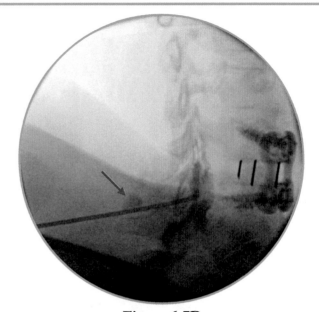

Figure 6-7D
Tilt: 0°
Oblique: 50° Right

Contralateral Oblique View. With a right CLO, the needle tip has now been advanced even further, with LOR obtained just anterior to the VILL, as expected. *Compare this appearance to Figure 6-7B (left CLO) where the needle tip appeared dangerously ventral to the VILL despite not obtaining LOR.*

Contralateral Oblique View. Administration of contrast now shows proper spread anterior to the VILL and in the posterior epidural space. *Compare this contrast spread to Figure 6-7B (when LOR was not achieved) – the extra-epidural contrast from Figure 6-7B is still seen in this view (red arrow).*

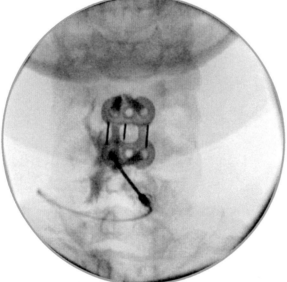

Figure 6-7E
Tilt: 0°
Oblique: 0°

A/P View. This view confirms that the needle tip has crossed midline – i.e., towards the left side. In addition, contrast is also noted to be flowing left of midline, which is opposite the intended side in ths case. **This example illustrates the importance of using intermittent A/P fluoroscopy to assess mediolateral needle positioning during needle advancement.**

Chapter 7
Lumbar Medial Branch Block

- Obtain an A/P view to locate the targeted vertebral levels.

- Next, apply an ipsilateral oblique (typically around 20°) and tilt as needed to square the endplates at the targeted level. *Of note, if both the superior and inferior endplates cannot be squared, preference should be given to squaring the superior endplate.* Identify the junction of the superior articular process and transverse process at the targeted medial branch.

- Place and advance the needle coaxially towards the junction of the superior articular process and transverse process, until contact with bone. Next, an additional ipsilateral oblique is applied (typically around 10° more) in order to see the entire length of the needle. In this view, the needle is further adjusted as needed until the tip is seen to be at the lateral border of the superior articular process, but still maintained at the junction of the superior articular process and transverse process. *Of note, for the L5 dorsal ramus, the needle is placed at the sacral ala, untl contact with bone, and just lateral to the S1 superior articular process – this can be done with an A/P view or with a lesser ipsilateral oblique angle if there is obstruction from the iliac crest.*

- Next, obtain an A/P view once again to ensure that the needle tip is seen to be at the expected location of the medial branch – i.e., the junction of the superior articular process and transverse process. *Similarly, for the L5 dorsal ramus, confirm that the needle tip is at the expected location – i.e., at the sacral ala and just lateral to the S1 superior articular process.* The needle can be slightly adjusted in this view as needed to obtain optimal needle positioning.

- Next, obtain a lateral view. The needle tip is adjusted as needed once again (typically mediolaterally) for placement just posterior to the foramen and at the junction of the superior articular process and transverse process. *Of note, cephalocaudal needle adjustment can also be made in the lateral view, but typically is not as frequently needed since this positioning can be adequately seen and performed in the prior A/P and oblique views.*

- Once the needle tip(s) is seen to be in the correct final position in the lateral view, an A/P view is obtained once again. After negative aspiration, contrast agent is administered under live fluoroscopy to verify flow at the expected location of the medial branch and/or dorsal ramus, without vascular uptake.

Right L3-L4, L4-L5, L5-S1
MBB

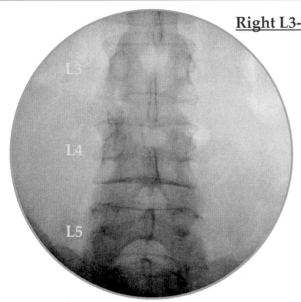

Figure 7-1A
Tilt: 0°
Oblique: 0°

A/P View. Note the vertebral levels in this view.

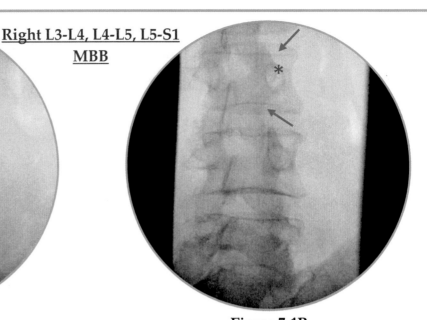

Figure 7-1B
Tilt: 0°
Oblique: 20° Right

Oblique View. Note the junction of the right L3 SAP and TP (red star). Without fluoroscopic tilting, the L3 endplates are not squared (blue arrows).

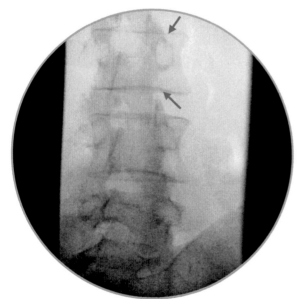

Figure 7-1C
Tilt: 10° Caudad
Oblique: 20° Right

Oblique View. Applying a caudal tilt better squares off the L3 endplates (blue arrows) – *compare to Figure 7-1B*. This is now a more ideal view for needle placement at this level.

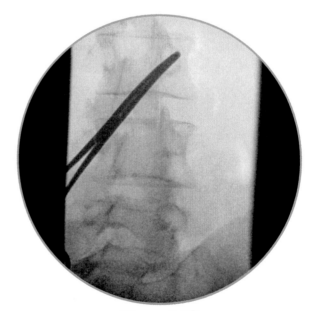

Figure 7-1D
Tilt: 10° Caudad
Oblique: 20° Right

Oblique View. Pointer showing the location of needle placement for the right L2 medial branch, at the junction of the right L3 SAP and TP.

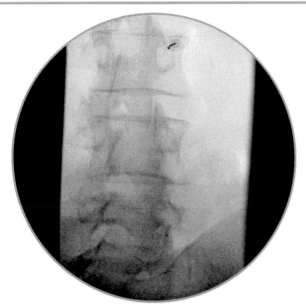

Figure 7-1E
Tilt: 10° Caudad
Oblique: 20° Right

Oblique View. Coaxial needle placement at the location of the right L2 medial branch – at the junction of the right L3 SAP and TP. Advance until contact with bone.

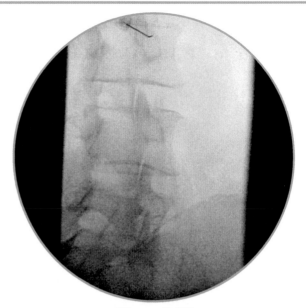

Figure 7-1F
Tilt: 10° Caudad
Oblique: 30° Right

Oblique View. After needle placement in the prior view, an additional ipsilateral oblique angle is applied and further needle adjustment is carried out as needed until the tip is at the lateral border of the right L3 SAP – and maintained at the junction of the right L3 SAP and TP.

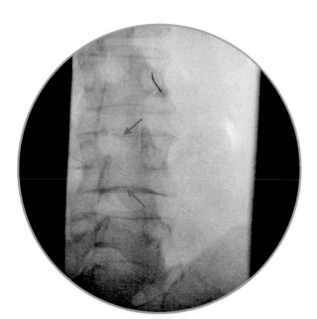

Figure 7-1G
Tilt: 0°
Oblique: 20° Right

Oblique View. For targeting the right L3 medial branch, note that by removing the fluoroscopic tilt, the L4 endplates become better squared (blue arrows) – *compare to Figure 7-1F where the L4 endplates are not optimally squared.*

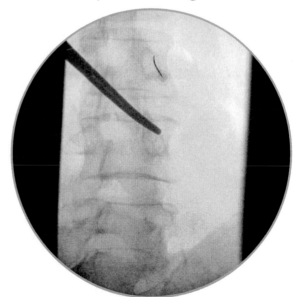

Figure 7-1H
Tilt: 0°
Oblique: 20° Right

Oblique View. Pointer showing the location of needle placement for the right L3 medial branch, at the junction of the right L4 SAP and TP.

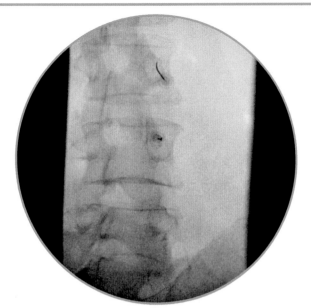

Figure 7-1I
Tilt: 0°
Oblique: 20° Right

Oblique View. Coaxial needle placement at the location of the right L3 medial branch – at the junction of the right L4 SAP and TP. Advance until contact with bone.

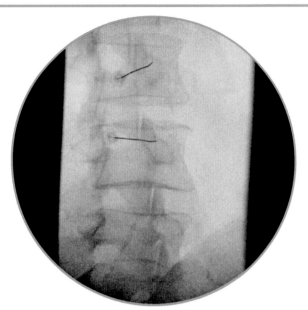

Figure 7-1J
Tilt: 0°
Oblique: 30° Right

Oblique View. After needle placement in the prior view, an additional ipsilateral oblique angle is applied and further needle adjustment is carried out as needed until the tip is at the lateral border of the right L4 SAP – and maintained at the junction of the right L4 SAP and TP.

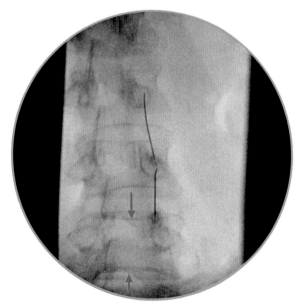

Figure 7-1K
Tilt: 15° Cephalad
Oblique: 20° Right

Oblique View. For the right L4 medial branch, note that by applying a cephalad fluoroscopic tilt, the L5 endplates become better squared (blue arrows) – *compare to Figure 7-1J where the L5 endplates are not optimally squared.*

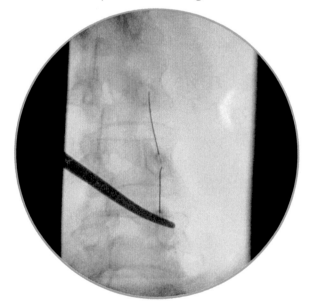

Figure 7-1L
Tilt: 15° Cephalad
Oblique: 20° Right

Oblique View. Pointer showing the location of needle placement for the right L4 medial branch, at the junction of the right L5 SAP and TP.

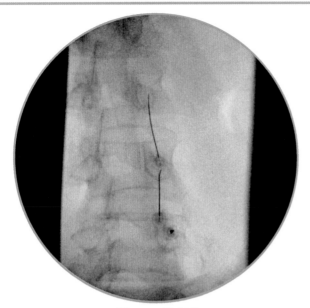

Figure 7-1M
Tilt: 15° Cephalad
Oblique: 20° Right

Oblique View. Coaxial needle placement at the location of the right L4 medial branch – at the junction of the right L5 SAP and TP. Advance until contact with bone.

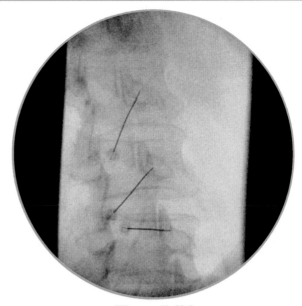

Figure 7-1N
Tilt: 15° Cephalad
Oblique: 30° Right

Oblique View. After needle placement in the prior view, an additional ipsilateral oblique angle is applied and further needle adjustment is carried out as needed until the tip is at the lateral border of the right L5 SAP – and maintained at the junction of the right L5 SAP and TP.

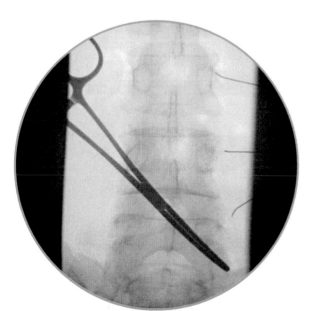

Figure 7-1O
Tilt: 0°
Oblique: 0°

A/P View. Pointer showing the location of needle placement for the right L5 dorsal ramus, at the right sacral ala just lateral to the right S1 SAP. *Of note, a slight ipsilateral oblique could have also been applied prior to needle placement.*

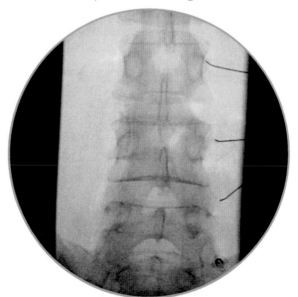

Figure 7-1P
Tilt: 0°
Oblique: 0°

A/P View. Needle placement at the location of the right L5 dorsal ramus – at the right sacral ala and just lateral to the right S1 SAP. Advance until contact with bone. *Next, a lateral view is taken where further needle adjustment at all levels may be carried out as needed.*

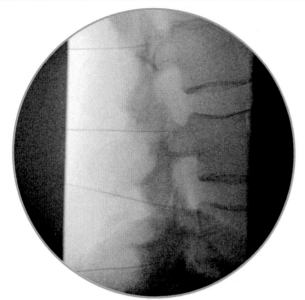

Figure 7-1Q
Tilt: 0°
Oblique: 90° Right

Lateral View. Each needle is adjusted mediolaterally and/or cephalocaudally as needed until the tip is seen to be at the junction of the SAP and TP *(or at the junction of the sacral ala and S1 SAP for the L5 dorsal ramus)*. Ensure that the needles are posterior to their respective IVF.

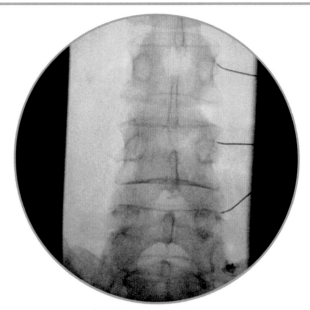

Figure 7-1R
Tilt: 0°
Oblique: 0°

A/P View. Needle positioning in the A/P view after further adjustments have been carried out in the prior lateral view. *Compare this final needle positioning to that of Figure 7-1P where needle adjustments had yet to be performed in the lateral view.*

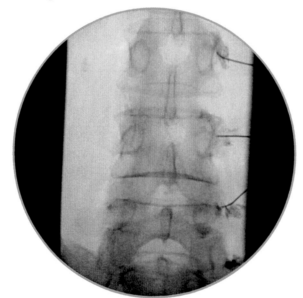

Figure 7-1S
Tilt: 0°
Oblique: 0°

A/P View. After negative aspiration, contrast is administered and shows proper spread at the location of each medial branch and the L5 dorsal ramus, without evidence of epidural flow or vascular uptake.

See Page 280

Bilateral L3-L4, L4-L5, L5-S1
MBB

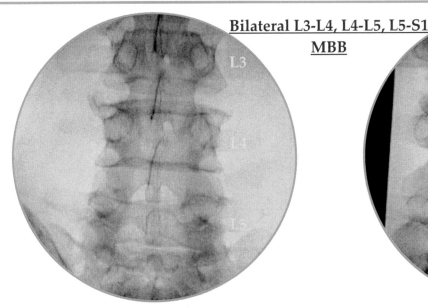

Figure 7-2A
Tilt: 0°
Oblique: 0°

A/P View. Note the vertebral levels in this view.

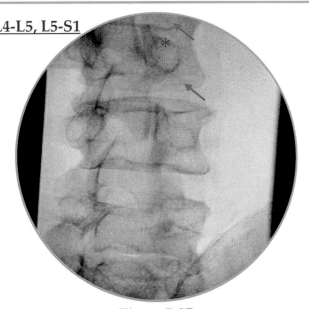

Figure 7-2B
Tilt: 0°
Oblique: 20° Right

Oblique View. Note the junction of the right L3 SAP and TP (red star). Without fluoroscopic tilting, the L3 endplates are not squared (blue arrows).

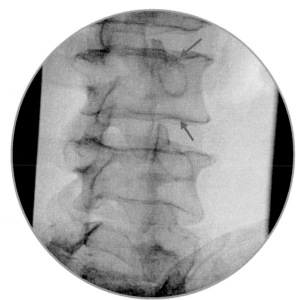

Figure 7-2C
Tilt: 15° Caudad
Oblique: 20° Right

Oblique View. Applying a caudal tilt better squares off the L3 endplates (blue arrows) – *compare to Figure 7-2B*. This is now a more ideal view for needle placement at this level.

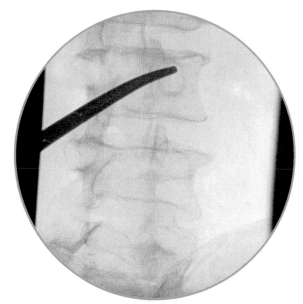

Figure 7-2D
Tilt: 15° Caudad
Oblique: 20° Right

Oblique View. Pointer showing the location of needle placement for the right L2 medial branch, at the junction of the right L3 SAP and TP.

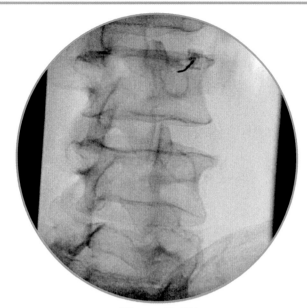

Figure 7-2E
Tilt: 15° Caudad
Oblique: 20° Right

Oblique View. Coaxial needle placement at the location of the right L2 medial branch – at the junction of the right L3 SAP and TP. *Further needle adjustment can be carried out by applying an additional ipsilateral oblique and ensuring the tip is at the lateral border of the right L3 SAP (see Figure 7-2K).*

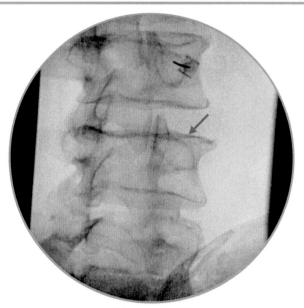

Figure 7-2F
Tilt: 10° Caudad
Oblique: 20° Right

Oblique View. For the right L3 medial branch, note that a lesser caudal fluoroscopic tilt better squares the L4 SEP (blue arrow) – *compare to Figure 7-2E where the L4 SEP is not optimally squared.*

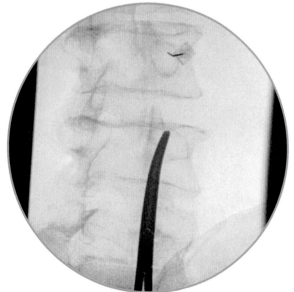

Figure 7-2G
Tilt: 10° Caudad
Oblique: 20° Right

Oblique View. Pointer showing the location of needle placement for the right L3 medial branch, at the junction of the right L4 SAP and TP.

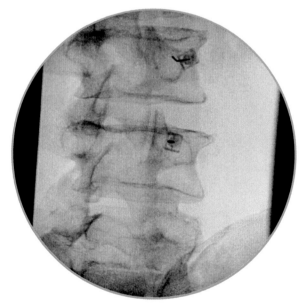

Figure 7-2H
Tilt: 10° Caudad
Oblique: 20° Right

Oblique View. Coaxial needle placement at the location of the right L3 medial branch – at the junction of the right L4 SAP and TP. *Further needle adjustment can be carried out by applying an additional ipsilateral oblique and ensuring the tip is at the lateral border of the right L4 SAP (see Figure 7-2K).*

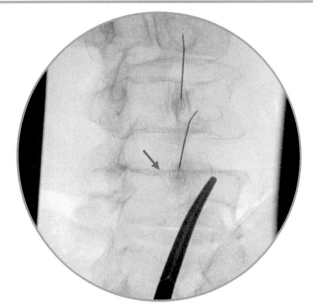

Figure 7-2I
Tilt: 10° Cephalad
Oblique: 20° Right

Oblique View. Pointer showing the location of needle placement for the right L4 medial branch, at the junction of the right L5 SAP and TP. Note that by applying a cephalad fluoroscopic tilt, the L5 SEP becomes better squared (blue arrow) – *compare to Figure 7-2B.*

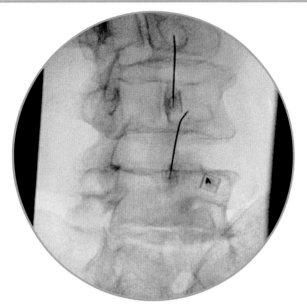

Figure 7-2J
Tilt: 10° Cephalad
Oblique: 20° Right

Oblique View. Coaxial needle placement at the location of the right L4 medial branch – at the junction of the right L5 SAP and TP. *Further needle adjustment can be carried out by applying an additional ipsilateral oblique and ensuring the tip is at the lateral border of the right L5 SAP (see Figure 7-2K).*

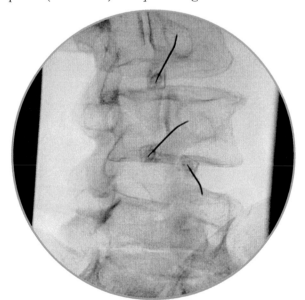

Figure 7-2K
Tilt: 0°
Oblique: 30° Right

Oblique View. After needle placement in the prior view, the fluoroscopic tilt is removed and an additional ipsilateral oblique is applied. Note that the needle tips at the L2 and L3 medial branches are not seen to be at the lateral border of their respective SAPs. *See next image.*

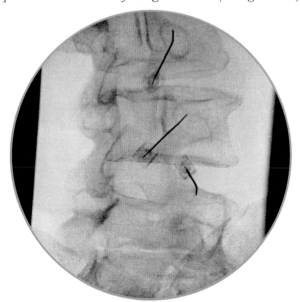

Figure 7-2L
Tilt: 0°
Oblique: 30° Right

Oblique View. The needles at the L2 and L3 medial branches are adjusted slightly until their tips are seen to be closer to the lateral border of their respective SAPs – while maintained at the junction of their respective right SAPs and TPs.

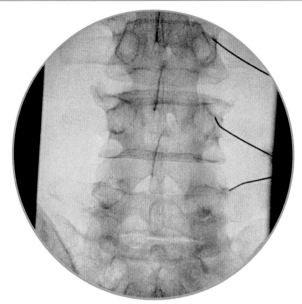

Figure 7-2M
Tilt: 0°
Oblique: 0°

A/P View. Needle positioning at the right L2, L3, and L4 medial branches after placement in the prior oblique views.

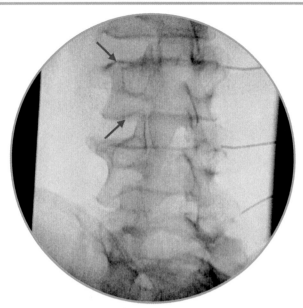

Figure 7-2N
Tilt: 15° Caudad
Oblique: 20° Left

Oblique View. Applying the same caudal tilt for the contralateral side again squares off the L3 endplates (red arrows). This is now a more ideal view for needle placement at this level.

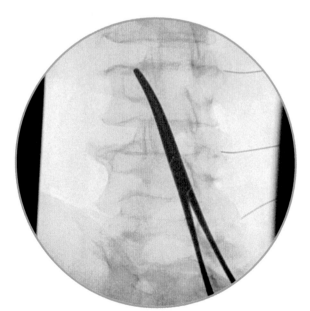

Figure 7-2O
Tilt: 15° Caudad
Oblique: 20° Left

Oblique View. Pointer showing the location of needle placement for the left L2 medial branch, at the junction of the left L3 SAP and TP.

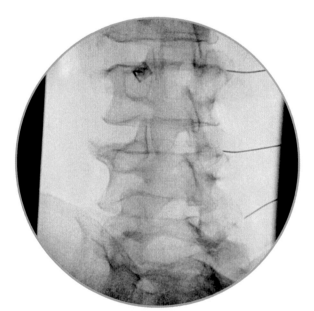

Figure 7-2P
Tilt: 15° Caudad
Oblique: 20° Left

Oblique View. Coaxial needle placement at the location of the left L2 medial branch – at the junction of the left L3 SAP and TP. Adance until contact with bone.

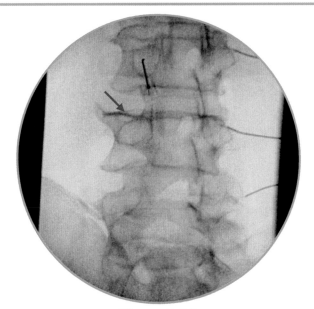

Figure 7-2Q
Tilt: 10° Caudad
Oblique: 20° Left

Oblique View. Applying the same caudal tilt for the contralateral side again better squares the L4 SEP (red arrow) – *compare to Figure 7-2P where the L4 SEP is not optimally squared.*

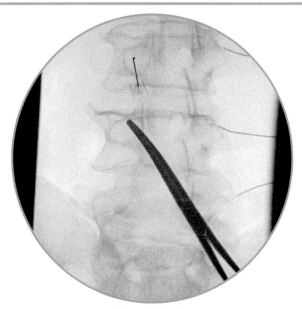

Figure 7-2R
Tilt: 10° Caudad
Oblique: 20° Left

Oblique View. Pointer showing the location of needle placement for the left L3 medial branch, at the junction of the left L4 SAP and TP.

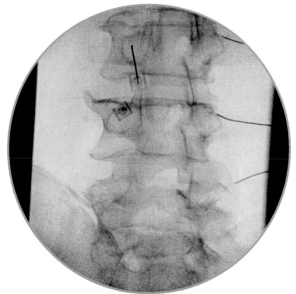

Figure 7-2S
Tilt: 10° Caudad
Oblique: 20° Left

Oblique View. Coaxial needle placement at the location of the left L3 medial branch – at the junction of the left L4 SAP and TP. Advance until contact with bone.

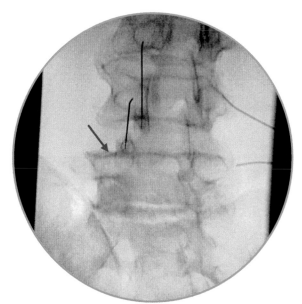

Figure 7-2T
Tilt: 10° Cephalad
Oblique: 20° Left

Oblique View. Applying the same cephalad tilt for the contralateral side again better squares the L5 SEP (red arrow) – *compare to Figure 7-2S where the L5 SEP is not optimally squared.*

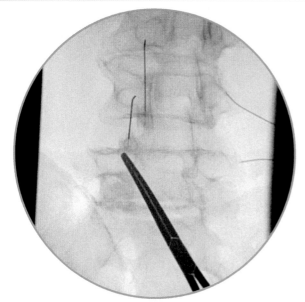

Figure 7-2U
Tilt: 10° Cephalad
Oblique: 20° Left

Oblique View. Pointer showing the location of needle placement for the left L4 medial branch, at the junction of the left L5 SAP and TP.

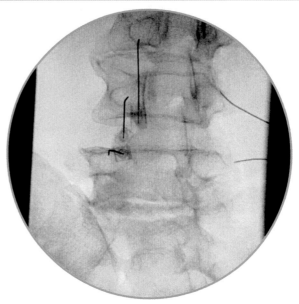

Figure 7-2V
Tilt: 10° Cephalad
Oblique: 20° Left

Oblique View. Coaxial needle placement at the location of the left L4 medial branch – at the junction of the left L5 SAP and TP. Advance until contact with bone.

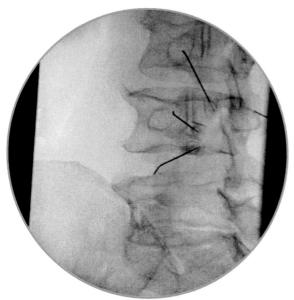

Figure 7-2W
Tilt: 0°
Oblique: 30° Left

Oblique View. After needle placement in the prior view, the tilt is removed and an additional ipsilateral oblique angle is applied. Note that the needles at the L2 and L3 medial branches are not seen to be at the lateral border of their respective SAPs – *further needle adjustment is needed.*

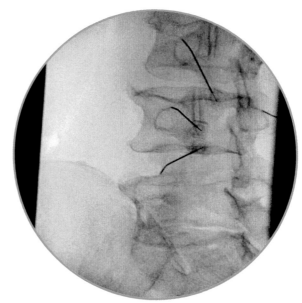

Figure 7-2X
Tilt: 0°
Oblique: 30° Left

Oblique View. After further needle adjustment, note that the needles at the L2, L3, and L4 medial branches are now at the lateral border of their corresponding SAPs – and maintained at the junction of the corresponding SAP and TP.

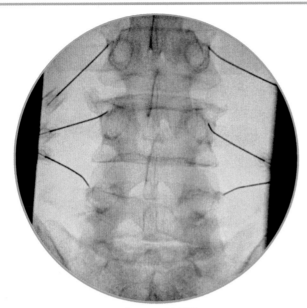

Figure 7-2Y
Tilt: 0°
Oblique: 0°

A/P View. Needle positioning in the A/P view after needle adjustments have been carried out in the prior oblique view.

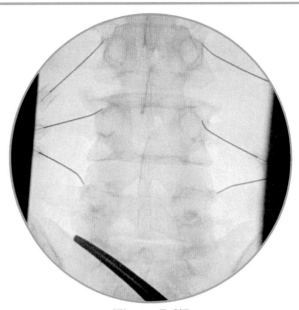

Figure 7-2Z
Tilt: 0°
Oblique: 0°

A/P View. Pointer showing the location of needle placement for the left L5 dorsal ramus, at the left sacral ala just lateral to the left S1 SAP. *Of note, a slight ipsilateral oblique could have also been applied prior to needle placement.*

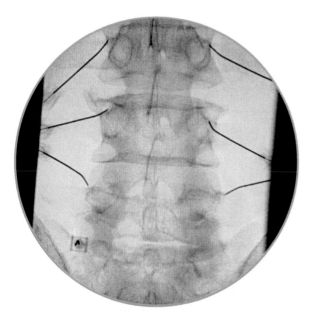

Figure 7-2A2
Tilt: 0°
Oblique: 0°

A/P View. Coaxial needle placement at the location of the left L5 dorsal ramus – at the left sacral ala just lateral to the left S1 SAP. Advance until contact with bone.

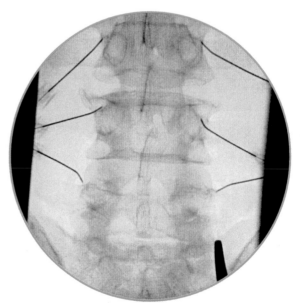

Figure 7-2B2
Tilt: 0°
Oblique: 0°

A/P View. Pointer showing the location of needle placement for the right L5 dorsal ramus, at the right sacral ala just lateral to the right S1 SAP. *Of note, a slight ipsilateral oblique could have also been applied prior to needle placement.*

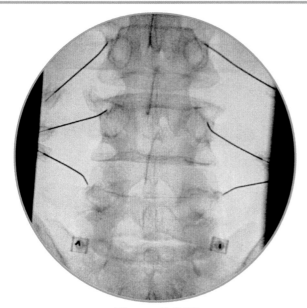

Figure 7-2C2
Tilt: 0°
Oblique: 0°

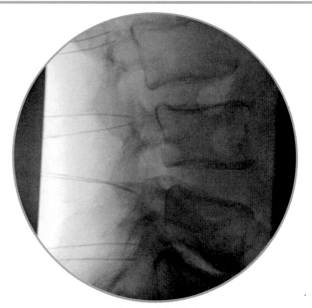

Figure 7-2D2
Tilt: 0°
Oblique: 90° Right

A/P View. Coaxial needle placement at the location of the right L5 dorsal ramus – at the right sacral ala just lateral to the right S1 SAP. Advance until contact with bone. *Next, further needle adjustment at all levels is carried out in the lateral view (see next Figure).*

Lateral View. Each needle is adjusted mediolaterally and/or cephalocaudally as needed until the tip is seen to be at the junction of the SAP and TP *(or at the junction of the sacral ala and S1 SAP for the L5 dorsal ramus).* Ensure that the needles are posterior to their respective IVF.

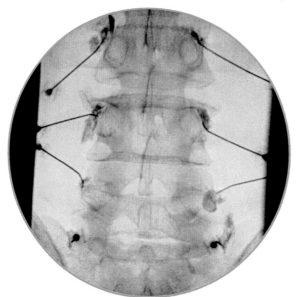

Figure 7-2E2
Tilt: 0°
Oblique: 0°

A/P View.   After negative aspiration, contrast is administered and shows proper spread at the location of each medial branch and L5 dorsal ramus, without evidence of epidural flow or vascular uptake.

See Page 281

**Bilateral L3-L4, L4-L5, L5-S1
MBB (Hardware)**

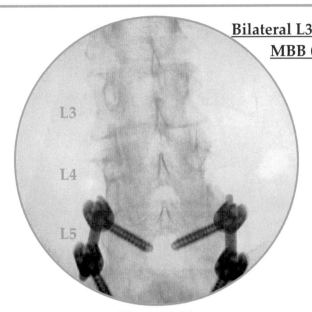

Figure 7-3A
Tilt: 0°
Oblique: 0°

A/P View. Note the vertebral levels in this view, and the PLIF and pedicle screws at L5-S1.

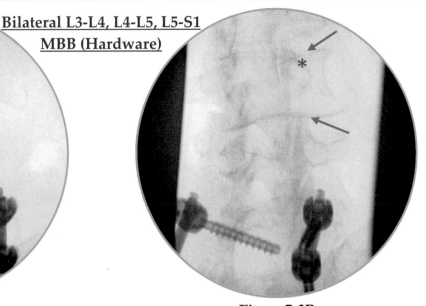

Figure 7-3B
Tilt: 0°
Oblique: 25° Right

Oblique View. Note the junction of the right L3 SAP and TP (red star). Without fluoroscopic tilting, note that the L3 endplates are fairly squared (blue arrows).

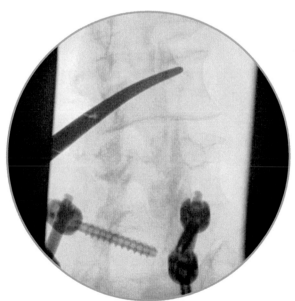

Figure 7-3C
Tilt: 0°
Oblique: 25° Right

Oblique View. Pointer showing the location of needle placement for the right L2 medial branch, at the junction of the right L3 SAP and TP.

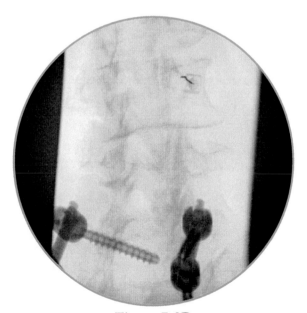

Figure 7-3D
Tilt: 0°
Oblique: 25° Right

Oblique View. Coaxial needle placement at the location of the right L2 medial branch – at the junction of the right L3 SAP and TP. Advance until contact with bone.

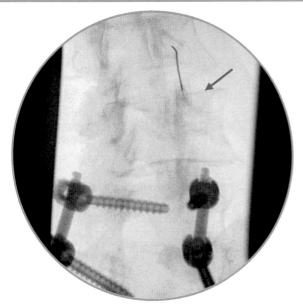

Figure 7-3E
Tilt: 10° Cephalad
Oblique: 25° Right

Oblique View. For targeting the right L3 medial branch, note that by applying a cephalad fluoroscopic tilt, this better squares the L4 SEP (blue arrow) – *compare to Figure 7-3D, where the L4 SEP is not optimally squared.*

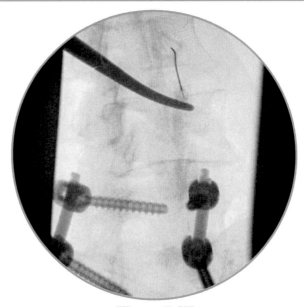

Figure 7-3F
Tilt: 10° Cephalad
Oblique: 25° Right

Oblique View. Pointer showing the location of needle placement for the right L3 medial branch, at the junction of the right L4 SAP and TP.

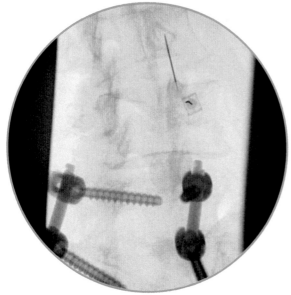

Figure 7-3G
Tilt: 10° Cephalad
Oblique: 25° Right

Oblique View. Coaxial needle placement at the location of the right L3 medial branch – at the junction of the right L4 SAP and TP. Advance until contact with bone.

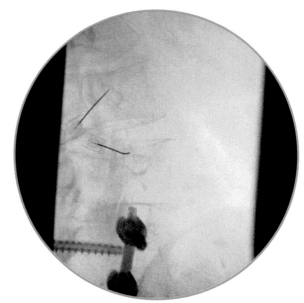

Figure 7-3H
Tilt: 10° Cephalad
Oblique: 35° Right

Oblique View. An additional ipsilateral oblique is applied to ensure that the needles for the right L2 and L3 medial branches are at the lateral border of their respective SAP – and maintained at the junction of the SAP and TP.

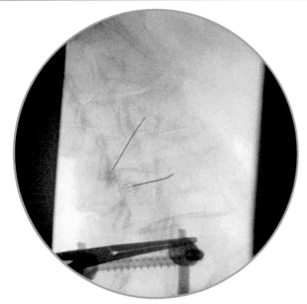

Figure 7-3I
Tilt: 20° Cephalad
Oblique: 35° Right

Oblique View. For targeting the right L4 medial branch, a further cephalad tilt is used to better square the L5 SEP. Pointer showing the location of needle placement for the right L4 medial branch, at the junction of the right L5 SAP and TP. *Note the pedicle screw at this level.*

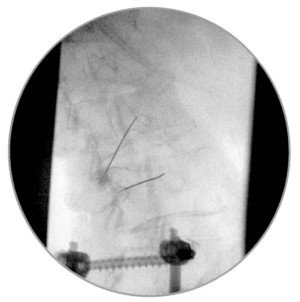

Figure 7-3J
Tilt: 20° Cephalad
Oblique: 35° Right

Oblique View. Coaxial needle placement at the location of the right L4 medial branch (just lateral to the right L5 pedicle screw) – at the junction of the right L5 SAP and TP. *It may be difficult to see the needle around hardware, as in this case, and intermittent multiplanar fluoroscopy should be used.*

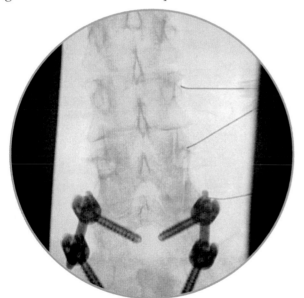

Figure 7-3K
Tilt: 0°
Oblique: 5° Right

A/P View. By applying a slight right ipsilateral oblique, you get a more "true" A/P view – *compare to Figure 7-3A.* Note needle placement at the right L2, L3, and L4 medial branches after placement in the prior oblique views.

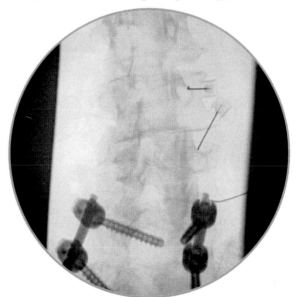

Figure 7-3L
Tilt: 0°
Oblique: 15° Right

Oblique View. Note the fluoroscopic obliquity for targeting the right L5 dorsal ramus at the right sacral ala and just lateral to the right S1 SAP and pedicle screw. *A lesser oblique angle is used for the dorsal ramus compared to the medial branch in order to remove obstruction from the iliac crest.*

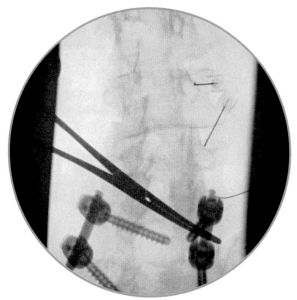

Figure 7-3M
Tilt: 0°
Oblique: 15° Right

Oblique View. Pointer showing the location of needle placement for the right L5 dorsal ramus, at the right sacral ala just lateral to the right S1 SAP and pedicle screw.

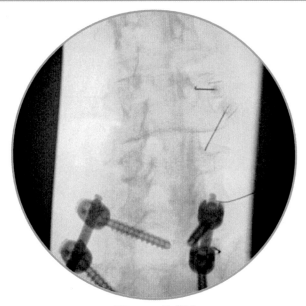

Figure 7-3N
Tilt: 0°
Oblique: 15° Right

Oblique View. Coaxial needle placement at the location of the right L5 dorsal ramus – at the right sacral ala just lateral to the right S1 SAP and pedicle screw. Advance until contact with bone.

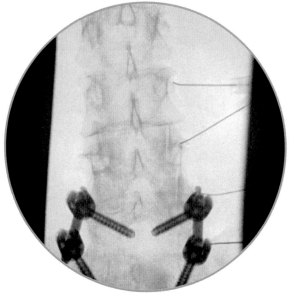

Figure 7-3O
Tilt: 0°
Oblique: 5° Right

A/P View. Needle positioning in the A/P view after needle placement has been performed in the prior oblique view.

Next, the contralateral side is targeted.

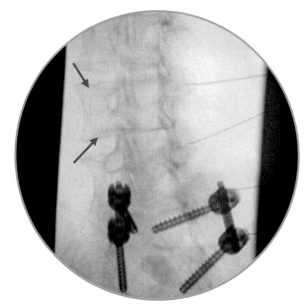

Figure 7-3P
Tilt: 5° Caudad
Oblique: 20° Left

Oblique View. Note that with the above fluoroscopic tilt, the L3 endplates are fairly squared (red arrows).

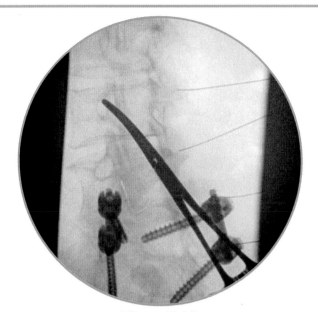

Figure 7-3Q
Tilt: 5° Caudad
Oblique: 20° Left

Oblique View. Pointer showing the location of needle placement for the left L2 medial branch, at the junction of the left L3 SAP and TP.

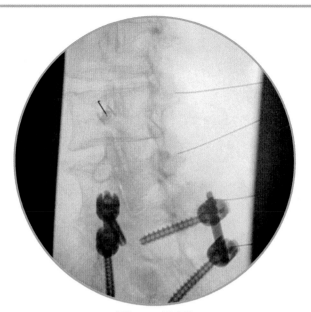

Figure 7-3R
Tilt: 5° Caudad
Oblique: 20° Left

Oblique View. Coaxial needle placement at the location of the left L2 medial branch – at the junction of the left L3 SAP and TP. Advance until contact with bone.

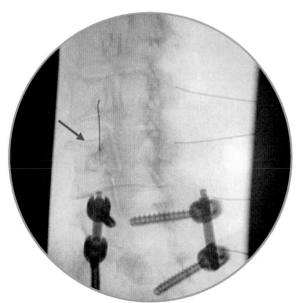

Figure 7-3S
Tilt: 10° Cephalad
Oblique: 20° Left

Oblique View. For targeting the left L3 medial branch, note that by applying a cephalad fluoroscopic tilt, this better squares the L4 SEP (red arrow) – *compare to Figure 7-3R, where the L4 SEP is not optimally squared.*

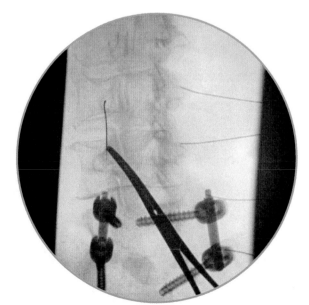

Figure 7-3T
Tilt: 10° Cephalad
Oblique: 20° Left

Oblique View. Pointer showing the location of needle placement for the left L3 medial branch, at the junction of the left L4 SAP and TP.

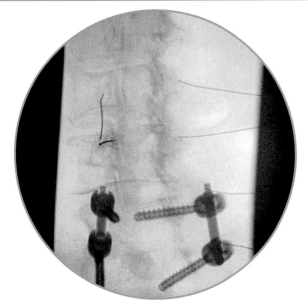

Figure 7-3U
Tilt: 10° Cephalad
Oblique: 20° Left

Oblique View. Coaxial needle placement at the location of the left L3 medial branch – at the junction of the left L4 SAP and TP. Advance until contact with bone.

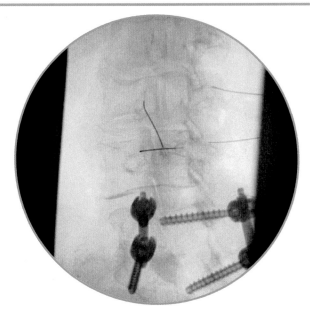

Figure 7-3V
Tilt: 10° Cephalad
Oblique: 30° Left

Oblique View. After needle placement in the prior view, an additional ipsilateral oblique angle is applied. Note that the needle at the left L2 medial branch is not seen to be at the lateral border of its respective SAP – *further needle adjustment is needed, see next image.*

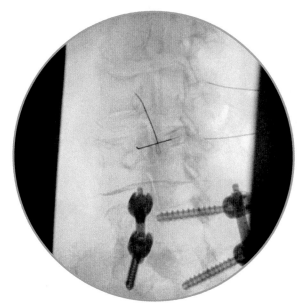

Figure 7-3W
Tilt: 10° Cephalad
Oblique: 30° Left

Oblique View. After needle adjustment, note that the needles at the left L2 and L3 medial branches are now at the lateral border of their corresponding SAPs – and maintained at the junction of the SAP and TP.

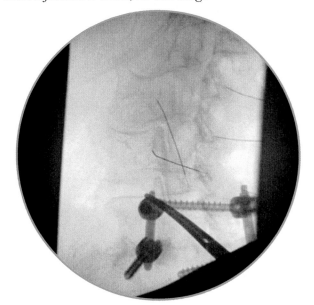

Figure 7-3X
Tilt: 20° Cephalad
Oblique: 30° Left

Oblique View. For targeting the left L4 medial branch, an additional cephalad tilt is needed to square the L5 SEP. Pointer showing the location of needle placement for the left L4 medial branch, at the junction of the left L5 SAP and TP and lateral to the pedicle screw.

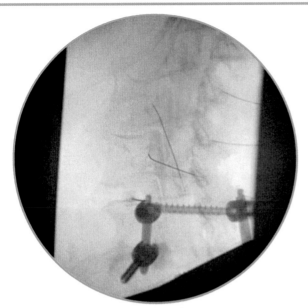

Figure 7-3Y
Tilt: 20° Cephalad
Oblique: 30° Left

Oblique View. Coaxial needle placement at the location of the left L4 medial branch, at the junction of the left L5 SAP and TP and just lateral to the pedicle screw. Advance until contact with bone.

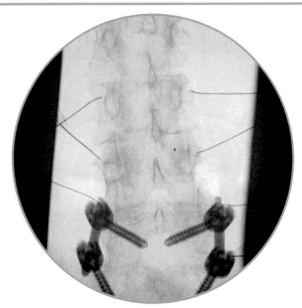

Figure 7-3Z
Tilt: 0°
Oblique: 0°

A/P View. Needle placement at the left L2, L3, and L4 medial branches after placement in the prior oblique views. Note that this is not a "true" A/P view, as the spinous processes are not midline – *compare to Figure 7-3K.*

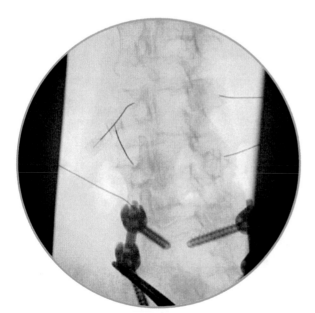

Figure 7-3A2
Tilt: 0°
Oblique: 10° Left

Oblique View. For targeting the left L5 dorsal ramus, a lesser oblique is used compared to that for targeting the medial branch. Pointer showing the location of needle placement for the left L5 dorsal ramus, near the left sacral ala and just lateral to the pedicle screw.

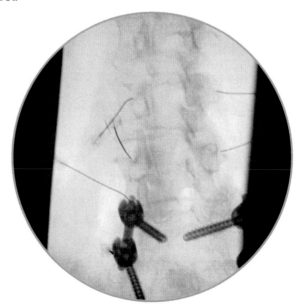

Figure 7-3B2
Tilt: 0°
Oblique: 10° Left

Oblique View. Coaxial needle placement at the location of the left L5 dorsal ramus – just lateral to the pedicle screw. Advance until contact with bone.

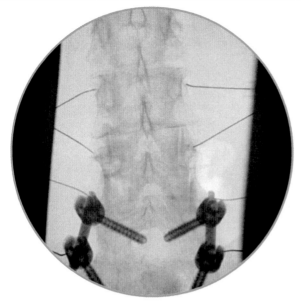

Figure 7-3C2
Tilt: 0°
Oblique: 0°

A/P View. Needle placement at the location of the left L5 dorsal ramus – at the left sacral ala just lateral to the left S1 SAP. *Next, further needle adjustment at all levels is carried out in the lateral view – see Figure 7-3D2.*

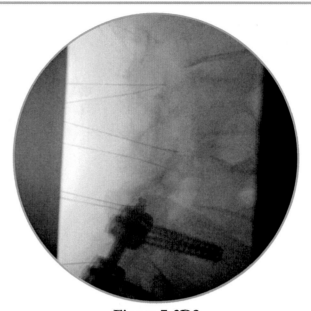

Figure 7-3D2
Tilt: 0°
Oblique: 90° Right

Lateral View. Each needle is adjusted mediolaterally and/or cephalocaudally as needed until the tip is seen to be at the junction of the SAP and TP (or sacral ala and S1 SAP for the L5 dorsal ramus). Ensure that each needle tip is posterior to its respective IVF.

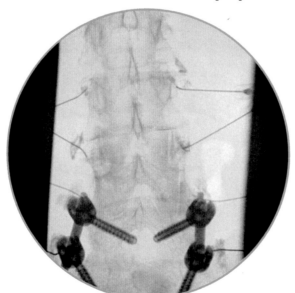

Figure 7-3E2
Tilt: 0°
Oblique: 5° Right

A/P View. After negative aspiration, contrast is administered and shows proper spread around the location of each medial branch and L5 dorsal ramus, without evidence of epidural flow or vascular uptake. *Note this is a more "true" A/P view – compare to Figure 7-3Z.*

Chapter 8
Lumbar Radiofrequency Nerve Ablation

☐ Obtain an A/P view to locate the targeted vertebral levels.

☐ Next, square the endplates and apply an ipsilateral oblique (typically around 20°) to identify the junction of the superior articular process (SAP) and transverse process (TP) for the targeted medial branch. *Of note, if both the superior and inferior endplate cannot be squared, preference should be given to squaring the superior endplate (SEP).*

☐ For placement of the RF needle to target the medial branch, the percutaneous entry site should be caudad and slightly lateral to the junction of the SAP and TP (as seen in the obique view) – *this needle trajectory allows for an ideal ablation along the length of the medial branch nerve.* As a rule of thumb, once the SEP of the targeted level has been squared, the caudal entry point for average-sized patients should be near the IEP (see page 135 for further details).

☐ The RF needle is advanced from the entry site towards the junction of the SAP and TP at the desired level. Once bone is gently contacted with the needle tip, an additional ipsilateral oblique is applied to see the entire length of the needle. In this view, the RF needle is further adjusted as needed until the tip is seen to be at the lateral border of the SAP – but still maintained at the junction of the SAP and TP. Of note, for the L5 dorsal ramus, the RF needle is placed in a similar fashion using the sacral ala and S1 SAP as anatomical landmarks (see page 137 for further details).

☐ Next, an A/P view is obtained to ensure that the needle tip is at the expected location of the medial branch (i.e., the junction of the SAP and TP). Similarly, for the L5 dorsal ramus, this view is obtained to ensure ideal placement at the sacral ala and just lateral to the S1 SAP.

☐ Next, a lateral view is obtained. The RF needle tip is adjusted as needed, typically mediolaterally, to get placement just posterior to the foramen and maintained at the junction of the SAP and TP. *Of note, cephalocaudal adjustment can also be made in the lateral view, but typically is not as frequently needed since this can be adequately seen and performed in the prior A/P and oblique views.*

☐ Once all needle tips are in their correct and final position, and after appropriate motor and/or sensory testing has been carried out, radiofrequency ablation at each level is performed. The RF cannulas are then rotated 180° and the ablation is carried out once again to account for any medial branch and/or L5 dorsal ramus anatomical variability.

**Left L3-L4, L4-L5, L5-S1
RFNA**

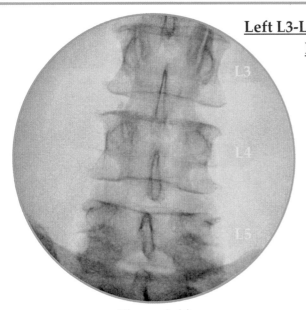

Figure 8-1A
Tilt: 0°
Oblique: 0°

A/P View. Note the vertebral levels in this view.

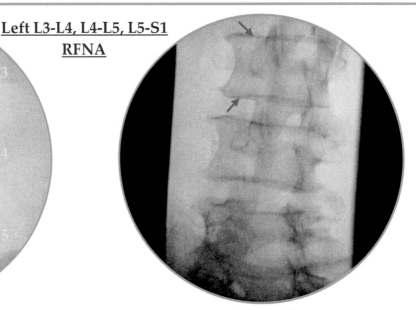

Figure 8-1B
Tilt: 5° Caudal
Oblique: 20° Left

Oblique View. Applying a caudal tilt better squares the L3 endplates (blue arrows). This is a more ideal view for needle placement targeting the left L2 medial branch.

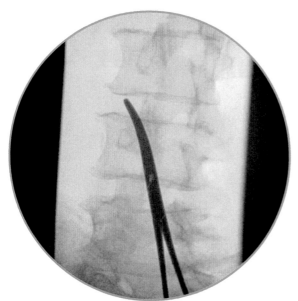

Figure 8-1C
Tilt: 5° Caudad
Oblique: 20° Left

Oblique View. Pointer showing the location of needle entry for the left L2 medial branch, near the L3 IEP. This entry point creates a shallow trajectory, which better approximates the length of the medial branch, allowing for a more effective ablation along the nerve.

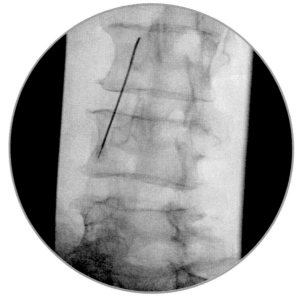

Figure 8-1D
Tilt: 5° Caudad
Oblique: 20° Left

Oblique View. RF needle placement at the location of the left L2 medial branch – at the junction of the left L3 SAP and TP. *The needle is advanced until gentle contact with bone at the junction.*

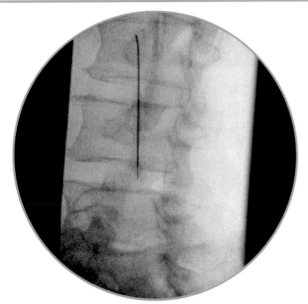

Figure 8-1E
Tilt: 5° Caudad
Oblique: 30° Left

Oblique View. After needle placement in the prior view, an additional ipsilateral oblique angle is applied and further needle adjustment is carried out as needed until the tip is at the lateral border of the left L3 SAP – and maintained at the junction of the left L3 SAP and TP.

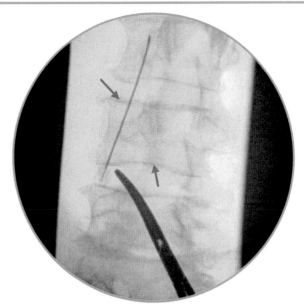

Figure 8-1F
Tilt: 0°
Oblique: 20° Left

Oblique View. For targeting the left L3 medial branch, removing the tilt better squares the L4 endplates (blue arrows). This is a more ideal view for needle placement. Pointer showing the location of needle entry for the left L3 medial branch, near the L4 IEP.

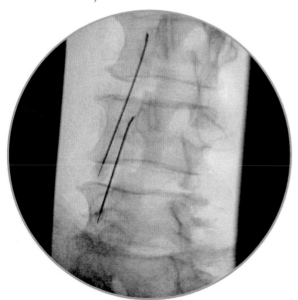

Figure 8-1G
Tilt: 0°
Oblique: 20° Left

Oblique View. RF needle placement at the location of the left L3 medial branch – at the junction of the left L4 SAP and TP. *The needle is advanced until gentle contact with bone at the junction.*

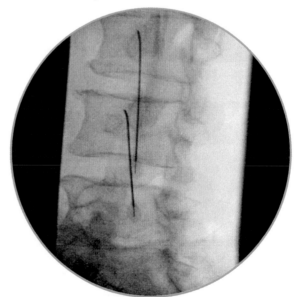

Figure 8-1H
Tilt: 0°
Oblique: 30° Left

Oblique View. After needle placement in the prior view, an additional ipsilateral oblique angle is applied and further needle adjustment is carried out as needed until the tip is at the lateral border of the left L4 SAP – and maintained at the junction of the left L4 SAP and TP.

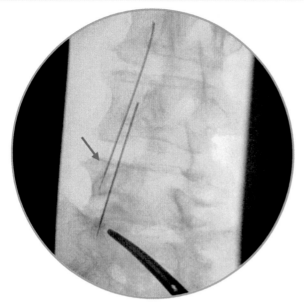

Figure 8-1I
Tilt: 5° Cephalad
Oblique: 20° Left

Oblique View. For targeting the left L4 medial branch, applying a cephalad tilt better squares the L5 SEP (blue arrow). This is a more ideal view for needle placement. Pointer showing the location of needle entry for the left L4 medial branch, near the L5 IEP.

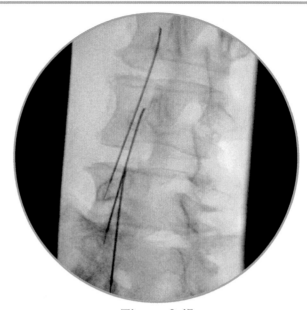

Figure 8-1J
Tilt: 5° Cephalad
Oblique: 20° Left

Oblique View. RF needle placement at the location of the left L4 medial branch – at the junction of the left L5 SAP and TP. *The needle is advanced until gentle contact with bone at the junction.*

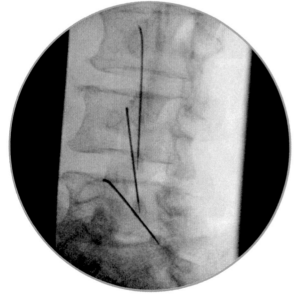

Figure 8-1K
Tilt: 5° Cephalad
Oblique: 30° Left

Oblique View. After needle placement in the prior view, an additional ipsilateral oblique angle is applied and further needle adjustment is carried out as needed until the tip is at the lateral border of the left L5 SAP – and maintained at the junction of the left L5 SAP and TP.

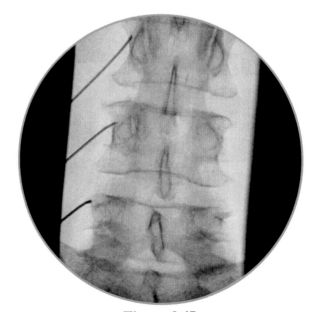

Figure 8-1L
Tilt: 0°
Oblique: 0°

A/P View. Needle positioning at the left L2, L3, and L4 medial branches after placement in the prior oblique views. In ths view, all needles appear to be at the expected location – i.e., the junction of the SAP and TP.

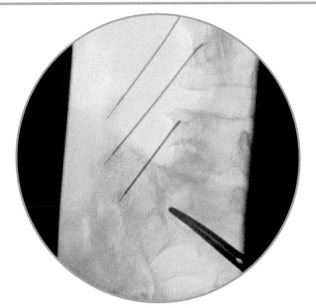

Figure 8-1M
Tilt: 0°
Oblique: 10° Left

Oblique View. Using less ipsilateral oblique removes the iliac crest from obstructing the needle trajectory. Pointer showing the location of needle entry for the left L5 dorsal ramus, inferior to the left sacral ala and slightly lateral to the left S1 SAP.

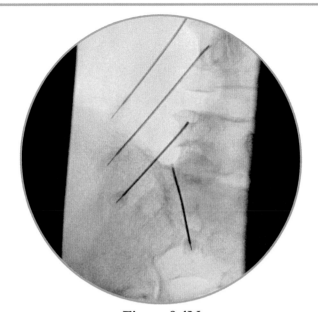

Figure 8-1N
Tilt: 0°
Oblique: 10° Left

Oblique View. RF needle placement at the location of the left L5 dorsal ramus – at the left sacral ala and just lateral to the left S1 SAP. *The needle is advanced until gentle contact with bone.*

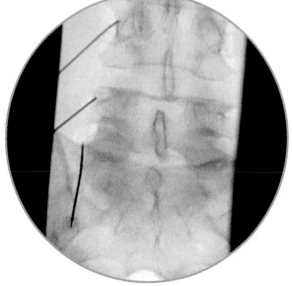

Figure 8-1O
Tilt: 0°
Oblique: 0°

A/P View. Note the needle positioning at the left L5 dorsal ramus after placement in the prior oblique view. Next, a lateral view is obtained where further adjustments are carried out as needed – *see Figure 8-1P.*

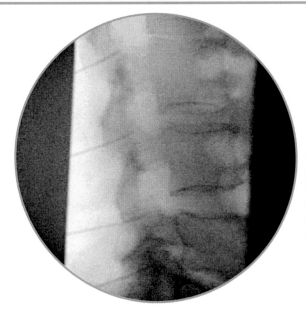

Figure 8-1P
Tilt: 0°
Oblique: 90° Right

Lateral View. Each needle is adjusted mediolaterally and/or cephalocaudally as needed until the tip is seen to be at the junction of the SAP and TP. Ensure that each needle tip is posterior to its respective IVF. Following appropriate motor and/or sensory stimulation, RFNA is carried out. *Note the cephalad curve of each needle tip.*

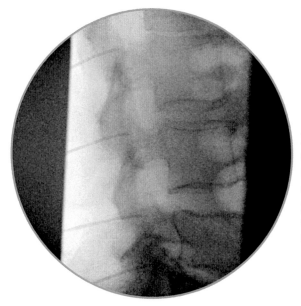

Figure 8-1Q
Tilt: 0°
Oblique: 90° Right

Lateral View. Next, the needles/probes are rotated 180° and a lateral view is taken once again to ensure no ventral needle advancement has occurred during rotation of each needle. After confirming that each needle tip is posterior to its respective IVF, RFNA is carried out once again to create a larger ablation, which accounts for anatomical variability. *Note the caudad curve of each needle tip.*

See Page 284

**Right L3-L4, L4-L5, L5-S1
RFNA**

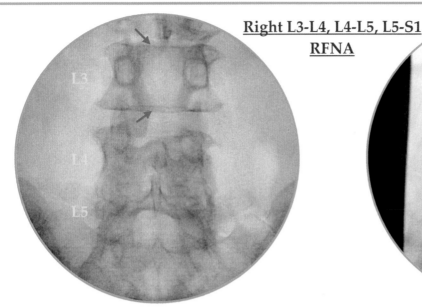

Figure 8-2A
Tilt: 0°
Oblique: 0°

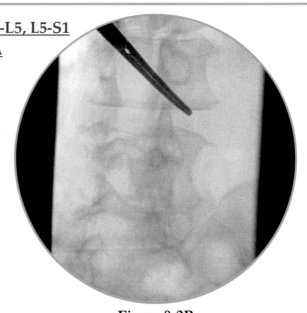

Figure 8-2B
Tilt: 0°
Oblique: 20° Right

A/P View. Note the vertebral levels in this view, and the prior laminectomy at L3. Without a fluoroscopic tilt, the L3 endplates appear to be fairly squared (blue arrows). Thus, no fluoroscopic tilting will be needed for targeting the L2 medial branch.

Oblique View. Pointer showing the location of needle entry for the right L2 medial branch, near the L3 IEP. This entry point creates a shallow trajectory, which better approximates the length of the medial branch and allows for a more effective ablation along the nerve.

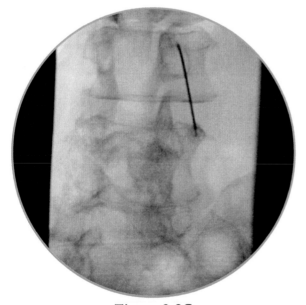

Figure 8-2C
Tilt: 0°
Oblique: 20° Right

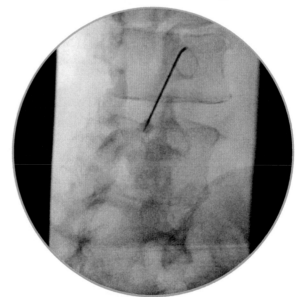

Figure 8-2D
Tilt: 0°
Oblique: 30° Right

Oblique View. RF needle placement at the location of the right L2 medial branch – at the junction of the right L3 SAP and TP. *The needle is advanced until gentle contact with bone at the junction.*

Oblique View. After needle placement in the prior view, an additional ipsilateral oblique angle is applied and further needle adjustment is carried out as needed until the tip is at the lateral border of the right L3 SAP – and maintained at the junction of the right L3 SAP and TP.

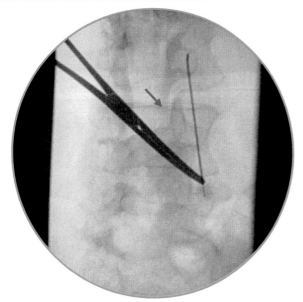

Figure 8-2E
Tilt: 10° Cephalad
Oblique: 20° Right

Oblique View. For targeting the right L3 medial branch, applying a cephalad tilt better squares the L4 SEP (blue arrow) – *compare to Figure 8-2C*. This is a more ideal view. Pointer showing the location of needle entry for the right L3 medial branch, near the L4 IEP.

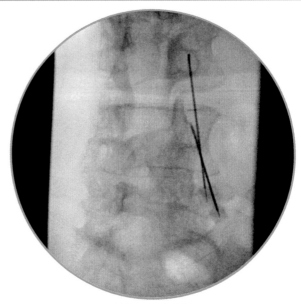

Figure 8-2F
Tilt: 10° Cephalad
Oblique: 20° Right

Oblique View. RF needle placement at the location of the right L3 medial branch – at the junction of the right L4 SAP and TP. *The needle is advanced until gentle contact with bone at the junction.*

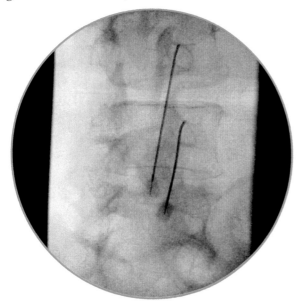

Figure 8-2G
Tilt: 10° Cephalad
Oblique: 30° Right

Oblique View. After needle placement in the prior view, an additional ipsilateral oblique angle is applied and further needle adjustment is carried out as needed until the tip is at the lateral border of the right L4 SAP – and maintained at the junction of the right L4 SAP and TP.

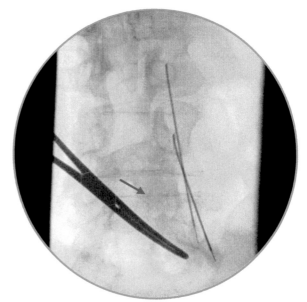

Figure 8-2H
Tilt: 25° Cephalad
Oblique: 20° Right

Oblique View. For targeting the right L4 medial branch, a greater cephalad tilt is used to better square the L5 SEP (blue arrow) – *compare to Figure 8-2F*. This is a more ideal view. Pointer showing the location of needle entry for the right L4 medial branch, near the L5 IEP.

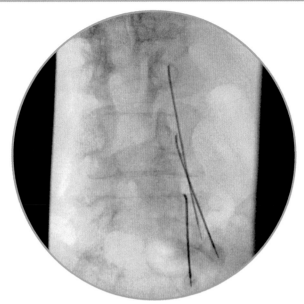

Figure 8-2I
Tilt: 25° Cephalad
Oblique: 20° Right

Oblique View. RF needle placement at the location of the right L4 medial branch – at the junction of the right L5 SAP and TP. *The needle is advanced until gentle contact with bone at the junction.*

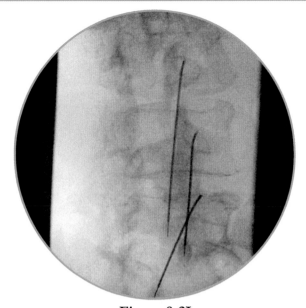

Figure 8-2J
Tilt: 25° Cephalad
Oblique: 30° Right

Oblique View. After needle placement in the prior view, an additional ipsilateral oblique angle is applied and further needle adjustment is carried out as needed until the tip is at the lateral border of the right L5 SAP – and maintained at the junction of the right L5 SAP and TP.

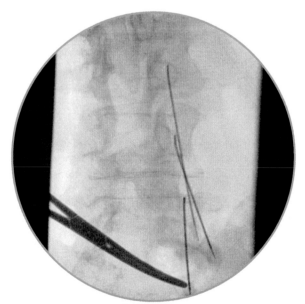

Figure 8-2K
Tilt: 25° Cephalad
Oblique: 10° Right

Oblique View. Using less ipsilateral oblique removes the iliac crest from obstructing the needle trajectory. Pointer showing the location of needle entry for the right L5 dorsal ramus, inferior to the right sacral ala and just lateral to the right S1 SAP.

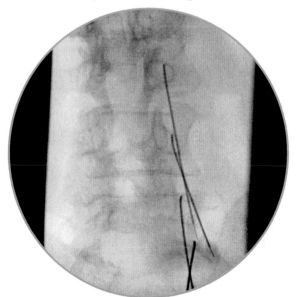

Figure 8-2L
Tilt: 25° Cephalad
Oblique: 10° Right

Oblique View. RF needle placement at the location of the right L5 dorsal ramus – at the right sacral ala and just lateral to the right S1 SAP. *The needle is advanced until gentle contact with bone.*

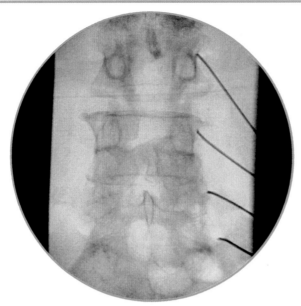

Figure 8-2M
Tilt: 0°
Oblique: 0°

A/P View. Note the needle positioning at the right L2, L3, and L4 medial branches & L5 dorsal ramus after placement in the prior oblique views – all RF needles are noted to be at their respective junctions. Next, a lateral view is obtained – *see Figure 8-2N*.

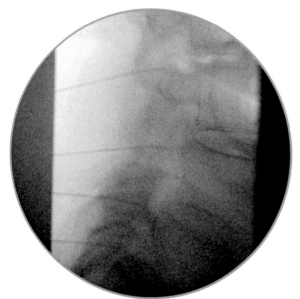

Figure 8-2N
Tilt: 0°
Oblique: 90° Right

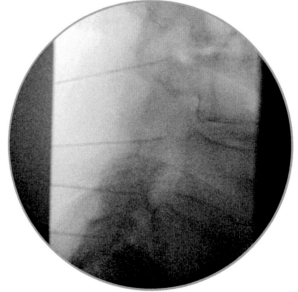

Figure 8-2O
Tilt: 0°
Oblique: 90° Right

Lateral View. Each needle is adjusted mediolaterally and/or cephalocaudally as needed until the tip is seen to be at the junction of the SAP and TP. Ensure that each needle tip is posterior to its respective IVF. Following appropriate motor and/or sensory stimulation, RFNA is carried out. *Note the caudad curve of each needle tip.*

Lateral View. Next, the needles/probes are rotated 180° and a lateral view is taken once again to ensure no ventral needle advancement has occurred during rotation. RFNA is carried out once again to create a larger ablation, which accounts for any anatomical variability. *Note the cephalad curve of each needle tip.*

See Page 284

Right L3-L4, L4-L5, L5-S1
RNFA (Hardware)

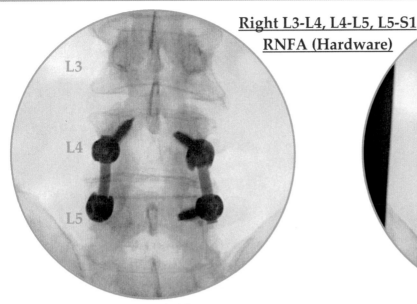

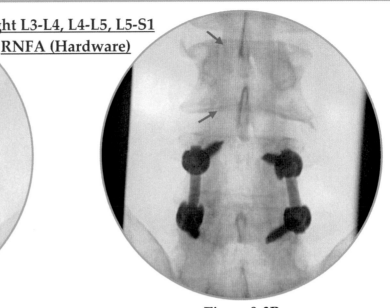

Figure 8-3A
Tilt: 0°
Oblique: 0°

Figure 8-3B
Tilt: 5° Caudad
Oblique: 0°

A/P View. Note the vertebral levels in this view, along with the laminectomy at L4 and placement of bilateral pedicle screws at L4 and L5. The L3 endplates are not adequately squared, and fluoroscopic tilting will be needed to target the L2 medial branch – *see next Figure.*

A/P View. For targeting the L2 medial branch, applying a caudal tilt better squares the L3 endplates (blue arrows) – *compare to Figure 8-3A.*

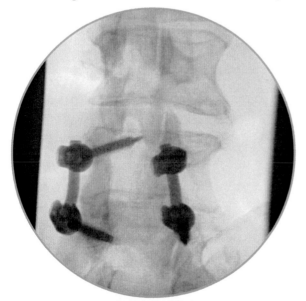

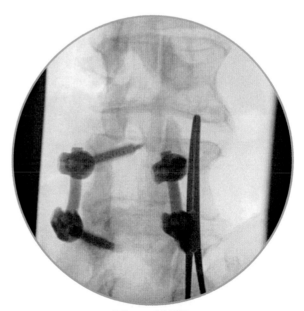

Figure 8-3C
Tilt: 5° Caudad
Oblique: 20° Right

Figure 8-3D
Tilt: 5° Caudad
Oblique: 20° Right

Oblique View. With the L3 endplates squared, a right ipsilateral oblique is applied to identify the location of the right L2 medial branch, at the junction of the right L3 SAP and TP.

Oblique View. Pointer showing the location of needle entry for the right L2 medial branch, near the L3 IEP. This entry point creates a shallow trajectory, which better approximates the length of the medial branch and allows for a more effective ablation along the nerve.

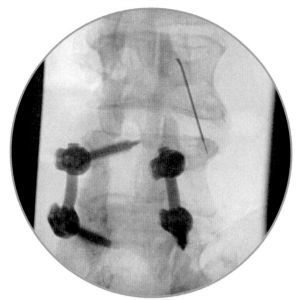

Figure 8-3E
Tilt: 5° Caudad
Oblique: 20° Right

Oblique View. RF needle placement at the location of the right L2 medial branch – at the junction of the right L3 SAP and TP. *The needle is advanced until gentle contact with bone at the junction.*

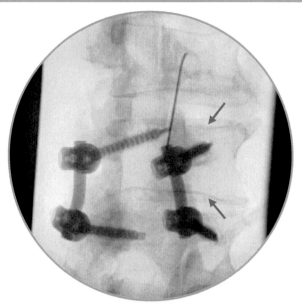

Figure 8-3F
Tilt: 0°
Oblique: 30° Right

Oblique View. For targeting the right L3 medial branch, removing the tilt better squares the L4 endplates (blue arrows) – *compare to Figure 8-3E*. Increasing the ipsilateral oblique angle allows for better visualization of the junction of the right L4 SAP and TP.

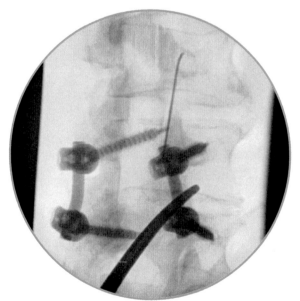

Figure 8-3G
Tilt: 0°
Oblique: 30° Right

Oblique View. Pointer showing the location of needle entry for the right L3 medial branch, near the L4 IEP. This entry point creates a shallow trajectory, which better approximates the length of the medial branch and allows for a more effective ablation along the nerve.

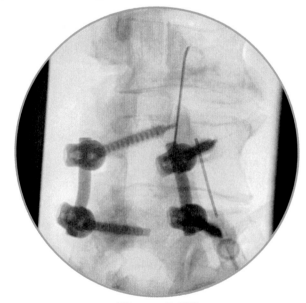

Figure 8-3H
Tilt: 0°
Oblique: 30° Right

Oblique View. RF needle placement at the location of the right L3 medial branch – at the junction of the right L4 SAP and TP. *The needle is advanced until gentle contact with bone at the junction.*

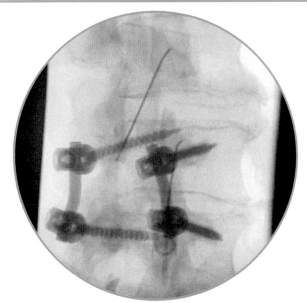

Figure 8-3I
Tilt: 0°
Oblique: 40° Right

Oblique View. After needle placement in the prior view, an additional ipsilateral oblique angle is applied and further needle adjustment is carried out as needed until the tips are at the lateral border of their respective SAPs – and maintained at the junction of the SAP and TP.

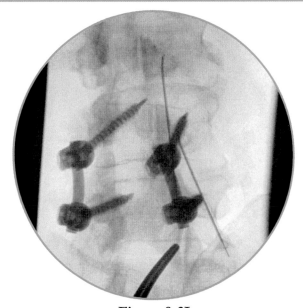

Figure 8-3J
Tilt: 5° Cephalad
Oblique: 25° Right

Oblique View. Pointer showing the location of needle entry for the right L4 medial branch, near the L5 IEP. Note the fluoroscopic adjustments used for visualizing the junction of the right L5 SAP and TP.

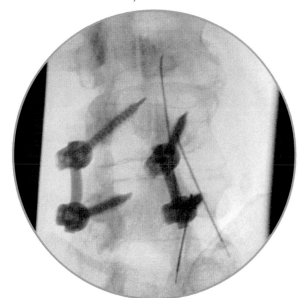

Figure 8-3K
Tilt: 5° Cephalad
Oblique: 25° Right

Oblique View. RF needle placement at the location of the right L4 medial branch – at the junction of the right L5 SAP and TP. *The needle is advanced until gentle contact with bone at the junction.*

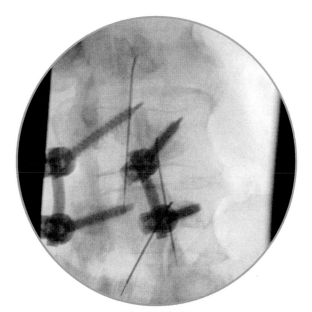

Figure 8-3L
Tilt: 5° Cephalad
Oblique: 35° Right

Oblique View. After needle placement in the prior view, an additional ipsilateral oblique angle is applied and further needle adjustment is carried out as needed until the tip is at the lateral border of the right L5 SAP – and maintained at the junction of the right L5 SAP and TP.

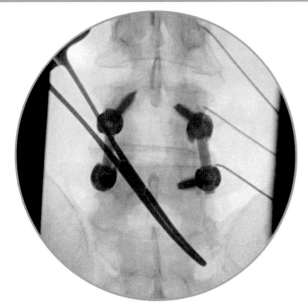

Figure 8-3M
Tilt: 0°
Oblique: 0°

A/P View. Pointer showing the location of needle entry for the right L5 dorsal ramus, inferior to the right sacral ala. *Note that due to obstruction from the right iliac crest, an ipsilateral oblique angle could not be used for needle placement.*

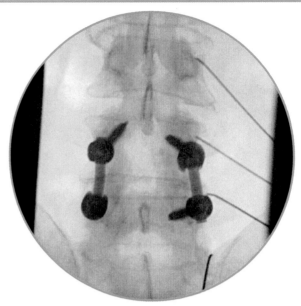

Figure 8-3N
Tilt: 0°
Oblique: 0°

A/P View. RF needle placement at the location of the right L5 dorsal ramus – at the right sacral ala and just lateral to the right S1 SAP. *The needle is advanced until gentle contact with bone.* Also note the positioning of the RF needles for the right L2, L3, and L4 medial branches.

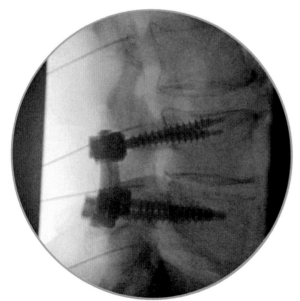

Figure 8-3O
Tilt: 0°
Oblique: 90° Right

Lateral View. Each needle is adjusted mediolaterally and/or cephalocaudally as needed until the tip is seen to be at the junction of the SAP and TP. Ensure that each needle tip is posterior to its respective IVF. Following appropriate motor and/or sensory stimulation, RFNA is carried out. *Note the caudad curve of each needle tip.*

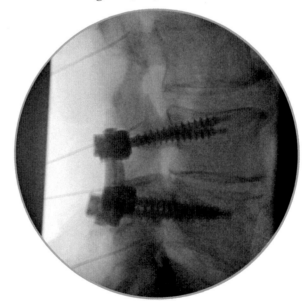

Figure 8-3P
Tilt: 0°
Oblique: 90° Right

Lateral View. Next, the needles/probes are rotated 180° and a lateral view is taken once again to ensure no ventral needle advancement has occurred during rotation. RFNA is carried out once again to create a larger ablation, which accounts for any anatomical variability. *Note the cephalad curve of each needle tip.*

Additional Discussion:
Needle Trajectory

Appropriate needle trajectory is essential for obtaining best outcomes during radiofrequency nerve ablation (RFNA). Unlike lumbar medial branch blocks, with RFNA the needle should be placed more parallel to the nerve rather than perpendicular *(see Figures 8-4 & 8-5).*

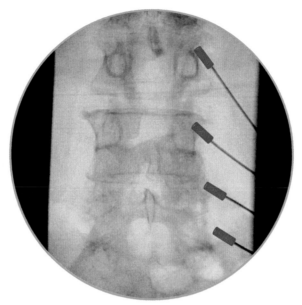

Figure 8-4
Tilt: 0°
Oblique: 0°
A/P View. *Figure 8-2M reproduced.*

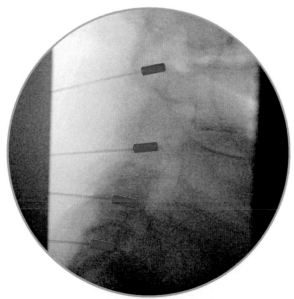

Figure 8-5
Tilt: 0°
Oblique: 90° Right
Lateral View. Figure 8-2N reproduced.

After applying the appropriate ipsilateral oblique to visualize the junction of the superior articular process (SAP) and transverse process (TP), the ideal needle trajectory for RFNA of the lumbar medial branch is created by first squaring the superior endplate (SEP) at the targeted level. Next, from the squared SEP, a caudal needle entry is performed so that the needle eventually lies in a parallel fashion along the length of the medial branch nerve, as depicted in Figures 8-4 & 8-5. For average sized patients, after squaring the SEP, the caudal needle entry point should be at approximately the inferior endplate (IEP). *For thinner patients, the needle entry point will be more cephalad, and for thicker patients the entry point will be more caudad.*

Of note, as an alternative to the described technique, one may also consider simply tilting the C-arm caudally 20-30° from the squared SEP and then placing the RF needle in a coaxial view towards the target (i.e., junction of SAP and TP for the lumbar medial branch *or* junction of sacral ala and S1 SAP for the L5 dorsal ramus). However, with this steep an angulation of the image intensifier, it may become more challenging to visualize the targeted structures. Thus, the aforementioned approach allows for a reliable method of placing a RF needle parallel to the nerve and with clear visualization of the target.

The ideal RF needle trajectory should be such that the needle ultimately forms an angle with the SEP/sacral endplate of approximately 20-30° (see Figure 8-6).

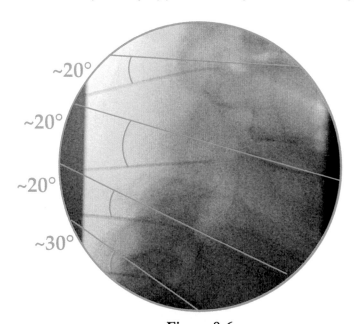

Figure 8-6
Tilt: 0°
Oblique: 90° Right

Lateral View. *Figure 8-5 Reproduced.* Note the "needle to SEP" angle at each level and the "needle to sacral endplate" angle.

Additional Discussion:
The L5 Dorsal Ramus Needle Entry

Radiofrequency (RF) needle placement for the L5 dorsal ramus may be done with or without first squaring the sacral endplate. In order to line up the sacral endplate, typically a cephalad fluoroscopic tilt is required as a result of the natural lumbar lordosis. Placing a RF needle without first lining up the sacral endplate requires more of an "estimate" of where to perform needle entry – a skill often acquired by more experienced proceduralists (see Figures 8-8A & 8-8B for further discussion). Due to the "c-shaped" curvature of the sacrum, having a solid understanding of the needle entry point is essential to ensure that the needle has access to the location of the L5 dorsal ramus.

Figures 8-7A through 8-8B compare ideal needle placement to that of using too caudal a needle entry when attempting to place the RF needle along the length of the L5 dorsal ramus...

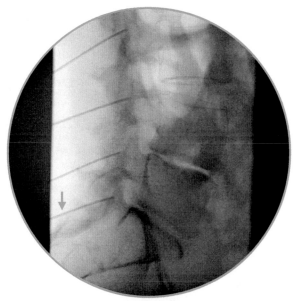

Figure 8-7A
Tilt: 0°
Oblique: 90° Right

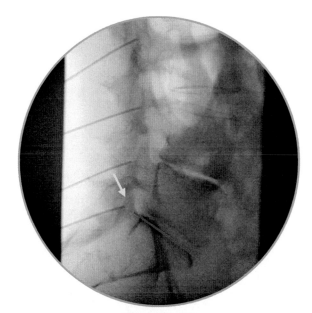

Figure 8-7B
Tilt: 0°
Oblique: 90° Right

Lateral View. This is ideal placement of the radiofrequency needle (green arrow) at the L5 dorsal ramus. *See next image for further anatomical details.*

Lateral View. *Figure 8-7A reproduced.* With this ideal placement for ablation of the L5 dorsal ramus, note how the needle tip is at the S1 SAP (yellow arrow). Additionally, note the cephalocaudal angulation of the sacral endplate (red line) as a result of the natural lumbar lordosis. By *NOT* using too caudal a needle entry, one may accurately place the RF needle tip at the location of the L5 dorsal ramus and along the nerve, as seen here.

However, if one were to have too caudal a needle entry point, challenges can be encountered which prevent accurate needle placement – *see Figure 8-8A for details.*

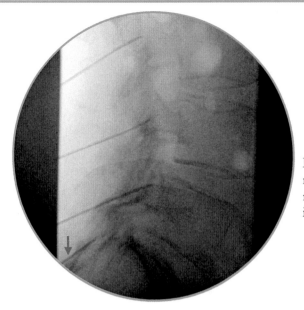

Figure 8-8A
Tilt: 0°
Oblique: 90° Right

Lateral View. This is NOT ideal placement of the radiofrequency needle (blue arrow) at the L5 dorsal ramus. In this example, the radiofrequency needle entry is too caudad. *See next image for further anatomical details.*

Figure 8-8B
Tilt: 0°
Oblique: 90° Right

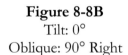

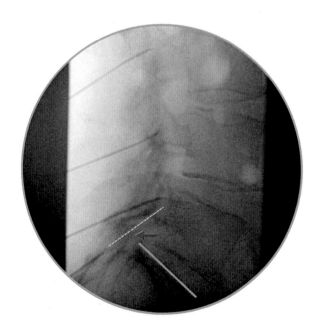

Lateral View. *Figure 8-8A reproduced.* With too caudad a needle entry, the RF needle in this image is on bone but cannot be advanced at a steeper angle towards the more anterior S1 SAP target (red arrow) due to the "c-shaped" curvature of the sacrum. If the RF needle is further advanced along its current trajectory, it will remain dorsal to the S1 SAP target – this can be visualized by extending out an imaginary line along the current needle trajectory (yellow dotted line). In addition, note that this current needle trajectory is nearly perpendicular to the sacral endplate (green line). Compare this "needle to sacral endplate" angle to that seen in Figure 8-7B. As discussed previously (reference Figure 8-6), the "needle to SEP/sacral endplate" angle should ideally be approximately 20-30°. In this example, the only option for correct RF needle placement will be to remove and replace it with a more cephalad entry point, in order to gain access to the S1 SAP – which will also create a more ideal "needle to sacral endplate" angle.

Of note, prior to RF needle placement for the L5 dorsal ramus, one may elect to first line up the sacral endplate to help determine the caudal needle entry point. If doing so, the entry point will be ~20-30° caudal to the squared sacral endplate (as discussed previously).

More experienced proceduralists may choose not to line up the sacral endplate prior to needle placement. In this case, the entry point is guided by both experience and with the principle: *the greater the cephalad angle needed to square the sacral endplate, the more cephalad the needle entry – and vice versa.*

Chapter 9
Cervical Medial Branch Block

___

- ☐ Obtain an A/P view to identify the targeted level. Although more important for cervical radiofrequency nerve ablation (see Chapter 10), if planning to place the needle parallel to the angle of the articular pillar (AP) for a cervical medial branch block, it is the author's preference to also obtain a scout lateral view prior to needle placement in order to clearly see the cephalocaudal angle of the AP – this helps to better estimate the caudal needle entry point needed to create the desired needle trajectory (see Figure 9-2A and page 165 for further discussion). *It is the author's preference to place the needle with a posterior approach (i.e. patient lying prone) rather than a lateral approach (i.e., patient in a lateral decubitus position). In the latter, if the bilateral articular pillars at the targeted level are not properly aligned, it is possible that the needle can unknowingly be advanced through the foramen and catastrophically towards the spinal cord.*

- ☐ In the A/P view, identify the waist of the targeted articular pillar (i.e., lateral mass). *Of note, in certain instances it may be challenging to get clear visualization of the target due to obstruction from the mandible, teeth, dental implants, etc. Applying a cephalad tilt can assist with removing these structures from obstruction and provide better visualization of the lateral mass (see Figure 9-1B).* Once the targeted lateral mass is clearly visualized, the needle is placed at the waist of the articular pillar, and contactng bone. Needle placement can be done in two ways.
    1. Sagittal Pass (see Figure 9-1D) – In the A/P view, advance the needle coaxially and ensure that the tip remains at the waist of the articular pillar at all times, until contact with bone. If there is any uncertainty regarding needle depth, use intermittent lateral and/or CLO views as needed. *Critical structures to avoid include the spinal cord (medially) and the vertebral artery, spinal nerve, and DRG (ventral aspect of the joint).*
    2. Oblique Pass (see Figure 9-2B) – In the A/P view, advance the needle from an oblique approach until contact is made with bone at the waist. Although this can be done by applying an ipsilateral oblique and advancing the needle with a coaxial approach, it is possible that rotation of the C-arm may lead to loss of clear visualization of the previously identified lateral mass. Thus, as an alternative, one may advance the needle using the aforementioned approach in a "non-coaxial" fashion towards the lateral mass. *This technique certainly requires more experience and a greater appreciation of needle depth (intermittent lateral and/or CLO views should be used frequently to assess depth).*

- ☐ After contact with bone, further minor needle adjustments are carried out in the lateral view until the tip is at the midpoint of the waist. *Of note, in the lower cervical segments it can often be difficult to clearly see the needle tip in the lateral view due to large shoulders and/or short necks. The CLO view should be used instead to assess depth and further advance the needle (see Figure 9-1R).*

- ☐ Next, obtain an A/P view once again to ensure that the needle tip is at waist of the AP and contacting bone. After negative aspiration, contrast is administered to ensure proper spread.

**Left C3-C4, C4-C5, C5-C6
MBB**

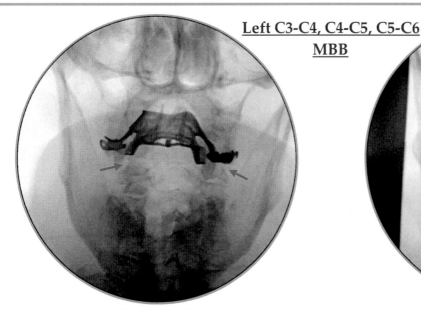

Figure 9-1A
Tilt: 0°
Oblique: 0°

A/P View. Identify the targeted level. Dental implants can often be present and cause obstruction of targeted structures. In this case, note the dental implant obstructing the view over the C2 & C3 levels (blue arrows showing waist of the bilateral C3 articular pillars).

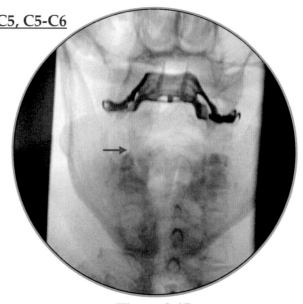

Figure 9-1B
Tilt: 5° Cephalad
Oblique: 0°

A/P View. By applying a cephalad tilt, note how both the jaw line and dental implant are removed from obstructing the targeted structures – *compare to Figure 9-1A*. There is now a clearer view of the waist of the left C3 articular pillar (red arrow).

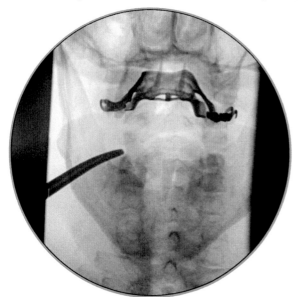

Figure 9-1C
Tilt: 5° Cephalad
Oblique: 0°

A/P View. Pointer at the location of the waist of the left C3 articular pillar.

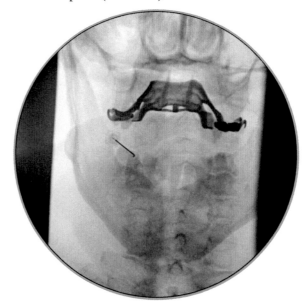

Figure 9-1D
Tilt: 5° Cephalad
Oblique: 0°

A/P View. Sagittal needle pass towards the waist of the left C3 articular pillar (C3 medal branch), until contact with bone. *Of note, intermittent lateral and/or CLO views should be used to assess needle depth throughout advancement if there is any question regarding needle depth (see Figure 9-1E).*

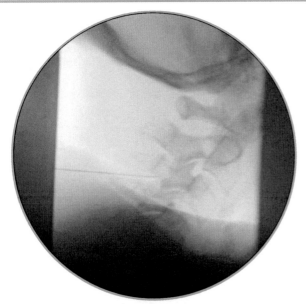

Figure 9-1E
Tilt: 5° Cephalad
Oblique: 90° Right

Lateral View. As the needle is being advanced in the A/P view towards the waist of the articular pillar, it is important to use intermittent lateral fluoroscopy to assess needle depth. In this case, note that the needle is approaching, but still posterior to, the C3 articular pillar.

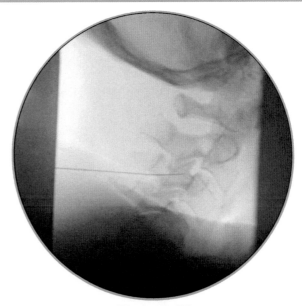

Figure 9-1F
Tilt: 5° Cephalad
Oblique: 90° Right

Lateral View. Once the needle has contacted bone in the A/P view, a lateral view is used to carry out further small adjustments until the tip is at the midpoint of the C3 waist, maintaining contact with bone. *Do NOT advance beyond the anterior margin of the articular pillar.*

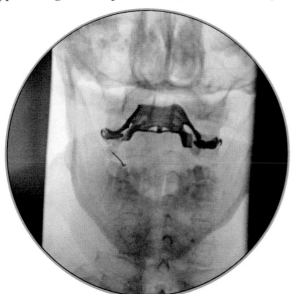

Figure 9-1G
Tilt: 5° Cephalad
Oblique: 0°

A/P View. Note the final needle position in the A/P view, after adjustments have been carried out in the prior lateral view. The tip is seen to be at the waist of the left C3 articular pillar, and contacting bone.

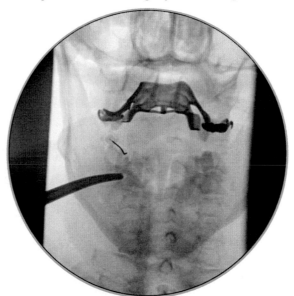

Figure 9-1H
Tilt: 5° Cephalad
Oblique: 0°

A/P View. Pointer at the location of the waist of the left C4 articular pillar.

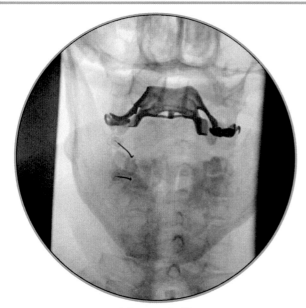

Figure 9-1I
Tilt: 5° Cephalad
Oblique: 0°

A/P View. Sagittal needle pass towards the waist of the left C4 articular pillar (C4 medal branch), until contact with bone. *Of note, intermittent lateral and/or CLO views should be used to assess needle depth throughout advancement if there is any question regarding needle depth.*

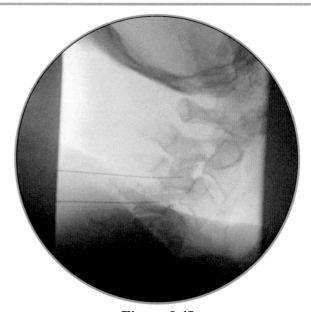

Figure 9-1J
Tilt: 5° Cephalad
Oblique: 90° Right

Lateral View. Once the needle has contacted bone in the A/P view, a lateral view is obtained to carry out further small adjustments until the tip is at the midpoint of the C4 waste, maintaining contact with bone. *Do NOT advance beyond the anterior margin of the articular pillar.*

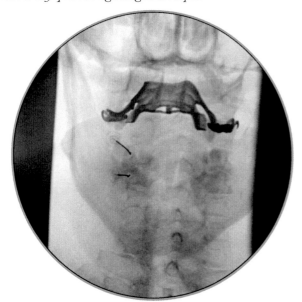

Figure 9-1K
Tilt: 5° Cephalad
Oblique: 0°

A/P View. Note the final needle position in the A/P view, after adjustments have been carried out in the prior lateral view. The tip is seen to be at the waist of the left C4 articular pillar, and contacting bone.

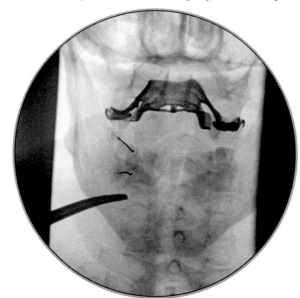

Figure 9-1L
Tilt: 5° Cephalad
Oblique: 0°

A/P View. Pointer at the location of the waist of the left C5 articular pillar.

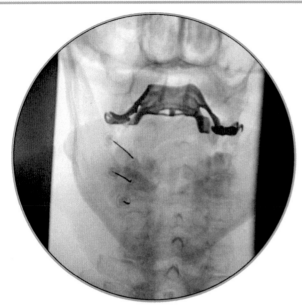

Figure 9-1M
Tilt: 5° Cephalad
Oblique: 0°

A/P View. Sagittal needle pass towards the waist of the left C5 articular pillar (C5 medal branch), until contact with bone. *Of note, intermittent lateral and/or CLO views should be used to assess needle depth throughout advancement if there is any question regarding needle depth.*

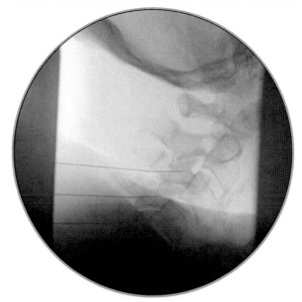

Figure 9-1N
Tilt: 5° Cephalad
Oblique: 90° Right

Lateral View. The needle tip at the C5 articular pillar is not clearly visualized due to obstruction from the patient's shoulders. *Thus, further needle advancement should not be carried out until an adequate view is obtained with a CLO view (see Figure 9-1R).*

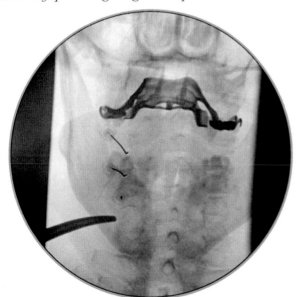

Figure 9-1O
Tilt: 5° Cephalad
Oblique: 0°

A/P View. Pointer at the location of the waist of the left C6 articular pillar.

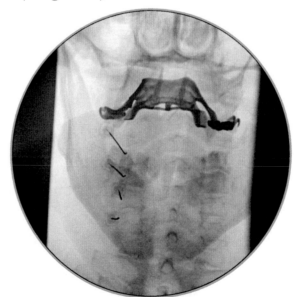

Figure 9-1P
Tilt: 5° Cephalad
Oblique: 0°

A/P View. Sagittal needle pass towards the waist of the left C6 articular pillar (C6 medal branch), until contact with bone. *Of note, intermittent lateral and/or CLO views should be used to assess needle depth throughout advancement if there is any question regarding needle depth.*

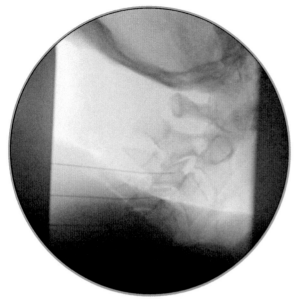

Figure 9-1Q
Tilt: 5° Cephalad
Oblique: 90° Right

Lateral View. The needle tip at the C6 articular pillar is not clearly visualized due to obstruction from the patient's shoulders. *Thus, further needle advancement should not be carried out until an adequate view is obtained with a CLO view (see Figure 9-1R).*

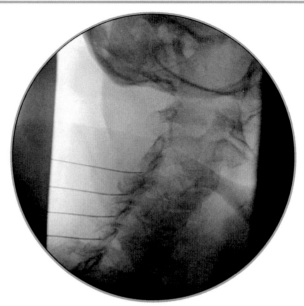

Figure 9-1R
Tilt: 5° Cephalad
Oblique: 45° Right

Contralateral Oblique View. The needle tips & articular pillars can be clearly seen at all levels in this view. *The inferior two needles (C5 and C6) have been advanced in this view to a depth that mirrors the superior two needles (C3 and C4), which were already placed at the desired target in the lateral view.*

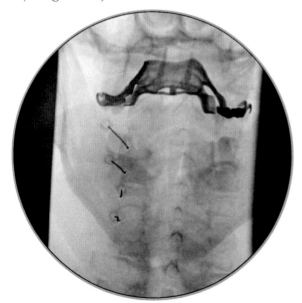

Figure 9-1S
Tilt: 5° Cephalad
Oblique: 0°

A/P View. Note the final A/P needle position at the left C3, C4, C5, and C6 medial branches. The needle tips are seen to be at the waist of each articular pillar, and contacting bone.

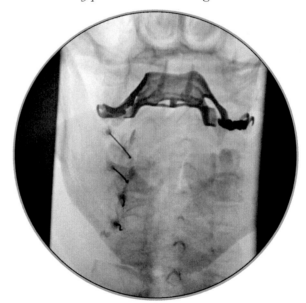

Figure 9-1T
Tilt: 5° Cephalad
Oblique: 0°

A/P View. After negative aspiration, contrast is administered with appropriate spread about the medial branches and without vascular uptake.

See Page 286

Left C2-C3, C3-C4, C4-C5
MBB

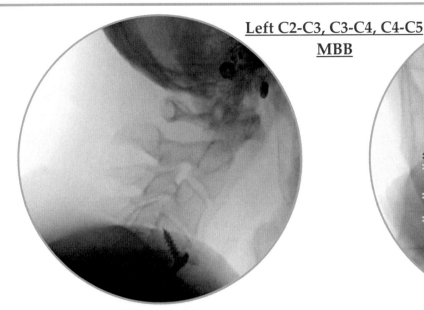

Figure 9-2A
Tilt: 0°
Oblique: 90° Right

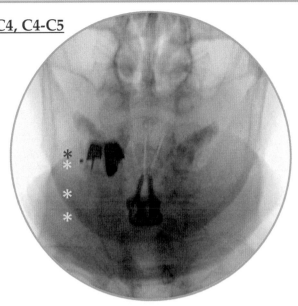

Figure 9-2B
Tilt: 0°
Oblique: 0°

Lateral View. In preparation for an oblique needle pass that is parallel to the angle of the articular pillar, a scout lateral view is obtained to assess the cephalocaudal angle of the lateral mass. This helps to determine the caudal entry point needed to create a parallel needle trajectory.

A/P View. Note the planned entry points for the TON (red star), C3, C4, and C5 medial branches (yellow stars) – which are lateral (for an oblique pass) and one level caudad (for a needle trajectory that is parallel to the cephalocaudal angulation of the articular pillars).

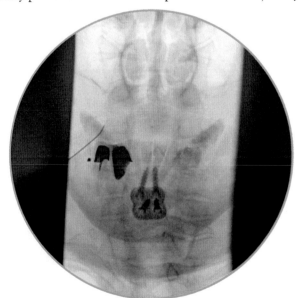

Figure 9-2C
Tilt: 0°
Oblique: 0°

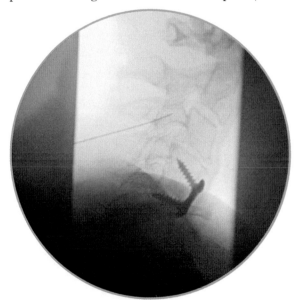

Figure 9-2D
Tilt: 0°
Oblique: 90° Right

A/P View. The C3 needle is advanced with an oblique pass towards the waist of the left C3 articular pillar. *Intermittent lateral and/or CLO views should be used throughout to assess needle depth, until contact is made with bone at the waist.*

Lateral View. Once the needle has contacted bone in the A/P view, a lateral view is obtained to carry out further small adjustments until the tip is at the midpoint of the C3 waist, maintaining contact with bone. *Note how the needle trajectory is parallel with the angle of the articular pillar.*

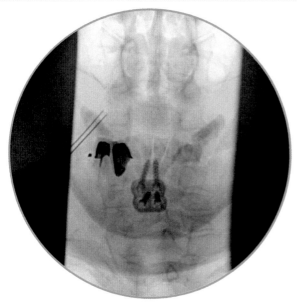

Figure 9-2E
Tilt: 0°
Oblique: 0°

A/P View. For the TON, the needle entry point is just cephalad to the C3 needle. The needle trajectory mirrors the previously placed C3 needle. *Intermittent lateral and/or CLO views should be used throughout to assess needle depth, until contact is made with bone.*

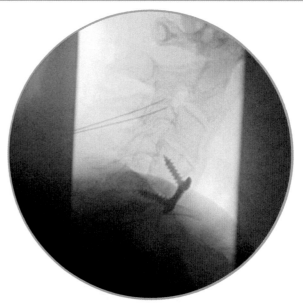

Figure 9-2F
Tilt: 0°
Oblique: 90° Right

Lateral View. Once the needle has contacted bone in the A/P view, a lateral view is obtained to carry out further small adjustments until the tip is at the midpoint of the C2-C3 joint, maintaining contact with bone. *Note that the needle trajectory is aligned with the articular pillar angle.*

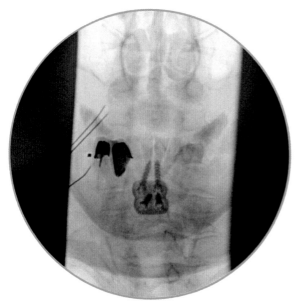

Figure 9-2G
Tilt: 0°
Oblique: 0°

A/P View. The C4 needle is advanced with an oblique pass towards the waist of the left C4 articular pillar. *Intermittent lateral and/or CLO views should be used throughout to assess needle depth, until contact is made with bone at the waist.*

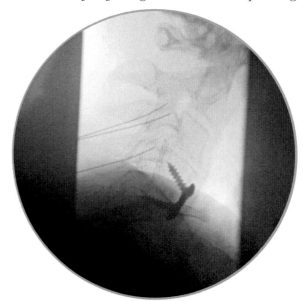

Figure 9-2H
Tilt: 0°
Oblique: 90° Right

Lateral View. Once the needle has contacted bone in the A/P view, a lateral view is obtained to carry out further small adjustments until the tip is at the midpoint of the C4 waist, maintaining contact with bone. *Note how the needle trajectory is parallel with the angle of the articular pillar.*

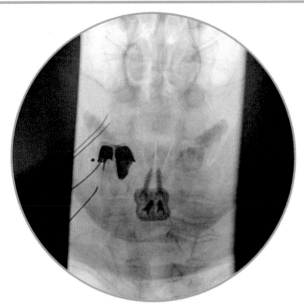

Figure 9-2I
Tilt: 0°
Oblique: 0°

A/P View. The C5 needle is advanced with an oblique pass towards the waist of the left C5 articular pillar. *Intermittent lateral and/or CLO views should be used throughout to assess needle depth, until contact is made with bone at the waist.*

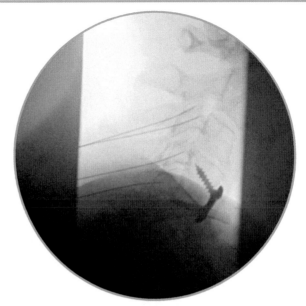

Figure 9-2J
Tilt: 0°
Oblique: 90° Right

Lateral View. Once the needle has contacted bone in the A/P view, a lateral view is obtained to carry out further small adjustments until the tip is at the midpoint of the C5 waist, maintaining contact with bone. *Note how the needle trajectory is aligned with the angle of the articular pillar.*

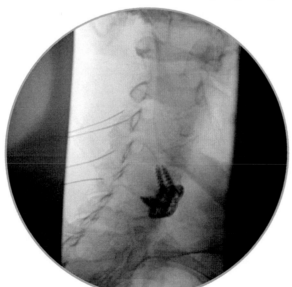

Figure 9-2K
Tilt: 0°
Oblique: 45° Right

Contralateral Obliqe View. The CLO view can be used as an additional confirmatory view for assessing needle depth. Note the final needle positioning at each level in this view.

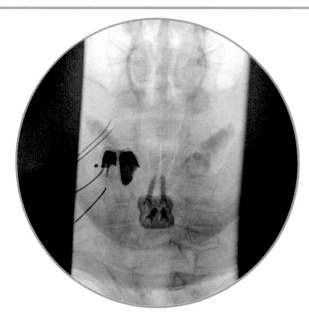

Figure 9-2L
Tilt: 0°
Oblique: 0°

A/P View. Note the final needle positioning at each level in the A/P view once the needles have been placed in their final position using the prior lateral/CLO views. Ensure that each needle tip is at the waist of its respective articular pillar, and contacting bone.

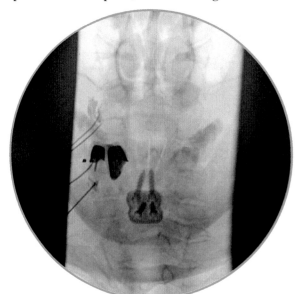

Figure 9-2M
Tilt: 0°
Oblique: 0°

A/P View. After negative aspiration, contrast is administered with appropriate spread about the medial branches and without vascular uptake.

Chapter 10
Cervical Radiofrequency Nerve Ablation

- Obtain an A/P view to identify the targeted level. For radiofrequency ablation, it is important that the needle trajectory be parallel to the cephalocaudal angle of the articular pillar (AP) in order to perform an ablation along the length of the nerve. Therefore, it is the author's preference to obtain a scout lateral view, prior to needle placement, to clearly see the cephalocaudal angle of the articular pillar and to estimate the caudal needle entry point needed to create the desired trajectory (see Figure 10-1B and page 165 for further discussion).

- In the A/P view, identify the waist of the targeted articular pillar (i.e., lateral mass). *Of note, in certain instances it may be challenging to get clear visualization of the target due to obstruction from the mandible, teeth, dental implants, etc. A cephalad tilt can assist with removing these structures from obstruction to provide better visualization of the targeted AP (compare Figures 10-1A & 10-1C).*

- Due to the advent of curved RF needles, it is possible to place a needle for ablation using the "sagittal pass" technique (see Figure 10-1E). However, it is the author's preference to use the "oblique pass" technique (*to get tight wrapping around the lateral mass and medial branch nerve)* with a <u>caudal</u> needle entry (*to match the cephalocaudal angle of the articular pillar and medial branch nerve)* – **see Figure 10-3D**. With this trajectory, one may theoretically reduce the risk of inadvertently ablating the lateral branch (located more laterally), which can cause unwanted neuritis and the classic "sunburn" complaint. *Of note, with this caudal & oblique needle pass, it is the author's preference not to perform caudal or ipsilateral oblique C-arm rotation (with coaxial needle placement), since this may cause loss of clear visualization of the targeted structure. This technique certainly requires more experience and a greater appreciation of needle depth, and intermittent lateral and/or CLO views should be used throughout with this approach to assess depth.*

- Once the needle tip has contacted the waist of the AP, further minor adjustments are carried out in the lateral view. In this view, ensure that the RF needle is parallel to the length of the medial branch at the middle of the waist, and advanced to (but not beyond) the ventral margin of the articular pillar. This allows for an ablation along the entire length of the cervical medial branch. *Of note, in the lower cervical segments it can often be difficult to clearly see the needle tip in the lateral view due to large shoulders and/or short necks. The CLO view should be used instead to assess depth and advance the needle (see Figure 10-1O & pages 166-168 for additional discussion).*

- Next, obtain an A/P view once again to ensure that the RF needle tip is at the waist of the targeted articular pillar and contacting bone. After appropriate motor and/or sensory testing, radiofrequency nerve ablation is performed.

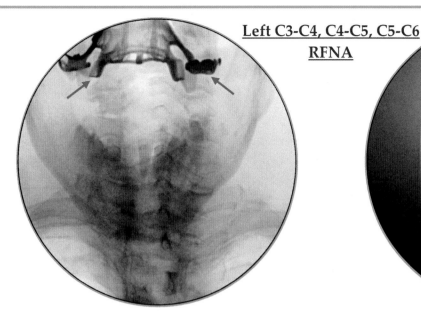

**Left C3-C4, C4-C5, C5-C6
RFNA**

Figure 10-1A
Tilt: 0°
Oblique: 0°

A/P View. Identify the targeted levels. Dental implants can often be present and cause obstruction of targeted structures. In this case, note that the inferior portion of the dental structure is seen to be overlying the C3 articular pillars (blue arrows).

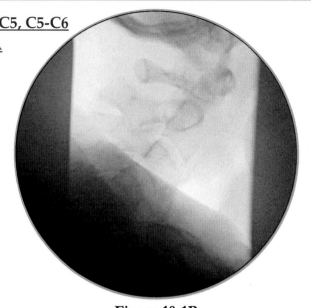

Figure 10-1B
Tilt: 0°
Oblique: 90° Right

Lateral View. This scout lateral view assists with pre-procedure preparation. Note that the articular pillars are not clearly seen at C5 and inferiorly. So, for needle placement at this level and inferior, a CLO view will be needed.

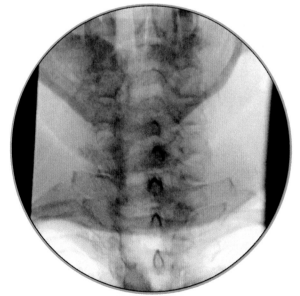

Figure 10-1C
Tilt: 10° Cephalad
Oblique: 0°

A/P View. By applying a cephalad tilt, note how both the jaw line and dental implant is removed from obstructing the targeted structures – *compare to Figure 10-1A.*

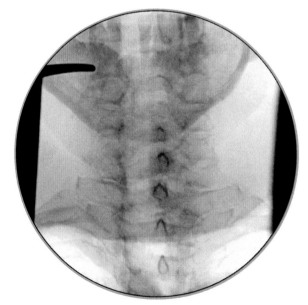

Figure 10-1D
Tilt: 10° Cephalad
Oblique: 0°

A/P View. Pointer at the location of the waist of the left C3 articular pillar.

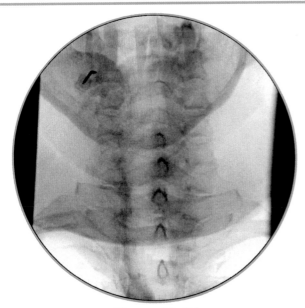

Figure 10-1E
Tilt: 10° Cephalad
Oblique: 0°

A/P View. Sagittal needle pass towards the waist of the left C3 articular pillar, until contact with bone. *Of note, intermittent lateral and/or CLO views should be used to assess needle depth throughout advancement if there is any question regarding needle depth.*

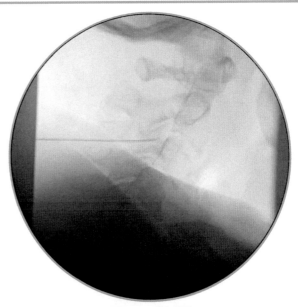

Figure 10-1F
Tilt: 10° Cephalad
Oblique: 90° Right

Lateral View. Once the needle has contacted bone in the prior A/P view, a lateral view is obtained to carry out further small needle adjustments until the tip is seen to be at the middle of the C3 waist and near the ventral margin, while maintaining contact with bone.

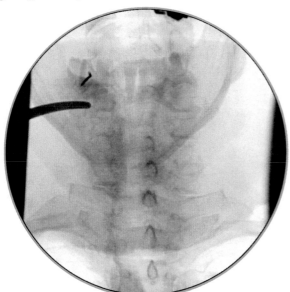

Figure 10-1G
Tilt: 10° Cephalad
Oblique: 0°

A/P View. Pointer at the location of the waist of the left C4 articular pillar.

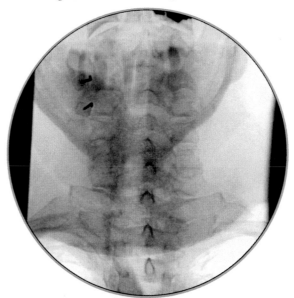

Figure 10-1H
Tilt: 10° Cephalad
Oblique: 0°

A/P View. Sagittal needle pass towards the waist of the left C4 articular pillar, until contact with bone. *Of note, intermittent lateral and/or CLO views should be used to assess needle depth throughout advancement if there is any question regarding needle depth.*

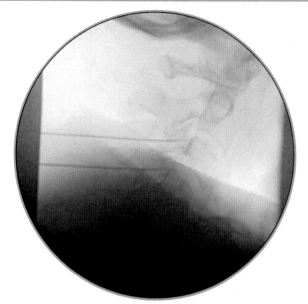

Figure 10-1I
Tilt: 10° Cephalad
Oblique: 90° Right

Lateral View. Once the needle has contacted bone in the prior A/P view, a lateral view is obtained to carry out further small needle adjustments until the tip is seen to be at the middle of the C4 waist and near the ventral margin, while maintaining contact with bone.

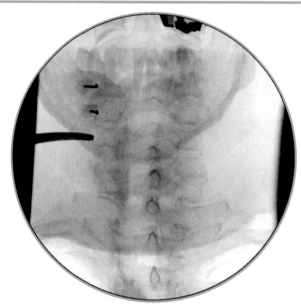

Figure 10-1J
Tilt: 10° Cephalad
Oblique: 0°

A/P View. Pointer at the location of the waist of the left C5 articular pillar. *The initial scout view (Figure 10-1B) showed the lack of clear visualization from C5 inferiorly. Thus, for subsequent depth assessment and needle advancement, the CLO view will be needed (see Figure 10-1O).*

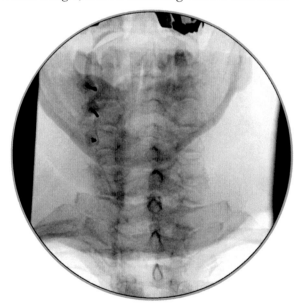

Figure 10-1K
Tilt: 10° Cephalad
Oblique: 0°

A/P View. Sagittal needle pass towards the waist of the left C5 articular pillar, until contact with bone. *Of note, intermittent lateral and/or CLO views should be used to assess needle depth throughout advancement if there is any question regarding needle depth.*

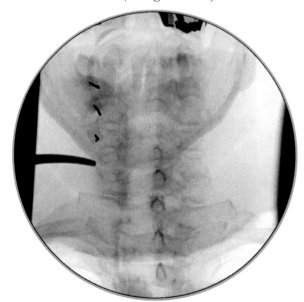

Figure 10-1L
Tilt: 10° Cephalad
Oblique: 0°

A/P View. Pointer at the location of the waist of the left C6 articular pillar.

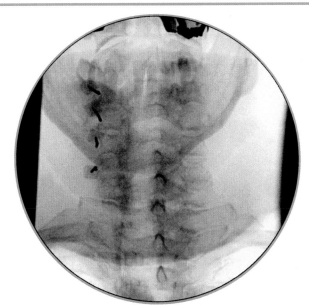

Figure 10-1M
Tilt: 10° Cephalad
Oblique: 0°

A/P View. Sagittal needle pass towards the waist of the left C6 articular pillar, until contact with bone. *Of note, intermittent lateral and/or CLO views should be used to assess needle depth throughout advancement if there is any question regarding needle depth.*

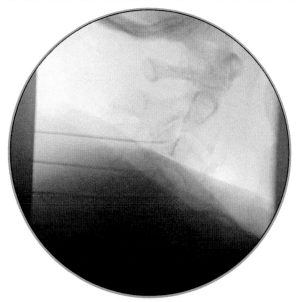

Figure 10-1N
Tilt: 10° Cephalad
Oblique: 90° Right

Lateral View. Unlike the more cephalad levels, the needle tips and articular pillars at C5 and C6 are not clearly seen. Thus, the CLO view will be needed to assess needle depth – *see Figure 10-1O.*

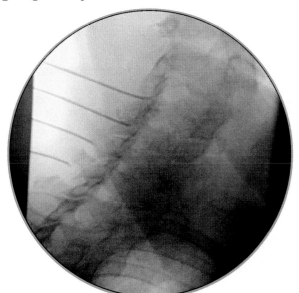

Figure 10-1O
Tilt: 0°
Oblique: 45° Right

Contralateral Oblique View. The needle tips & articular pillars can be clearly seen at all levels in this view. *The inferior two needles (C5 and C6) may be advanced in this view to a depth that mirrors the superior two needles (C3 and C4), which were already placed at the desired target in the lateral view.*

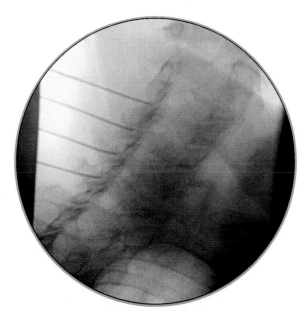

Figure 10-1P
Tilt: 0°
Oblique: 45° Right

Contralateral Oblique View. The needles at the C5 & C6 articular pillars are advanced to a depth relative to the PILL that matches the superior two needles (see pages 166-167 for further discussion). *Ensure needle contact with bone at all times.*

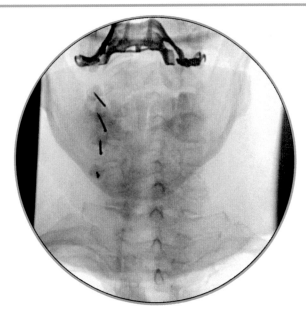

Figure 10-1Q
Tilt: 10° Cephalad
Oblique: 0°

A/P View. Note the final needle position at the left C3, C4, C5, and C6 medial branches. Ensure that each needle is at the waist of the articular pillar and contacting bone.

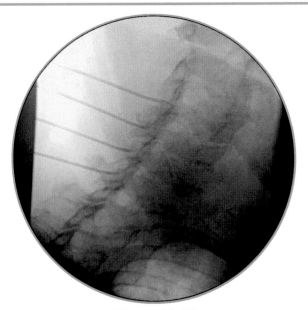

Figure 10-1R
Tilt: 0°
Oblique: 45° Right

Contralateral Oblique View. Final needle positioning at the left C3, C4, C5, and C6 medial branches. After appropriate motor and/or sensory testing, RFNA is carried out. *Note the cephalad curve of each needle.*

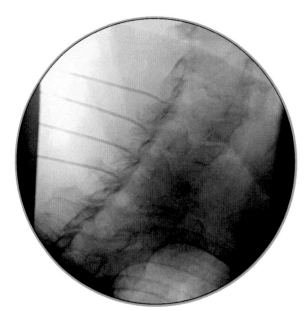

Figure 10-1S
Tilt: 0°
Oblique: 45° Right

Contralateral Oblique View. Each RF needle/probe is rotated 180° and a CLO view is obtained once again to ensure no further ventral needle advancement has occurred during rotation. Next, RFNA is carried out once again to account for any anatomical variability. *Note the caudad curve of each needle.*

See Page 290

Left C3-C4, C4-C5, C5-C6
RFNA

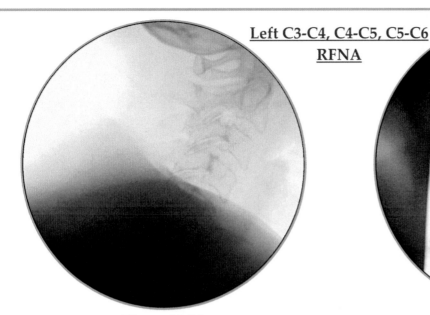

Figure 10-2A
Tilt: 0°
Oblique: 90° Right

Lateral View. This scout lateral view assists with pre-procedure preparation. Note that the articular pillars are not clearly seen at C5 and inferiorly. So, for needle placement at this level and inferior, a CLO view will be needed.

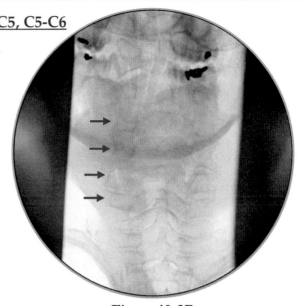

Figure 10-2B
Tilt: 0°
Oblique: 0°

A/P View. The waists of the left C3-C6 articular pillars are clearly visualized in this view (purple arrows).

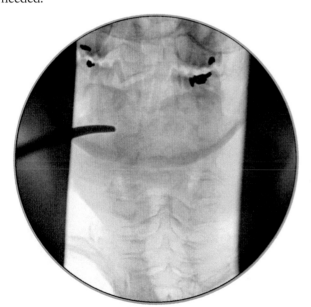

Figure 10-2C
Tilt: 0°
Oblique: 0°

A/P View. Pointer at the waist of the left C3 articular pillar.

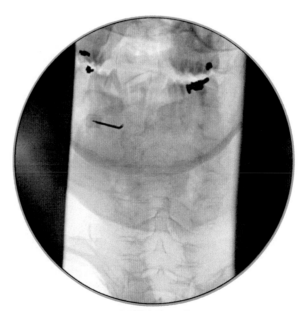

Figure 10-2D
Tilt: 0°
Oblique: 0°

A/P View. Sagittal needle pass towards the waist of the left C3 articular pillar, until contact with bone. *Of note, intermittent lateral and/or CLO views should be used to assess needle depth throughout advancement if there is any question regarding needle depth.*

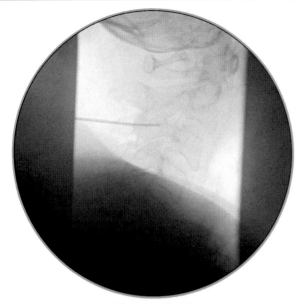

Figure 10-2E
Tilt: 0°
Oblique: 90° Right

Lateral View. Once the needle has contacted bone in the prior A/P view, a lateral view is obtained to carry out further small needle adjustments until the tip is seen to be at the middle of the C3 waist and near the ventral margin, while maintaining contact with bone.

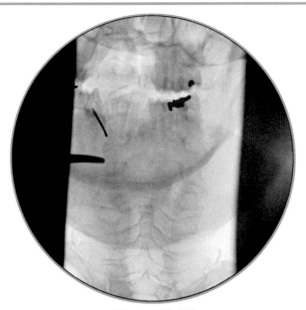

Figure 10-2F
Tilt: 0°
Oblique: 0°

A/P View. Pointer at the waist of the left C4 articular pillar.

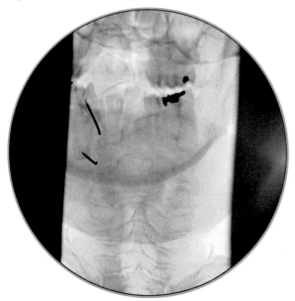

Figure 10-2G
Tilt: 0°
Oblique: 0°

A/P View. Sagittal needle pass towards the waist of the left C4 articular pillar, until contact with bone. *Of note, intermittent lateral and/or CLO views should be used to assess needle depth throughout advancement if there is any question regarding needle depth.*

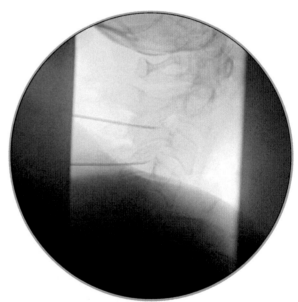

Figure 10-2H
Tilt: 0°
Oblique: 90° Right

Lateral View. Once the needle has contacted bone in the prior A/P view, a lateral view is obtained to carry out further small needle adjustments until the tip is seen to be at the middle of the C4 waist and near the ventral margin, while maintaining contact with bone.

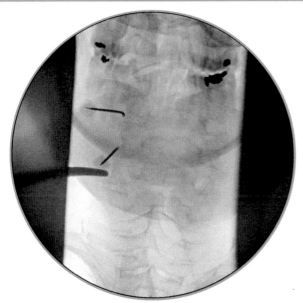

Figure 10-2I
Tilt: 0°
Oblique: 0°

A/P View. Pointer at the waist of the left C5 articular pillar. *The initial scout view (Figure 10-2A) showed the lack of clear visualization from C5 inferiorly. Thus, for subsequent depth assessment and needle advancement, the CLO view will be needed (see Figure 10-2N).*

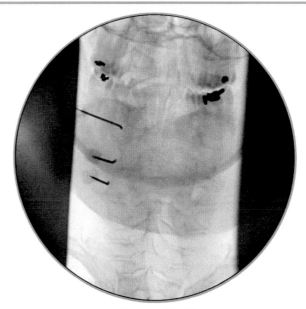

Figure 10-2J
Tilt: 0°
Oblique: 0°

A/P View. Sagittal needle pass towards the waist of the left C5 articular pillar, until contact with bone. *Of note, intermittent lateral and/or CLO views should be used to assess needle depth throughout advancement if there is any question regarding needle depth.*

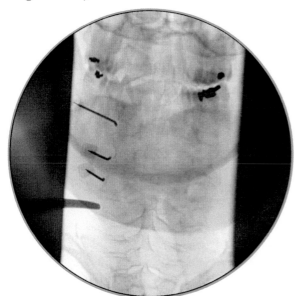

Figure 10-2K
Tilt: 0°
Oblique: 0°

A/P View. Pointer at the waist of the left C6 articular pillar.

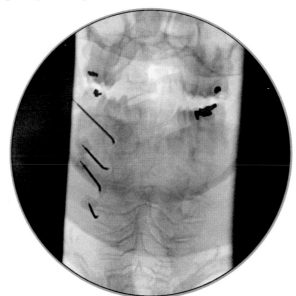

Figure 10-2L
Tilt: 0°
Oblique: 0°

A/P View. Sagittal needle pass towards the waist of the left C6 articular pillar, until contact with bone. *Of note, intermittent lateral and/or CLO views should be used to assess needle depth throughout advancement if there is any question regarding needle depth.*

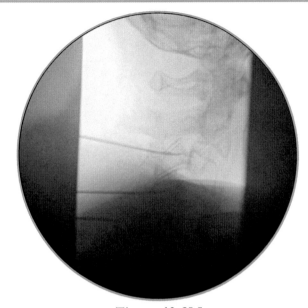

Figure 10-2M
Tilt: 0°
Oblique: 90° Right

Lateral View. Note that that there is poor visualization of the needles at C5 and C6 due to the shoulders. Therefore, the CLO view will be needed to assess needle depth and perform further needle advancement – *see next Figure.*

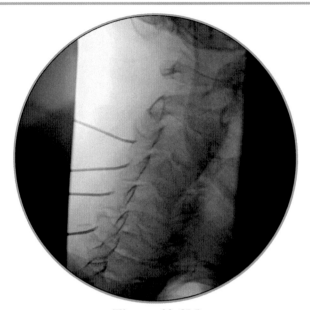

Figure 10-2N
Tilt: 0°
Oblique: 30° Right

Contralateral Oblique View. The needles at C5 & C6 are advanced to a depth relative to the PILL that matches the superior two needles. *Of note, this is NOT the ideal CLO angle to use the PILL as an approximation of the ventral margin of the AP (see pages 166-168 for further discussion).*

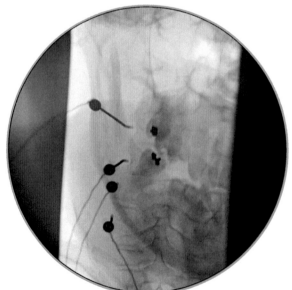

Figure 10-2O
Tilt: 0°
Oblique: 0°

A/P View. Final needle placement at the waist of the left C3-C6 articular pillars, targeting the left C3-C6 medial branches. After appropriate motor and/or sensory testing, RFNA of the targeted medial branches is carried out.

**Left C2-C3, C3-C4, C4-C5
RFNA**

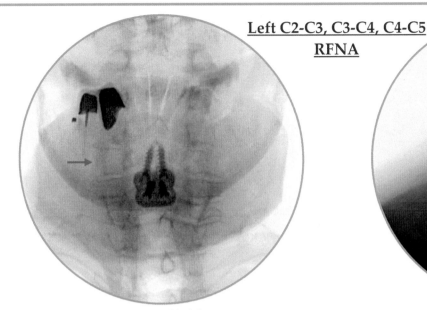

Figure 10-3A
Tilt: 0°
Oblique: 0°

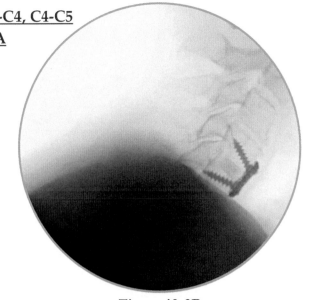

Figure 10-3B
Tilt: 0°
Oblique: 90° Right

A/P View. The waists of the articular pillars are identified in this view. *For reference, the waist of the left C5 articular pillar is indicated by the blue arrow.*

Note the ACDF at C4-C5.

Lateral View. In this scout lateral view, note the cephalocaudal angle of the articular pillars. This assists with pre-procedure preparation and estimating the caudal needle entry point (for an oblique pass and caudal approach). *The APs are not clearly seen from C6 inferiorly.*

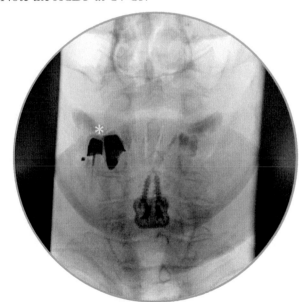

Figure 10-3C
Tilt: 0°
Oblique: 0°

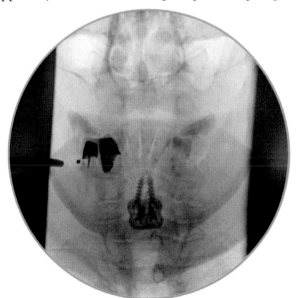

Figure 10-3D
Tilt: 0°
Oblique: 0°

A/P View. To target the left C3 medial branch, the needle tip will need to be placed at the waist of the left C3 articular pillar (yellow star).

A/P View. Pointer showing the needle entry point for a caudal (approximately one level below) and oblique pass approach for targeting the left C3 medial branch. *This needle trajectory best approximates the length of the C3 medial branch for an effective ablation.*

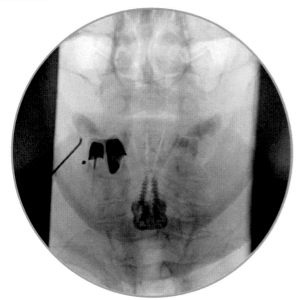

Figure 10-3E
Tilt: 0°
Oblique: 0°

A/P View. The needle is advanced in a trajectory towards the targeted left C3 medial branch at the waist of the left C3 articular pillar. *It is imperative to frequently use intermittent CLO and/or lateral views to assess needle depth throughout in order to avoid critical structures (see Figure 10-3F).*

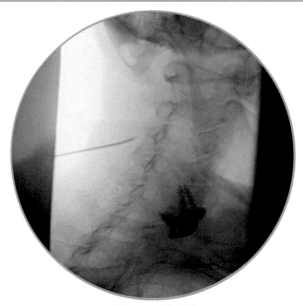

Figure 10-3F
Tilt: 0°
Oblique: 45° Right

Contralateral Oblique View. Intermittent CLO views are taken to ensure that the needle does not travel ventrally (*anterior to the joint lie the spinal nerve, DRG, and vertebral artery*). The proceduralist should go back and forth with A/P and CLO views, until contact with bone.

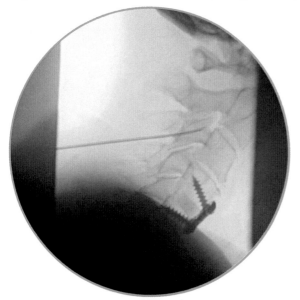

Figure 10-3G
Tilt: 0°
Oblique: 90° Right

Lateral View. Once the needle has contacted bone in the prior A/P view, a lateral view is obtained to carry out further small needle adjustments until the tip is seen to be at the middle of the C3 waist and near the ventral margin of the AP, while maintaining contact with bone.

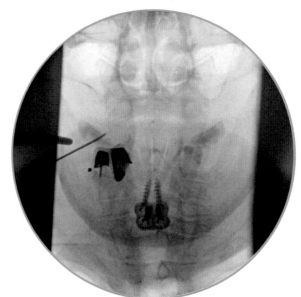

Figure 10-3H
Tilt: 0°
Oblique: 0°

A/P View. Pointer showing the needle entry point for a caudal (approximately one level below) and oblique pass approach for targeting the left TON. *This needle trajectory best approximates the length of the TON for an effective ablation.*

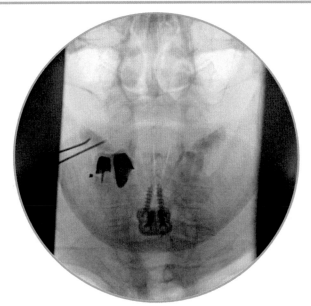

Figure 10-3I
Tilt: 0°
Oblique: 0°

A/P View. The needle is advanced in a trajectory towards the targeted left TON at the left C2-C3 joint line. *It is imperative to frequently use intermittent CLO and/or lateral views to assess needle depth throughout in order to avoid critical structures located anterior to the joint (see Figure 10-3J).*

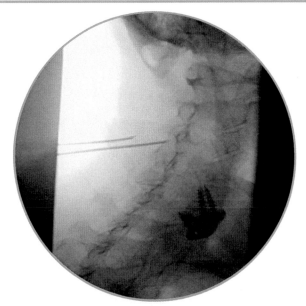

Figure 10-3J
Tilt: 0°
Oblique: 45° Right

Contralateral Oblique View. Intermittent CLO views are used to assess needle depth during advancement. Note that this needle tip is still quite posterior to the articular pillar. Alternating A/P and CLO views should be used for further advancement.

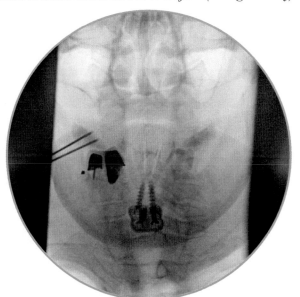

Figure 10-3K
Tilt: 0°
Oblique: 0°

A/P View. The needle is advanced further towards the target using frequent intermittent CLO views to assess needle depth, until contact with bone.

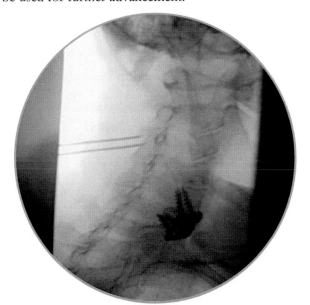

Figure 10-3L
Tilt: 0°
Oblique: 45° Right

Contralateral Oblique View. Once the needle has contacted bone in the prior A/P view, an additional CLO view is checked to assess depth. Note that the needle tip is now seen to be approaching the targeted C2-C3 joint.

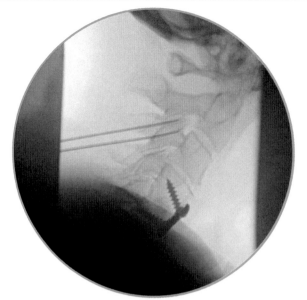

Figure 10-3M
Tilt: 0°
Oblique: 90° Right

Lateral View. Once the needle has contacted bone in the prior A/P view, a lateral view is obtained to carry out further small needle adjustments until the tip is seen to be at the C2-C3 joint line and near the ventral margin, while maintaining contact with bone.

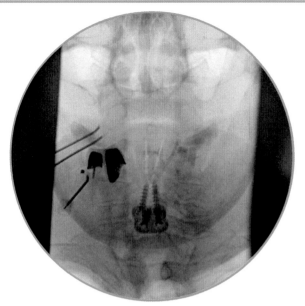

Figure 10-3N
Tilt: 0°
Oblique: 0°

A/P View. The entry point for targeting the C4 medial branch is carried out in a similar fashion, lateral and caudal to the waist of the left C4 articular pillar. *The needle is advanced in a trajectory towards the targeted left C4 medial branch using intermittent CLO and/or lateral views.*

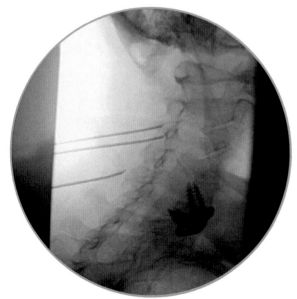

Figure 10-3O
Tilt: 0°
Oblique: 45° Right

Contralateral Oblique View. Intermittent CLO views are used to assess needle depth during advancement. Note the needle tip positioning relative to the lateral mass. Further advancement using A/P and CLO views is carried out until contact with bone.

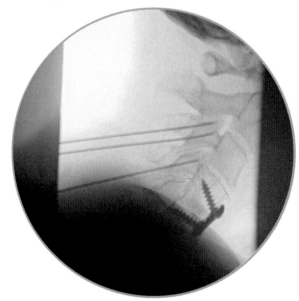

Figure 10-3P
Tilt: 0°
Oblique: 90° Right

Lateral View. Once the needle has contacted bone in the prior A/P view, a lateral view is obtained to carry out further small needle adjustments until the tip is seen to be at the middle of the C4 waist and near the ventral margin of the AP, while maintaining contact with bone.

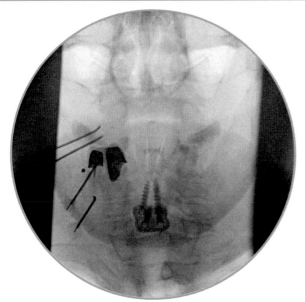

Figure 10-3Q
Tilt: 0°
Oblique: 0°

A/P View. The entry point for the targeting the C5 medial branch is carried out in a similar fashion, lateral and caudal to the waist of the left C5 articular pillar. *The needle is advanced in a trajectory towards the targeted left C5 medial branch using intermittent CLO and/or lateral views.*

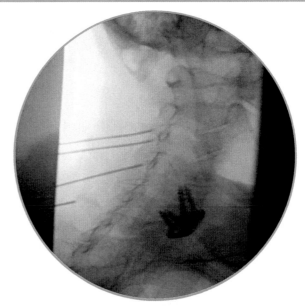

Figure 10-3R
Tilt: 0°
Oblique: 45° Right

Contralateral Oblique View. Intermittent CLO views are used to assess needle depth during advancement. Note that the C5 needle tip is still quite posterior to the articular pillar. Alternating A/P and CLO views are taken for further needle advancement.

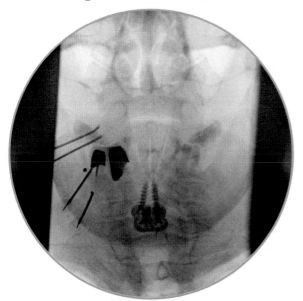

Figure 10-3S
Tilt: 0°
Oblique: 0°

A/P View. The needle is advanced further towards the target using frequent intermittent A/P and CLO views, until contact with bone.

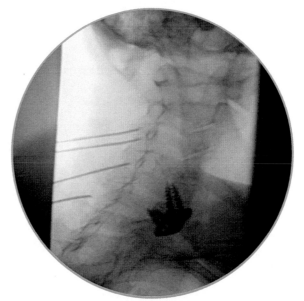

Figure 10-3T
Tilt: 0°
Oblique: 45° Right

Contralateral Oblique View. The needle is now seen to be approaching the lateral mass, and is advanced until contact with bone.

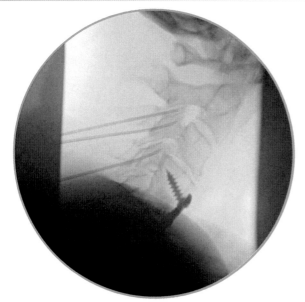

Figure 10-3U
Tilt: 0°
Oblique: 90° Right

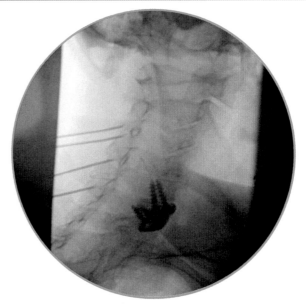

Figure 10-3V
Tilt: 0°
Oblique: 45° Right

Lateral View. Once the needle has contacted bone in the prior A/P and CLO views, a lateral view is obtained to carry out further small needle adjustments until the tip is seen to be at the middle of the C5 waist and near the ventral margin, while maintaining contact with bone.

Contralateral Oblique View. Use this view if there is any question regarding the visualization of the needle tip. *Note the similar positioning of each needle tip relative to the PILL (see pages 166-168 for additional discussion regarding the PILL).* After motor/sensory testing, RFNA is performed.

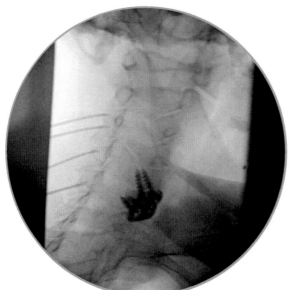

Figure 10-3W
Tilt: 0°
Oblique: 45° Right

Contralateral Oblique View. The RF needles/probes are rotated 180°, and a CLO view is taken again to confirm no further ventral advancement has occurred during rotation. After motor and/or sensory testing, RFNA is performed to account for nerve anatomical variability.

Additional Discussion:
Understanding the Articular Pillar Angle

If the natural cervical lordosis is maintained, the articular pillars have a pronounced superoinferior angulation (see Figure 10-4A). For radiofrequency (RF) ablation of the cervical medial branches, it is ideal to have the RF needle trajectory approximate this superoinferior angle, so that it covers the entire length of the nerve during ablation. Although curved RF needles have helped with better approximating this angle, it is still ideal to have a good appreciation of this superoinferior angle prior to needle placement. Thus, taking a scout lateral image can be helpful in estimating how far caudal the needle entry point will need to be to create the inferior-to-superior trajectory needed to match the angle of the articular pillar, and in turn the targeted medial branch.

Note that by placing pillows under the patient's chest, this lessens the cervical lordosis and in turn reduces the superoinferior angle as seen on the lateral view (see Figure 10-4B). By lessening the superoinferior angle of the articular pillar, the needle entry point need not be as caudal. It is the author's experience that by placing two pillows under the chest, most often the ideal needle trajectory can be created by entering no more than one level caudal to the targeted medial branch.

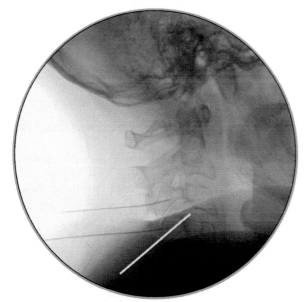

Figure 10-4A
Tilt: 0°
Oblique: 90° Right

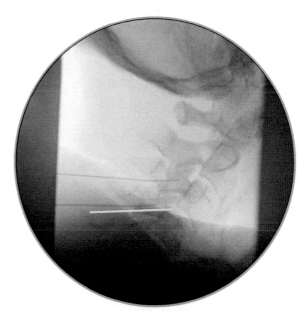

Figure 10-4B
Tilt: 0°
Oblique: 90° Right

Lateral View. No pillows have been placed under the patient's chest, and the cervical lordosis has not been removed. Note the superoinferior angle of the C4 articular pillar (yellow line). With this patient positioning, for the RF needle to match the angulation of the articular pillar, a significantly caudal needle entry point will be required.

Lateral View. Two pillows have been placed under the patient's chest, which lessens the natural cervical lordosis. Now note the lesser superoinferior angle of the C4 articular pillar (yellow line) compared to Figure 10-4A. With this patient positioning, for the RF needle to match the angulation of the articular pillar, a lesser caudal needle entry point will be required.

Additional Discussion:
Using the PILL to Approximate the Ventral Articular Pillar
In the Contralateral Oblique View

During cervical needle placement in the higher cervical segments, the CLO view is not needed since the needle tip can be clearly visualized in the lateral view. However, in the lower cervical segments, it can be challenging, or even impossible, to see the needle tip due to the shoulders. This is even more evident in those with short necks or larger shoulders. When the needle tip cannot be visualized in the lateral view, the CLO view must be relied upon for assessing depth and performing needle advancement. Thus, during cervical radiofrequency ablation, it is imperative that the proceduralist clearly understand the CLO view, and how the needle tip depth visually changes with changing the CLO angle. This understanding will assist in avoiding injury to critical neurovascular structures.

As previously discussed in Chapter 6 (see Page 95), during placement of a needle in the cervical epidural space, with respect to the VILL:

- Decreasing the CLO angle causes the needle tip to appear more ventral.
- Increasing the CLO angle causes the needle tip to appear more dorsal.

However, the opposite relationship is seen when performing cervical RFNA (a more lateral needle than with cervical epidural placement), with respect to the PILL (see Figures 10-7 through 10-10):

- **Decreasing the CLO angle causes the needle tip to appear more dorsal.**
- **Increasing the CLO angle causes the needle tip to appear more ventral.**

It is the author's experience that by using a CLO angle of approximately 45°, the posterior interlaminar line (PILL) will roughly correlate with the ventral margin of the articular pillar. In other words, at a CLO angle of 45°, when the needle tip is approximately at, or near, the PILL, this will correspond to the needle being at the ventral margin of the articular pillar (see Figures 10-5A & 10-5B). However, with lesser CLO angles, despite being at the ventral margin of the articular pillar, the needle tip will appear quite posterior to the PILL (see Figures 10-6A & 10-6B) – *at this lesser CLO angle, if the needle is advanced towards the PILL, this will lead to a needle tip that approaches the danger zone of critical neurovascular structures (e.g., exiting nerve root, DRG, vertebral artery).*

> *In the CLO view, if the PILL is to be used as an anatomical landmark to correlate with the ventral margin of the articular pillar, it is the author's experience that a <u>CLO angle of approximately 45°</u> should be considered.*

It should be noted that the CLO view **CANNOT** guarantee appropriate needle positioning as it relates to the PILL and ventral margin of the articular pillar. Therefore, when relying solely upon the CLO view in the lower cervical segments, motor and/or sensory testing must be performed for additional verification of needle depth prior to carrying out radiofrequency nerve ablation.

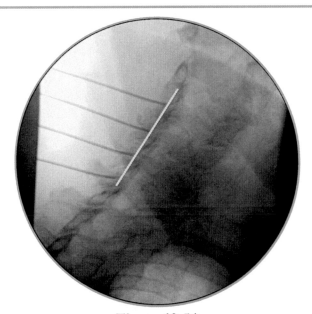

Figure 10-5A
Tilt: 0°
Oblique: 45° Right

Contralateral Oblique View. *Figure 10-1R reproduced.* Note the PILL (yellow line).

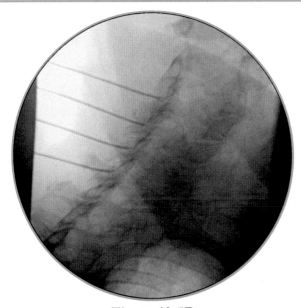

Figure 10-5B
Tilt: 0°
Oblique: 45° Right

Contralateral Oblique View. *Figure 10-5A reproduced (with the PILL line removed).* All needles have been placed and confirmed to be at the ventral margin of the articular pillar using the lateral view (not shown here). Note that all needle tips are seen to be at approximately the PILL.

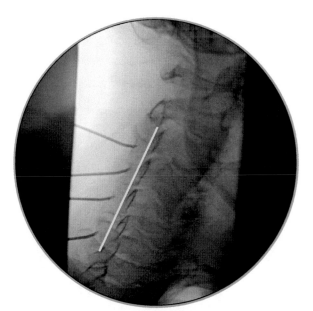

Figure 10-6A
Tilt: 0°
Oblique: 30° Right

Contralateral Oblique View. *Figure 10-2N reproduced.* Note the PILL (yellow line).

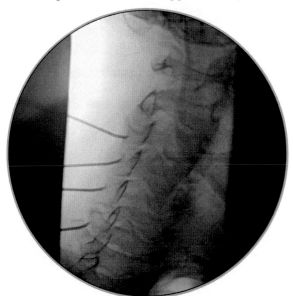

Figure 10-6B
Tilt: 0°
Oblique: 30° Right

Contralateral Oblique View. *Figure 10-6A reproduced (with the PILL line removed).* All needles have been placed and confirmed to be at the ventral margin of the articular pillar using the lateral view (not shown here). Note that all needle tips are seen to be quite dorsal to the PILL.

Additional Discussion:
Visual Changes of Needle Depth with Changing CLO Angles

In the following images, the superior two needles (i.e., at the C3 and C4 medial branches) have already been placed at the ventral margin of the articular pillar using lateral fluoroscopy, where they could be clearly seen. We can use these superior needles as a reference to see how the visual relationship between the needle tips and PILL changes with increasing CLO angles (*note that there has been no adjustment to the superior two needles and only the CLO angle is being changed*) …

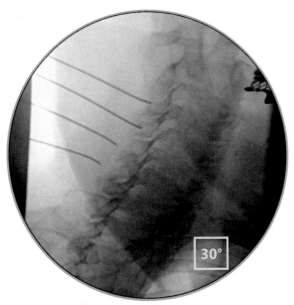

Figure 10-7

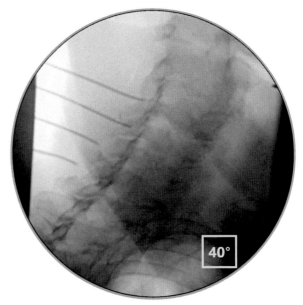

Figure 10-8

CLO angle of 30°. C3 and C4 needle tips appear posterior to the PILL.

CLO angle of 40°. C3 and C4 needle tips appear to be approaching, but not at, the PILL.

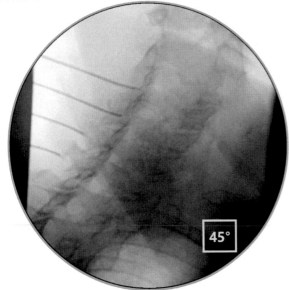

Figure 10-9

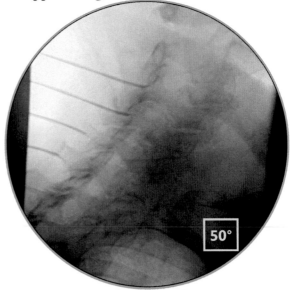

Figure 10-10

***CLO angle of 45°. C3 and C4 needle tips appear to be at the PILL

CLO angle of 50°. C3 and C4 needle tips appear to be heading just beyond the PILL.

Chapter 11
Sacroiliac Joint Radiofrequency Neve Ablation

- Obtain an A/P view to locate the targeted joint. *Of note, due to anatomic variation of the nerves innervating the sacroiliac (SI) joint (i.e., L5 dorsal ramus, lateral branches of S1-S3 dorsal rami), there can be significant challenges with effective denervation during radiofrequency ablation. Consequently, a bipolar lesion approach is recommended using a palisade guide block technique.*

- A palisade guide block (see Figure 11-1B) is placed over the nerves innervating the targeted joint for purposes of creating a continuous and controlled strip lesion using bipolar radiofrequency ablation. The guide block should be placed on the skin such that it covers the sacral ala (just lateral to the base of the S1 SAP) down to the S3 foramen (lateral to the lateral border). The guide block is designed in a way that all needles placed through it are parallel and 10 mm apart – with this configuration, most average sized patients will require approximately 6-7 needles to cover the innervation from L5-S3.

- The RF needles are placed through each through-hole in the guide block, which are sized in a way that minimizes lateral movement of the needles. The through-holes facilitate parallel and equally spaced RF needles, which is imperative for creating a controlled strip lesion using bipolar radiofrequency ablation. Once placed within the through-hole, each needle is subsequently advanced to the dorsal surface of the sacrum, until contact with bone. Ensure that no needle enters the sacral foramen.

- Next, obtain a lateral view to confirm correct needle placement over the dorsal sacrum, and not on the iliac crest or within the sacral foramen. *Of note, the sacrum is somewhat c-shaped with an uneven surface. Thus, the proceduralist will often see varying needle depths in the lateral view despite all needles being correctly placed on the posterior sacrum (see Figures 11-1E & 11-2C).*

- After confirmation of correct needle placement, bipolar radiofrequency ablation is carried out. It is the author's preference to create a strip radiofrequency lesion using the parameters 85° C for 150 seconds. *With placement of 7 needles, a total of 3 sets of two bipolar lesions at a time (i.e., 4 electrodes at a time) will be required to create a continuous strip lesion across all needles (see Figures 11-1B & 11-2D). This large strip will cover the L5 dorsal ramus and the lateral branches of the S1-S3 dorsal rami, while accounting for anatomic variation of the nerves.*

<u>Right SI RFNA</u>

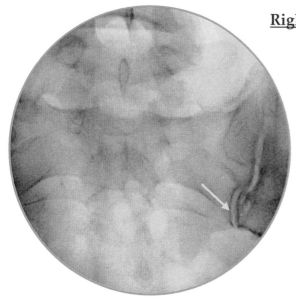

Figure 11-1A
Tilt: 0°
Oblique: 0°

A/P View. Note the right SI joint (yellow arrow).

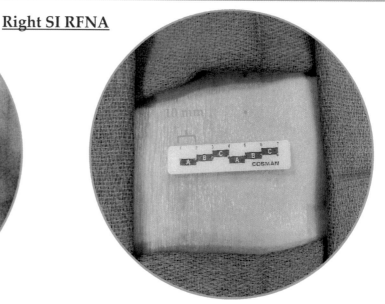

Figure 11-1B

A palisade guide block is placed on the skin over the nerves innervating the right SI joint, from the sacral ala down to at least the S3 foramen. The guide block has 7 through-holes spaced 10 mm apart, which facilitate parallel and equally spaced needles that create a controlled strip-lesion using bipolar radiofrequency ablation.

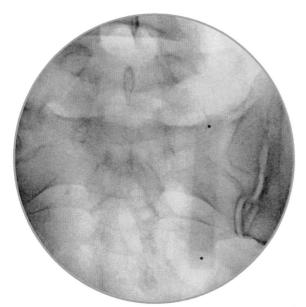

Figure 11-1C
Tilt: 0°
Oblique: 0°

A/P View. Fluoroscopy is used to adjust the guide block such that the superior radiopaque marker is on top of the sacral ala just lateral to the S1 SAP, and the inferior radiopaque marker is lateral and distal to the lateral border of the S3 foramen.

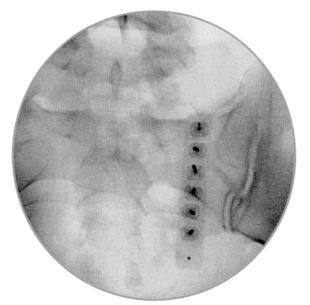

Figure 11-1D
Tilt: 0°
Oblique: 0°

A/P View. A RF needle is placed coaxially through each through-hole and advanced until contact with bone. *Ensure that no needle inadvertently enters the sacral foramen or lies on top of the iliac crest.*

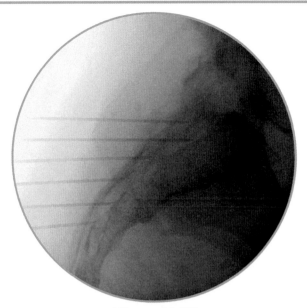

Figure 11-1E
Tilt: 0°
Oblique: 90° Right

Lateral View. Note the RF needles on the dorsal surface of the sacrum, and contacting bone. Due to the "c-shaped" surface of the sacrum, with multiple elevations and depressions, the RF needles will be noted to have varying depths as seen above.

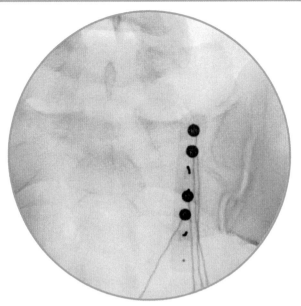

Figure 11-1F
Tilt: 0°
Oblique: 0°

A/P View. Next, bipolar radiofrequency ablation is carried out at the needles placed within both sets of the "A" through-holes (see Figure 11-1B).

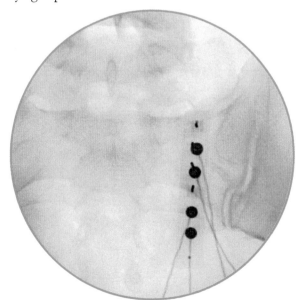

Figure 11-1G
Tilt: 0°
Oblique: 0°

A/P View. Next, bipolar radiofrequency ablation is carried out at the needles placed within both sets of the "B" through-holes (see Figure 11-1B).

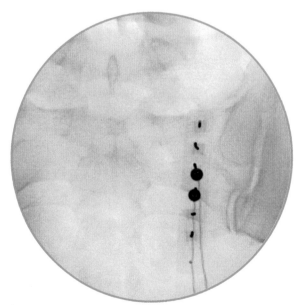

Figure 11-1H
Tilt: 0°
Oblique: 0°

A/P View. Next, bipolar radiofrequency ablation is carried out at the needles placed within the single superior set of "C" through-holes (see Figure 11-1B). *Of note, placement of 7 RF needles (instead of 6) would require ablation at both sets of the "C" through-holes.*

See Page 292

Right SI RFNA

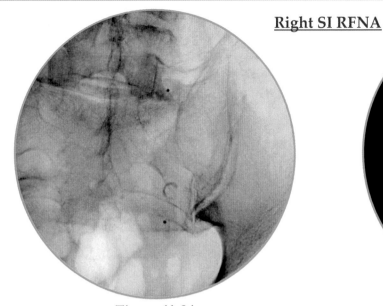

Figure 11-2A
Tilt: 0°
Oblique: 5° Left

A/P View. *A slight contralateral oblique is applied to remove the iliac crest from obstructing the target.* The guide block is placed with the superior radiopaque marker on top of the sacral ala just lateral to the S1 SAP, and the inferior marker lateral and distal to the S3 foramen.

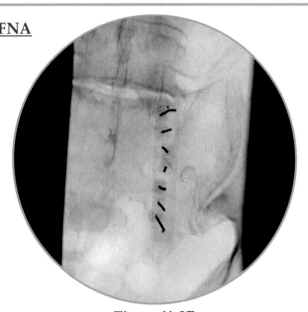

Figure 11-2B
Tilt: 0°
Oblique: 5° Left

A/P View. A RF needle is placed coaxially through each through-hole and advanced until contact with bone. Note that for this particular patient, a total of 7 needles were required to cover the entirety of the joint. *Ensure that no needle inadvertently enters the sacral foramen.*

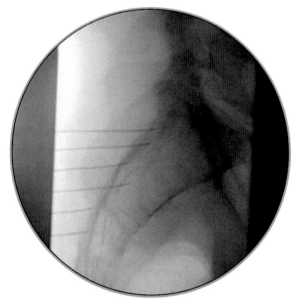

Figure 11-2C
Tilt: 0°
Oblique: 90° Right

Lateral View. Note the RF needles on the dorsal surface of the sacrum, and contacting bone. Due to the "c-shaped" surface of the sacrum, with multiple elevations and depressions, the RF needles will be noted to have varying depths as seen above.

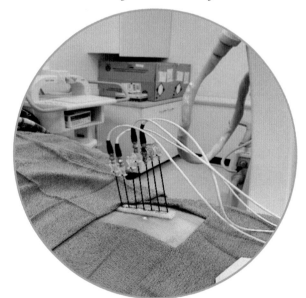

Figure 11-2D

Note the setup for carrying out RFNA using the palisade guide block technique. Four probes are used to make 2 bipolar lesions at a time. In this case, there will be a total of three sets of 2 bipolar lesions:
(1) Start with ablation at the two "A" through-holes
(2) Followed by ablation of the two "B" through-holes
(3) Followed by ablation of the two "C" through-holes
(see Figure 11-1B for labeling of the through-holes)

Chapter 12
Sacroiliac Intraarticular Joint Injection

Although the SI joint is characterized as a large diarthrodial synovial joint, in actuality its synovial characteristic is limited to the inferior and anterior third. *Described below are 3 methods to properly place the needle into the inferior third – and preferably towards the anterior third (when able) – of the joint.*

METHOD 1: (*Author's preferred approach – most time efficient and least technically challenging*)
☐ Obtain an A/P view over the targeted SI joint, focusing on the inferior aspect of the joint.
☐ Place the needle coaxially towards the inferior aspect of the medial joint space, as this typically (but not always) represents the posterior joint (the lateral joint space typically represents the anterior joint – see Figure 12-1A). If needed, apply an ipsilateral oblique to separate the anterior and posterior joint spaces for better visualization of the targeted medial joint space.
☐ Once the needle tip approaches/enters the inferior joint, obtain a lateral view to assess needle depth. Advance the needle in this view towards the anterior third of the joint (if able).
☐ After negative aspiration, administer contrast and look for spread that outlines the joint space.
☐ Obtain an A/P view once again and confirm that contrast spreads cephalad along the joint line and within the joint space.

METHOD 2:
☐ Obtain an A/P view over the targeted SI joint, focusing on the inferior aspect of the joint.
☐ Place a marker over the inferior aspect of the medial joint space.
☐ Next, tilt the C-arm approximately 20-25° cephalad – this projects the posterior portion of the SI joint in a caudal direction, while the anterior joint is projected cephalad (see Figure 12-2C). Note that the marker has not been moved from its original position.
☐ At the location of the marker, place the needle perpendicular to the skin (i.e., non-coaxial fashion) until it enters the posteroinferior aspect of the joint.
☐ Once the needle tip approaches/enters the inferior joint, take a lateral view to assess needle depth. Next, advance the needle towards the anterior third of the joint (if able).
☐ Follow the steps in "Method 1" for administering contrast in the lateral and A/P views.

METHOD 3:
☐ Obtain an A/P view over the targeted SI joint, focusing on the inferior aspect of the joint.
☐ Apply a contralateral oblique until there is alignment of the anterior and posterior joint spaces, particularly inferiorly. Place the needle coaxially towards the inferior aspect of this hyperlucency.
☐ Once the needle tip approaches/enters the inferior joint, take a lateral view to assess needle depth. Next, advance the needle towards the anterior third of the joint (if able).
☐ Follow the steps in "Method 1" for administering contrast in the lateral and A/P views.

"Method 1" – Straight A/P
<u>**Left SI**</u>

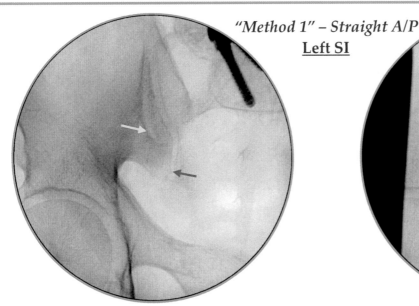

Figure 12-1A
Tilt: 0°
Oblique: 0°

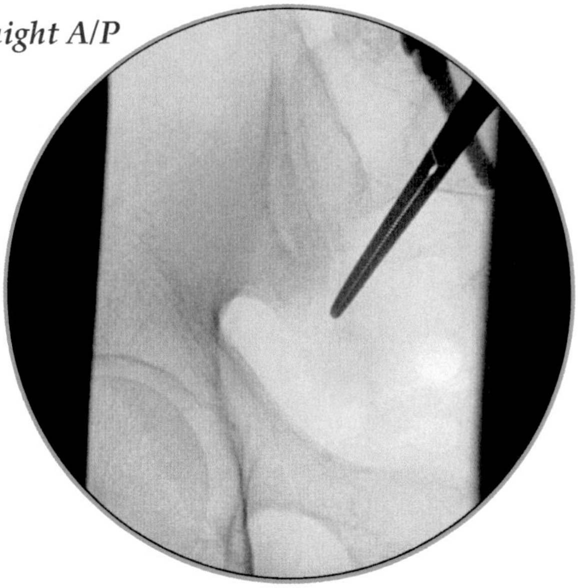

Figure 12-1B
Tilt: 0°
Oblique: 0°

A/P View. Left SI joint. Note the targeted medial joint space (blue arrow), corresponding to the posterior aspect of the joint. *The anterior aspect of the joint is typically represented by the lateral joint space (yellow arrow).*

A/P View. Pointer showing location of needle placement, at the inferior third of the medial joint space (posterior aspect of the joint).

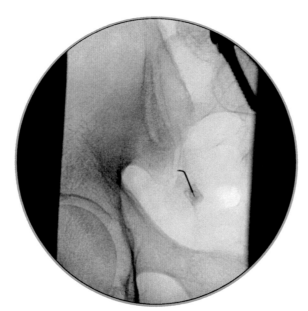

Figure 12-1C
Tilt: 0°
Oblique: 0°

A/P View. Coaxial needle placement approaching the medial joint space (i.e, posterior aspect of the joint). One may feel a subtle increase in resistance as the needle begins to enter the joint. Next, obtain a lateral view to perform further needle advancement.

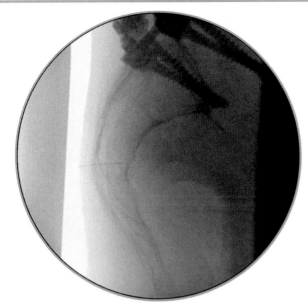

Figure 12-1D
Tilt: 0°
Oblique: 90° Right

Lateral View. The needle is further advanced in this view towards the anterior third of the joint.

Note the bilateral pedicle screws at L5-S1.

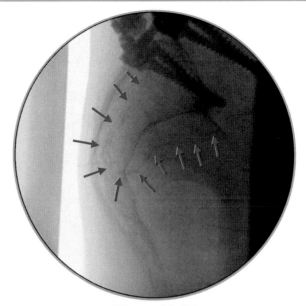

Figure 12-1E
Tilt: 0°
Oblique: 90° Right

Lateral View. Following needle placement, and after negative aspiration, contrast agent is administered. Note how the contrast outlines the joint space (red arrows), and does not flow posterior or outside of the joint space.

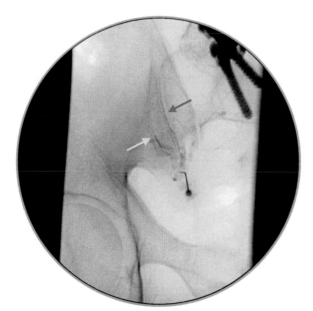

Figure 12-1F
Tilt: 0°
Oblique: 0°

A/P View. In this view, note how the contrast spreads cephalad, and outlines the medial (blue arrow) and lateral (yellow arrow) joint spaces, corresponding to the posterior and anterior joint, respectively.

See Page 294

"Method 2" – Cephalad Tilt
Bilateral SI

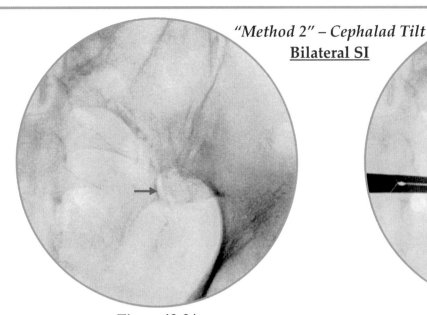

Figure 12-2A
Tilt: 0°
Oblique: 0°

A/P View. Right SI joint. Note the medial joint space (blue arrow), corresponding to the posterior aspect of the joint.

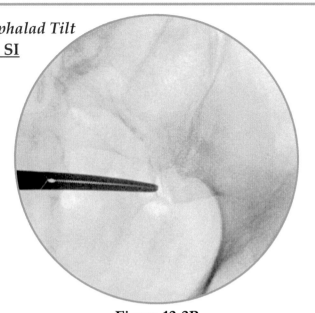

Figure 12-2B
Tilt: 0°
Oblique: 0°

A/P View. Pointer at the inferior third of the posterior joint.

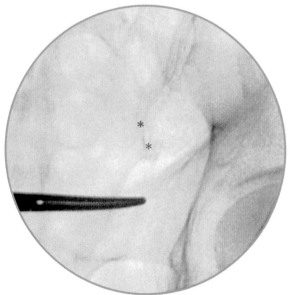

Figure 12-2C
Tilt: 20° Cephalad
Oblique: 0°

A/P View. After tilting cephalad, the posterior joint is projected caudad (blue star), while the anterior joint is projected cephalad (red star). *With a cephalad tilt, note the position of the pointer (which has not been moved) relative to the medial joint space.* The needle is placed at the location of the pointer, but perpendicular to the skin *(non-coaxially)*.

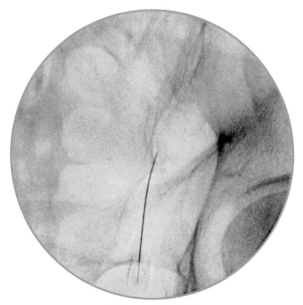

Figure 12-2D
Tilt: 20° Cephalad
Oblique: 0°

A/P View. While advancing the needle perpendicular to the skin, it should be placed into the clearly visible medial joint space (projected caudally in this view), corresponding to the posterior aspect of the joint.

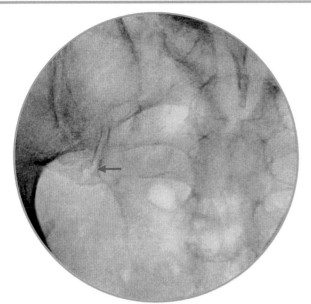

Figure 12-2E
Tilt: 0°
Oblique: 0°

A/P View. Left SI joint. Note the medial joint space (blue arrow), corresponding to the posterior aspect of the joint.

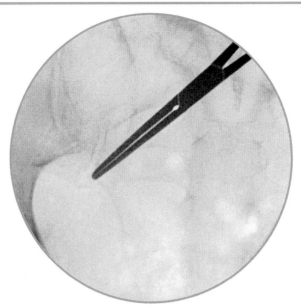

Figure 12-2F
Tilt: 0°
Oblique: 0°

A/P View. Pointer at the inferior third of the posterior joint.

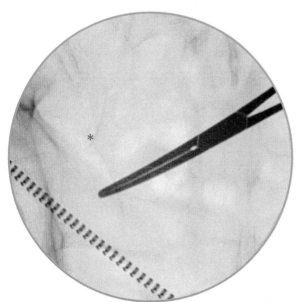

Figure 12-2G
Tilt: 20° Cephalad
Oblique: 0°

A/P View. After tilting cephalad, the posterior joint is projected caudad (blue star). *With a cephalad tilt, note the position of the pointer (which has not been moved) relative to the medial joint space.* The needle is placed at the location of the pointer, perpendicular to the skin *(non-coaxially).*

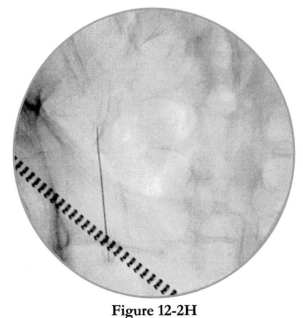

Figure 12-2H
Tilt: 20° Cephalad
Oblique: 0°

A/P View. While advancing the needle perpendicular to the skin, it should be placed into the clearly visible medial joint space (projected caudally in this view), corresponding to the posterior aspect of the joint.

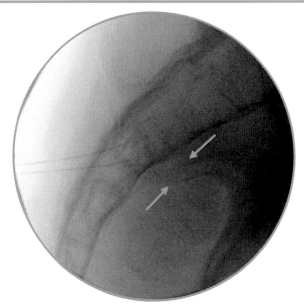

Figure 12-2I
Tilt: 0°
Oblique: 90° Right

Lateral View. The needles are further advanced anteriorly into the joints. Contrast agent is administered and outlines the bilateral joint spaces (green arrows). Note that in this particular case the needles could not be advanced further towards the anterior third of the joint.

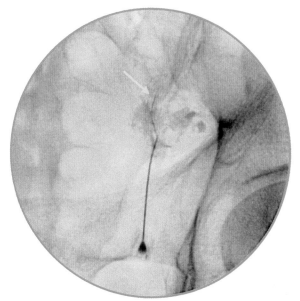

Figure 12-2J
Tilt: 20° Cephalad
Oblique: 0°

A/P View. Right SI joint. After negative aspiration, contrast is administered. Note how it spreads cephalad and outlines the joint space, corresponding to proper intra-articular spread.

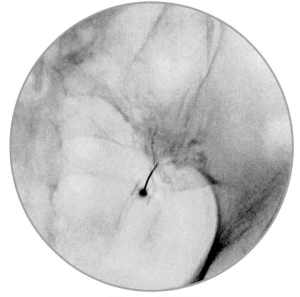

Figure 12-2K
Tilt: 0°
Oblique: 0°

A/P View. Right SI joint. After removing the tilt, and taking a "Straight A/P" view, note how the contrast outlines the joint space, corresponding to proper intra-articular spread. *Also, note how the view of the needle changes after removing the cephalad tilt – compare to Figure 12-2J.*

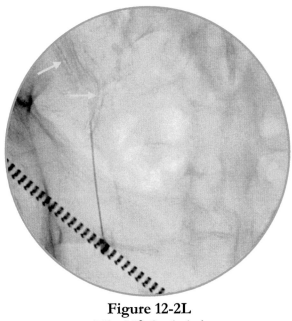

Figure 12-2L
Tilt: 20° Cephalad
Oblique: 0°

A/P View. Left SI joint. After negative aspiration, contrast is administered. Note how it spreads cephalad (yellow arrows) and outlines the joint space, indicating proper intra-articular spread.

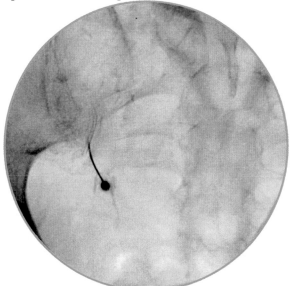

Figure 12-2M
Tilt: 0°
Oblique: 0°

A/P View. Left SI joint. After removing the tilt, and taking a "Straight A/P" view, note how the contrast outlines the joint space, corresponding to proper intra-articular spread. *Also, note how the view of the needle changes after removing the cephalad tilt – compare to Figure 12-2L.*

See Page 295

"Method 3" – Contralateral Oblique
Bilateral SI

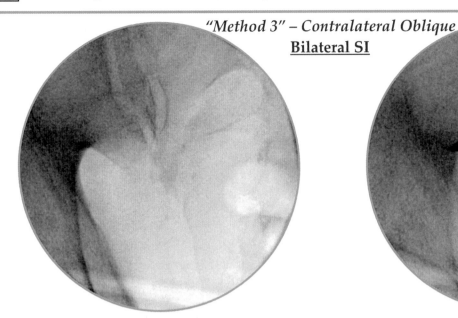

Figure 12-3A
Tilt: 0°
Oblique: 0°

A/P View. Left SI joint. Note how inferiorly there are two separate joint spaces seen, both medial and lateral – corresponding to the posterior and anterior aspect of the joint, respectively.

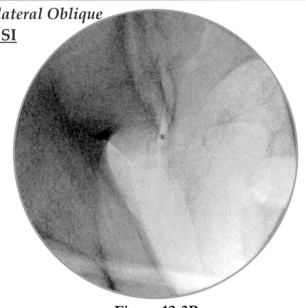

Figure 12-3B
Tilt: 0°
Oblique: 10° Right

Contralateral Oblique View. By applying a contralateral oblique, note how the medial and lateral joint spaces overlap at the inferior aspect, forming a hyperlucency (blue star) – *compare to Figure 12-3A.*

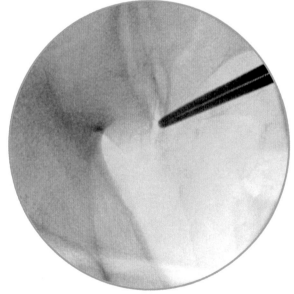

Figure 12-3C
Tilt: 0°
Oblique: 10° Right

Contralateral Oblique View. Pointer showing the location of needle placement, at the inferior third of the posterior joint.

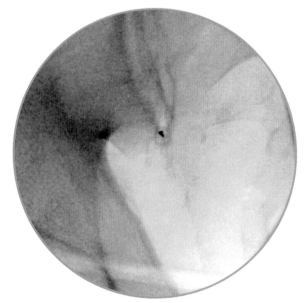

Figure 12-3D
Tilt: 0°
Oblique: 10° Right

Contralateral Oblique View. Coaxial needle placement approaching the inferior aspect of the joint.

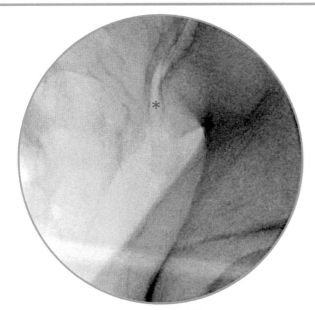

Figure 12-3E
Tilt: 0°
Oblique: 10° Left

Contralateral Oblique View. Right SI joint. By applying a contralateral oblique, note how the medial and lateral joint spaces overlap at the inferior aspect, forming a hyperlucency (blue star).

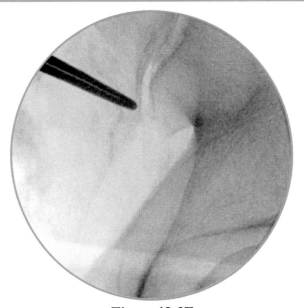

Figure 12-3F
Tilt: 0°
Oblique: 10° Left

Contralateral Oblique View. Pointer showing the location of needle placement, at the inferior third of the posterior joint.

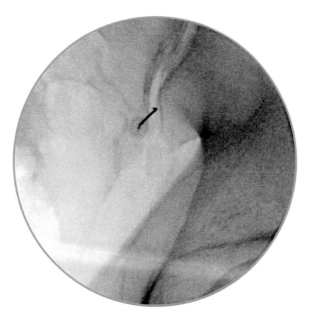

Figure 12-3G
Tilt: 0°
Oblique: 10° Left

Contralateral Oblique View. Coaxial needle placement approaching the inferior joint.

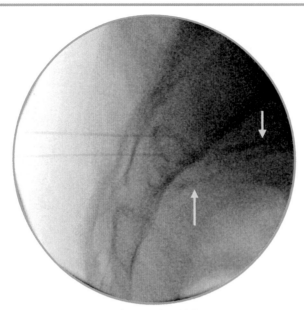

Figure 12-3H
Tilt: 0°
Oblique: 90° Right

Lateral View. The needle is advanced anteriorly into the joint. After negative aspiration, contrast agent is administered. Note the spread outlining the joint spaces (yellow arrows), without flow posterior or outside of the joint space.

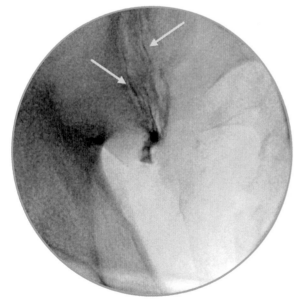

Figure 12-3I
Tilt: 0°
Oblique: 10° Right

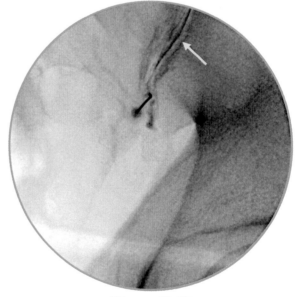

Figure 12-3J
Tilt: 0°
Oblique: 10° Left

Contralateral Oblique View. Left SI joint. In this view, note how the contrast spreads cephalad, and outlines the medial and lateral joint spaces (yellow arrows), corresponding to the posterior and anterior joint, respectively.

Contralateral Oblique View. Right SI joint. In this view, note how the contrast spreads cephalad (yellow arrow), and outlines the joint space.

Additional "Method 1" Examples:

Bilateral SI

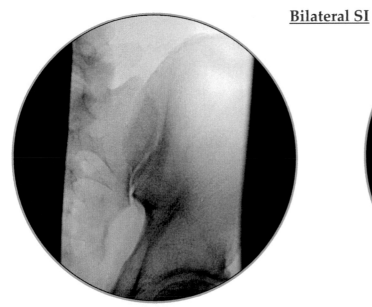

Figure 12-4A
Tilt: 0°
Oblique: 0°

A/P View. Right SI joint.

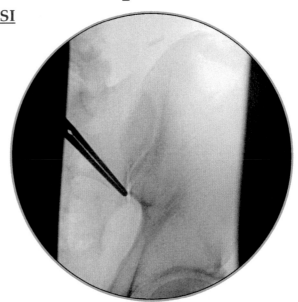

Figure 12-4B
Tilt: 0°
Oblique: 0°

A/P View. Pointer showing the location of needle placement at the inferior aspect of the right SI joint.

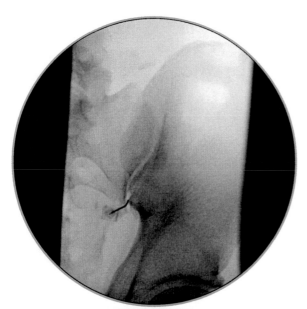

Figure 12-4C
Tilt: 0°
Oblique: 0°

A/P View. Coaxial needle placement at the inferior aspect of the right SI joint.

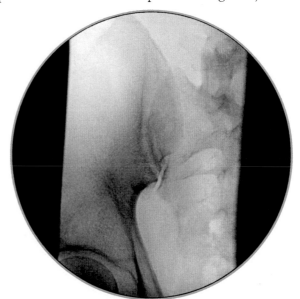

Figure 12-4D
Tilt: 0°
Oblique: 0°

A/P View. Left SI joint.

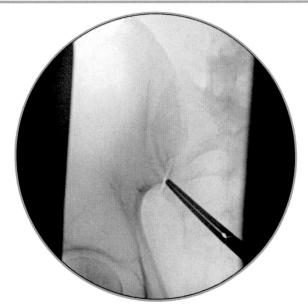

Figure 12-4E
Tilt: 0°
Oblique: 0°

A/P View. Pointer showing the location of needle placement at the inferior aspect of the left SI joint.

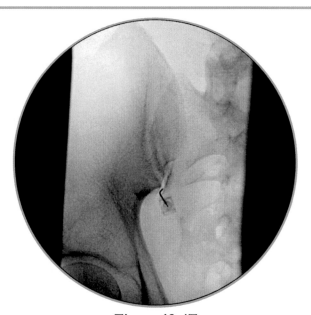

Figure 12-4F
Tilt: 0°
Oblique: 0°

A/P View. Coaxial needle placement at the inferior aspect of the left SI joint.

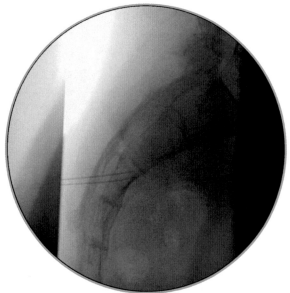

Figure 12-4G
Tilt: 0°
Oblique: 90° Right

Lateral View. The needles are further advanced in this view towards the anterior third of the joint.

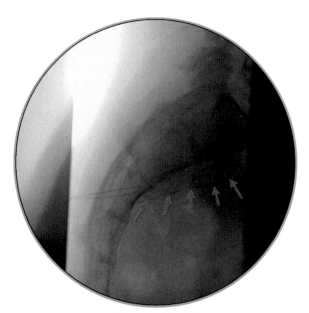

Figure 12-4H
Tilt: 0°
Oblique: 90° Right

Lateral View. After negative aspiration, contrast is administered through the left needle and shows proper spread outlining the left joint space (red arrows).

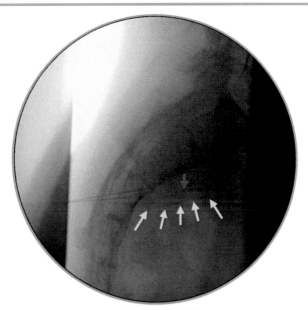

Figure 12-4I
Tilt: 0°
Oblique: 90° Right

Lateral View. After negative aspiration, contrast administration through the right needle shows proper spread outlining the right joint space (yellow arrows). *Note the prior contrast spread through the left SI joint space (red arrow).*

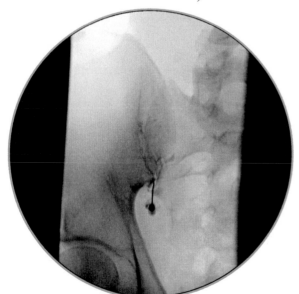

Figure 12-4J
Tilt: 0°
Oblique: 0°

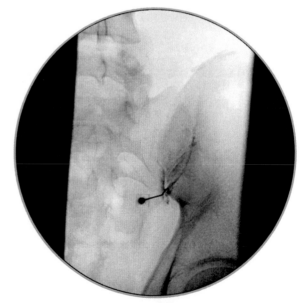

Figure 12-4K
Tilt: 0°
Oblique: 0°

A/P View. Contrast administration through the left needle shows proper spread traveling cephalad and outlining the joint space.

A/P View. Contrast administration through the right needle shows proper spread traveling cephalad and outlining the joint space.

Left SI

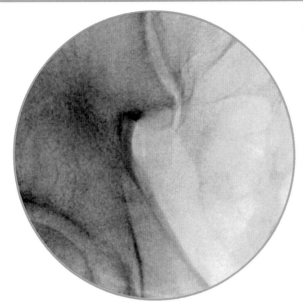

Figure 12-5A
Tilt: 0°
Oblique: 0°

A/P View. Left SI joint.

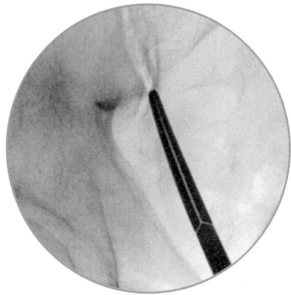

Figure 11-2B
Tilt: 0°
Oblique: 0°

A/P View. Pointer showing the location of needle placement at the inferior aspect of the left SI joint.

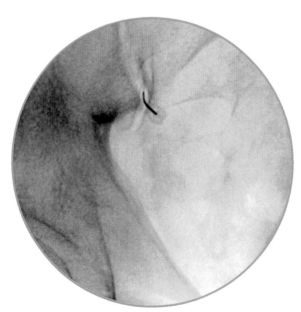

Figure 12-5C
Tilt: 0°
Oblique: 0°

A/P View. Coaxial needle placement at the inferior aspect of the left SI joint.

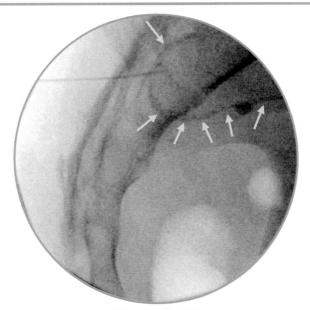

Figure 12-5D
Tilt: 0°
Oblique: 90° Right

Lateral View. The needle is further advanced in this view, but note that it could not be advanced to the anterior third of the joint. After negative aspiration, contrast administration shows proper spread outlining the joint space.

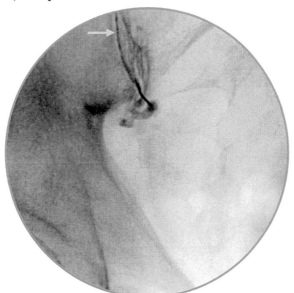

Figure 12-5E
Tilt: 0°
Oblique: 0°

A/P View. Contrast administration shows proper spread traveling cephalad (yellow arrow) and outlining the joint space.

Bilateral SI

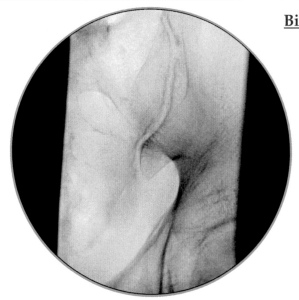
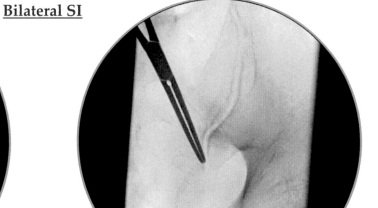

Figure 12-6A
Tilt: 0°
Oblique: 0°

A/P View. Right SI joint.

Figure 12-6B
Tilt: 0°
Oblique: 0°

A/P View. Pointer showing the location of needle placement at the inferior aspect of the right SI joint.

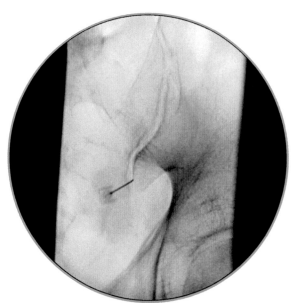
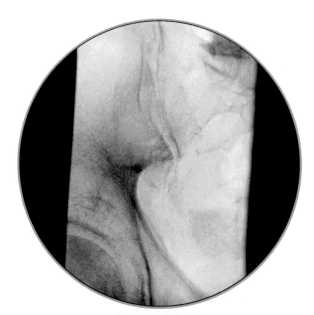

Figure 12-6C
Tilt: 0°
Oblique: 0°

A/P View. Coaxial needle placement at the inferior aspect of the right SI joint.

Figure 12-6D
Tilt: 0°
Oblique: 0°

A/P View. Left SI joint.

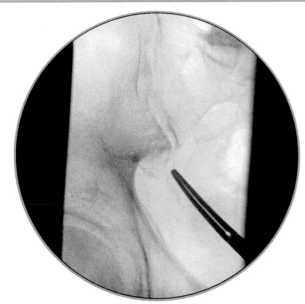

Figure 12-6E
Tilt: 0°
Oblique: 0°

A/P View. Pointer showing the location of needle placement at the inferior aspect of the left SI joint.

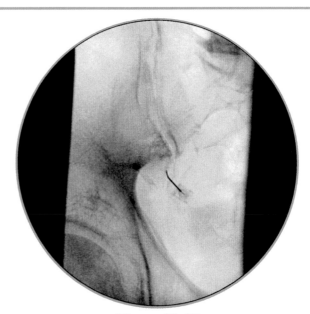

Figure 12-6F
Tilt: 0°
Oblique: 0°

A/P View. Coaxal needle placement at the inferior aspect of the left SI joint.

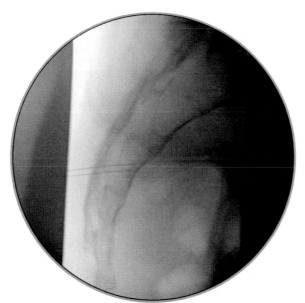

Figure 12-6G
Tilt: 0°
Oblique: 90° Right

Lateral View. The needles are further advanced in this view towards the anterior third of the joint.

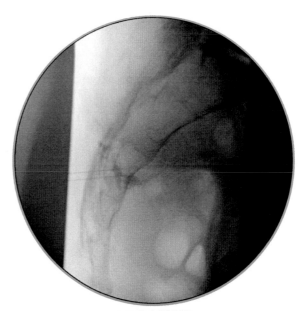

Figure 12-6H
Tilt: 0°
Oblique: 90° Right

Lateral View. After negative aspiration, contrast administration through each needle shows proper spread outlining the joint spaces.

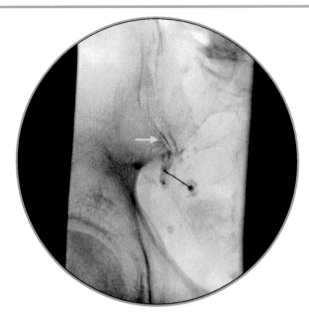

Figure 12-6I
Tilt: 0°
Oblique: 0°

A/P View. Contrast administration through the left needle shows proper spread traveling cephalad (yellow arrow) and outlining the joint space.

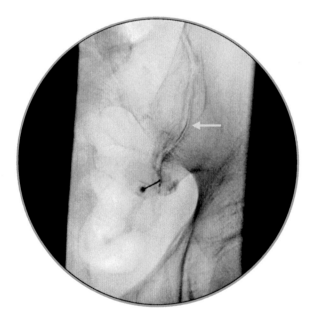

Figure 12-6J
Tilt: 0°
Oblique: 0°

A/P View. Contrast administration through the right needle shows proper spread traveling cephalad (yellow arrow) and outlining the joint space.

Left SI

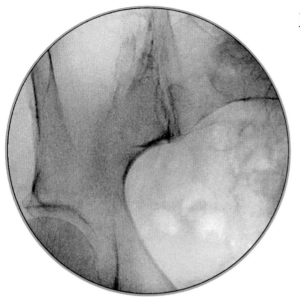

Figure 12-7A
Tilt: 0°
Oblique: 0°

A/P View. Left SI joint.

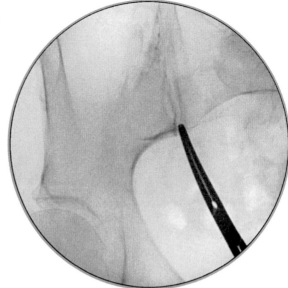

Figure 12-7B
Tilt: 0°
Oblique: 0°

A/P View. Pointer showing the location of needle placement at the inferior aspect of the left SI joint.

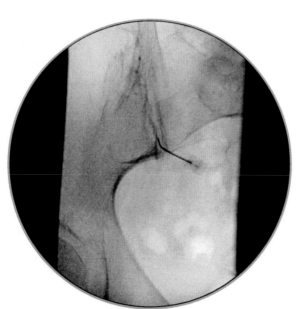

Figure 12-7C
Tilt: 0°
Oblique: 0°

A/P View. Coaxial needle placement at the inferior aspect of the left SI joint.

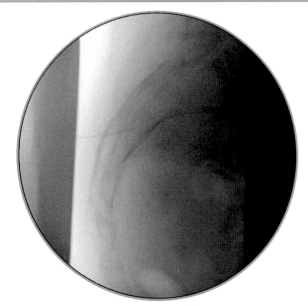

Figure 12-7D
Tilt: 0°
Oblique: 90° Right

Lateral View. The needle is further advanced in this view towards the anterior joint.

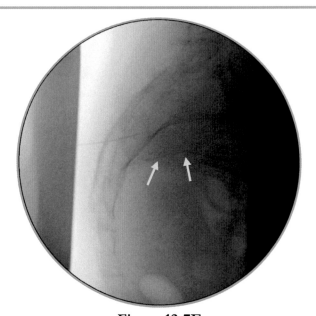

Figure 12-7E
Tilt: 0°
Oblique: 90° Right

Lateral View. After negative aspiration, contrast administration shows proper spread outlining the joint space (yellow arrows).

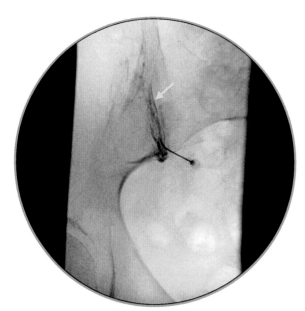

Figure 12-7F
Tilt: 0°
Oblique: 0°

A/P View. Contrast administration shows proper spread traveling cephalad (yellow arrow) and outlining the joint space.

Right SI

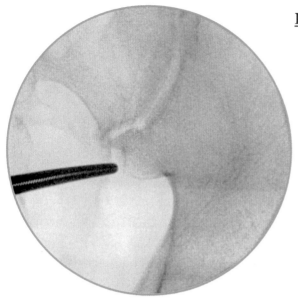

Figure 12-8A
Tilt: 0°
Oblique: 0°

A/P View. Pointer showing the location of needle placement at the inferior aspect of the right SI joint.

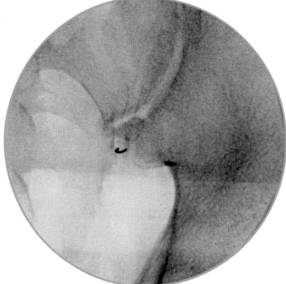

Figure 12-8B
Tilt: 0°
Oblique: 0°

A/P View. Coaxial needle placement at the right SI joint.

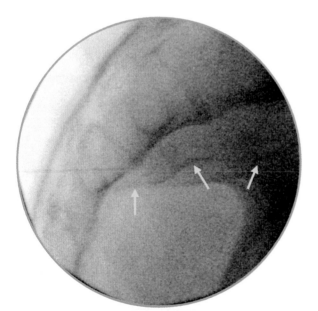

Figure 12-8C
Tilt: 0°
Oblique: 90°

Lateral View. After negative aspiration, contrast administration shows proper spread outlining the joint space (yellow arrows).

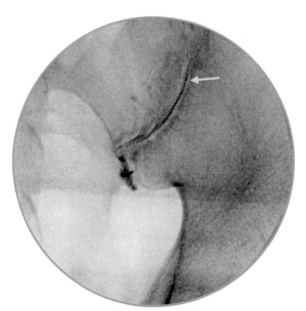

Figure 12-8D
Tilt: 0°
Oblique: 0°

A/P View. Contrast administration shows proper spread traveling cephalad (yellow arrow) and outlining the joint space.

See Page 294

Bilateral SI

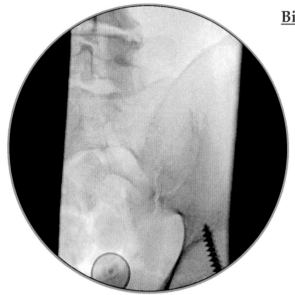

Figure 12-9A
Tilt: 0°
Oblique: 0°

A/P View. Right SI joint.

Note the right total hip arthroplasty hardware.

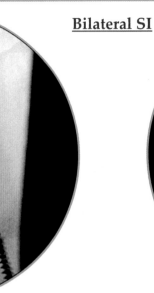

Figure 12-9B
Tilt: 0°
Oblique: 0°

A/P View. Pointer showing the location of needle placement at the inferior aspect of the right SI joint.

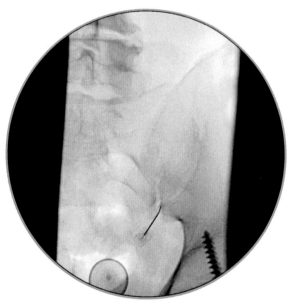

Figure 12-9C
Tilt: 0°
Oblique: 0°

A/P View. Coaxial needle placement at the inferior aspect of the right SI joint.

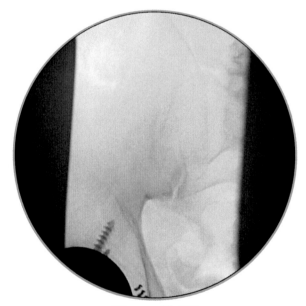

Figure 12-9D
Tilt: 0°
Oblique: 0°

A/P View. Left SI joint.

Note the left total hip arthroplasty hardware.

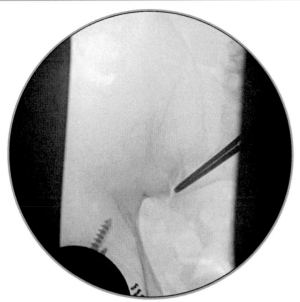

Figure 12-9E
Tilt: 0°
Oblique: 0°

A/P View. Pointer showing the location of needle placement at the inferior aspect of the left SI joint.

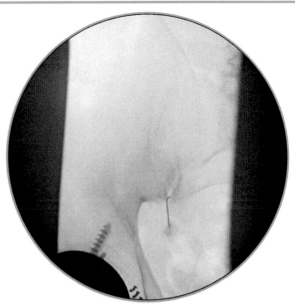

Figure 12-9F
Tilt: 0°
Oblique: 0°

A/P View. Coxial needle placement at the inferior aspect of the left SI joint.

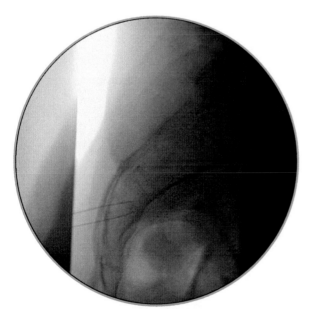

Figure 12-9G
Tilt: 0°
Oblique: 90° Right

Lateral View. The needles are further advanced in this view towards the anterior third of the joint.

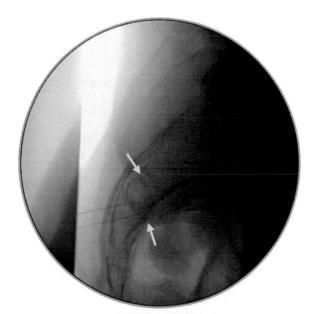

Figure 12-9H
Tilt: 0°
Oblique: 90° Right

Lateral View. After negative aspiration, contrast administration through the left needle shows proper spread outlining the joint space (yellow arrows).

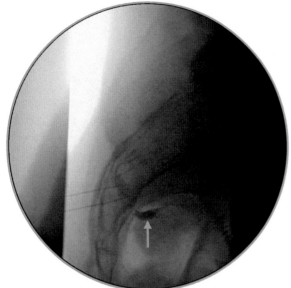

Figure 12-9I
Tilt: 0°
Oblique: 90° Right

Lateral View. After negative aspiration, contrast administration through the right needle shows proper spread outlining the joint space. Note the contrast in the inferior recess of the joint (green arrow).

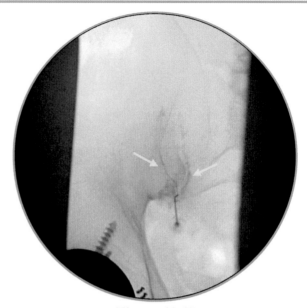

Figure 12-9J
Tilt: 0°
Oblique: 0°

A/P View. Contrast administration through the left needle shows proper spread traveling cephalad and outlining the joint spaces (yellow arrows).

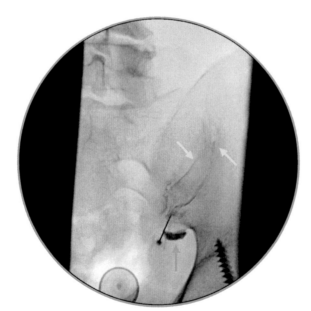

Figure 12-9K
Tilt: 0°
Oblique: 0°

A/P View. Contrast administration through the right needle shows proper spread traveling cephalad and outlining the joint spaces (yellow arrows). Once again, note the contrast in the inferior recess of the joint (green arrow).

Chapter 13
Lumbar Facet Joint Injection

- Obtain an A/P view to locate the targeted level(s). Oblique the C-arm ipsilaterally as needed to identify the posterior joint space. Note that the lumbar facet joint is "C-shaped" with the posterior portion of the joint oriented in a more sagittal plane and the anterior portion in a more coronal plane (see Image 1). Due to this shape, if the C-arm is obliqued too far ipsilaterally, the joint space may appear open and accessible, when in fact the anterior portion of the joint is what is actually being visualized. In order to access the posterior portion of the joint, typically an ipsilateral oblique of approximately 10-20° is all that is needed. *However, it should be noted that this is just a rule of thumb. At times it may be necessary to use an ipsilateral oblique angle of 30-45° to enter the posterior portion of the joint, while in other instances no oblique whatsoever will be needed if the joint is completely sagitally oriented. Additionally, if there is significant facet hypertrophy leading to overgrowth (usually off the SAP), needle entry into the posterior joint may be obstructed despite the appearance of a fluoroscopically accessible joint – in this case a more medial-to-lateral needle trajectory (i.e., less ipsilateral oblique or possibly even contralateral oblique) may be used to facilitate entry into the joint (see Image 2).* Of note, cephalad or caudal tilting may be applied as needed, but is typically not necessary.

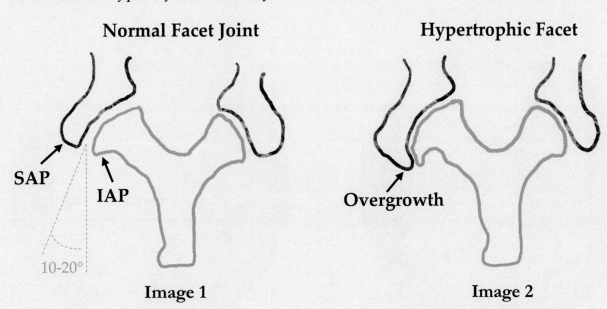

Normal Facet Joint   **Hypertrophic Facet**

SAP   IAP   Overgrowth

10-20°

Image 1   **Image 2**

- The needle is advanced in a coaxial view into the posterior joint. After placement within the joint, an additional oblique angle may be applied to confirm that the needle tip is within the joint silhouette.

- Next, A/P and lateral views are taken to confirm needle positioning in multi-planar views.

- After negative aspiration, contrast is administered to confirm intra-articular spread.

Bilateral L3-L4, L4-L5, L5-S1
Facet Joint Injection

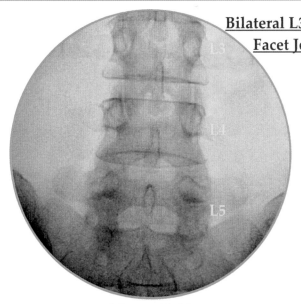

Figure 13-1A
Tilt: 0°
Oblique: 0°

A/P View. Note the vertebral levels.

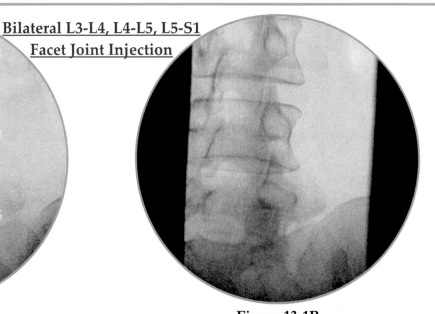

Figure 13-1B
Tilt: 0°
Oblique: 20° Right

Oblique View. Note the right sided facet joint spaces.

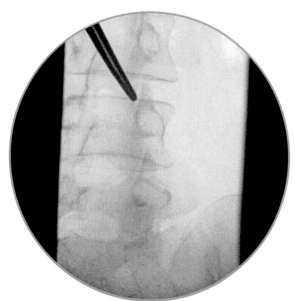

Figure 13-1C
Tilt: 0°
Oblique: 20° Right

Oblique View. Pointer showing the location of needle placement at the right L3-L4 facet joint. Aim to be in the superior half of the joint space.

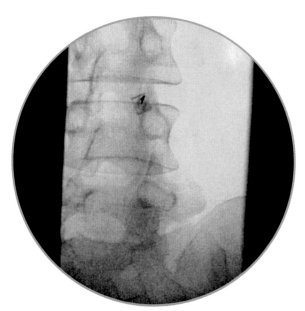

Figure 13-1D
Tilt: 0°
Oblique: 20° Right

Oblique View. Coaxial needle placement within the right L3-L4 facet joint. Often a subtle resistance can be felt as the needle tip pierces the facet joint capsule and enters the joint space.

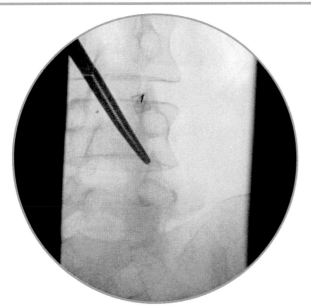

Figure 13-1E
Tilt: 0°
Oblique: 20° Right

Oblique View. Pointer showing the location of needle placement at the right L4-L5 facet joint. Aim to be in the superior half of the joint space.

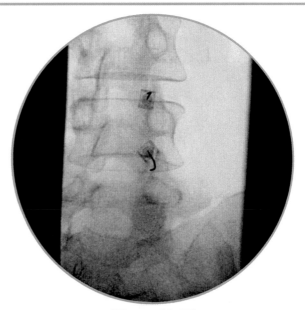

Figure 13-1F
Tilt: 0°
Oblique: 20° Right

Oblique View. Coaxial needle placement in the right L4-L5 facet joint. Often a subtle resistance can be felt as the needle tip pierces the facet joint capsule and enters the joint space.

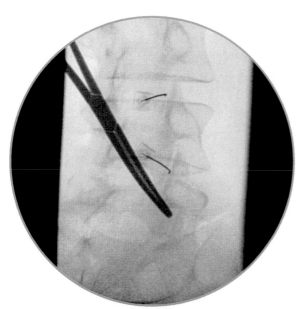

Figure 13-1G
Tilt: 0°
Oblique: 25° Right

Oblique View. Pointer showing the location of needle placement at the right L5-S1 facet joint. Note that an additional ipsilateral oblique provides better visualization of the joint space (*compare to Figure 13-1E*).

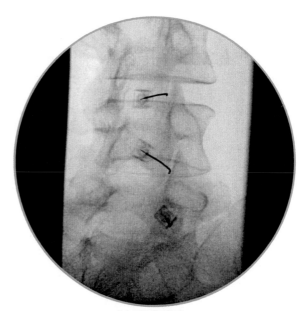

Figure 13-1H
Tilt: 0°
Oblique: 25° Right

Oblique View. Coaxial needle placement in the right L5-S1 facet joint. Often a subtle resistance can be felt as the needle tip pierces the facet joint capsule and enters the joint space.

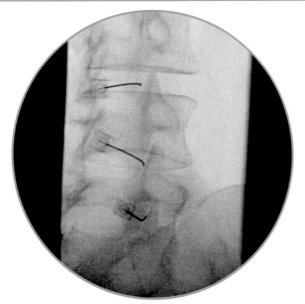

Figure 13-1I
Tilt: 0°
Oblique: 30° Right

Oblique View. Applying an additional ipsilateral oblique provides confirmation that the needle is in the facet joint, by noting that the tip remains in the joint space as seen above.

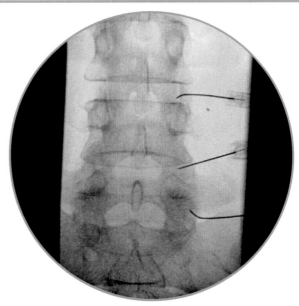

Figure 13-1J
Tilt: 0°
Oblique: 0°

A/P View. Final needle positioning after placement within the right L3-L4, L4-L5, and L5-S1 facet joints.

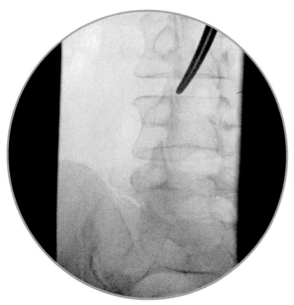

Figure 13-1K
Tilt: 0°
Oblique: 20° Left

Oblique View. Pointer showing the location of needle placement at the left L3-L4 facet joint. Aim to be in the superior half of the joint space.

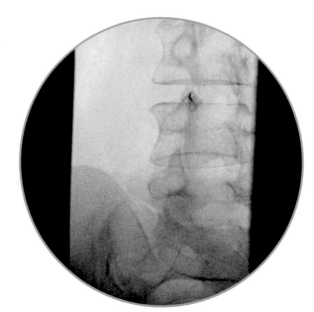

Figure 13-1L
Tilt: 0°
Oblique: 20° Left

Oblique View. Coaxial needle placement in the left L3-L4 facet joint. Often a subtle resistance can be felt as the needle tip pierces the facet joint capsule and enters the joint space.

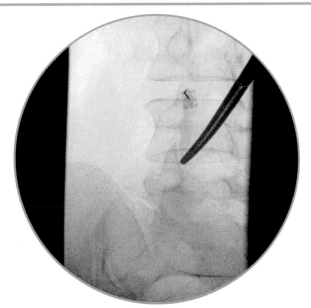

Figure 13-1M
Tilt: 0°
Oblique: 20° Left

Oblique View. Pointer showing the location of needle placement at the left L4-L5 facet joint. Aim to be in the superior half of the joint space.

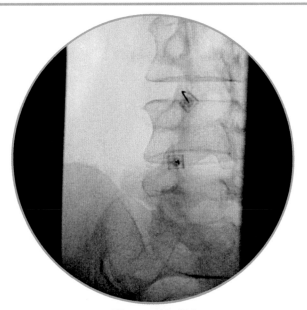

Figure 13-1N
Tilt: 0°
Oblique: 20° Left

Oblique View. Coaxial needle placement in the left L4-L5 facet joint. Often a subtle resistance can be felt as the needle tip pierces the facet joint capsule and enters the joint space.

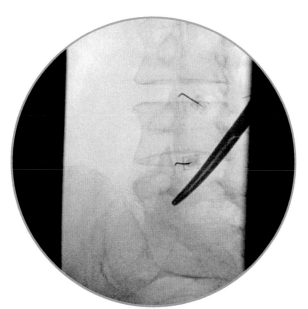

Figure 13-1O
Tilt: 0°
Oblique: 25° Left

Oblique View. Pointer showing the location of needle placement at the left L5-S1 facet joint. Note that an additional ipsilateral oblique provides better visualization of the joint space (*compare to Figure 13-1M*).

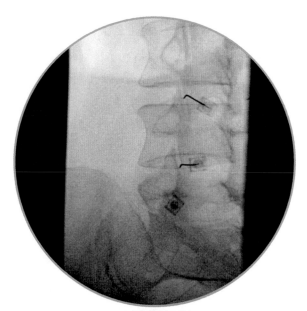

Figure 13-1P
Tilt: 0°
Oblique: 25° Left

Oblique View. Coaxial needle placement in the left L5-S1 facet joint. Often a subtle resistance can be felt as the needle tip pierces the facet joint capsule and enters the joint space.

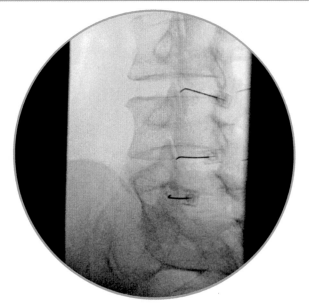

Figure 13-1Q
Tilt: 0°
Oblique: 30° Left

Oblique View. Applying a further ipsilateral oblique provides confirmation that the needle is in the facet joint, by noting that the tip remains in the joint space as seen above.

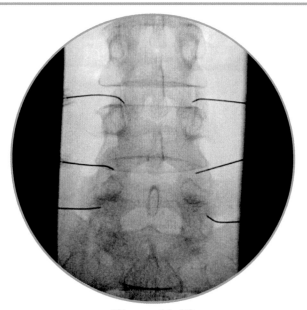

Figure 13-1R
Tilt: 0°
Oblique: 0°

A/P View. Final needle positioning after placement within the bilateral L3-L4, L4-L5, and L5-S1 facet joints.

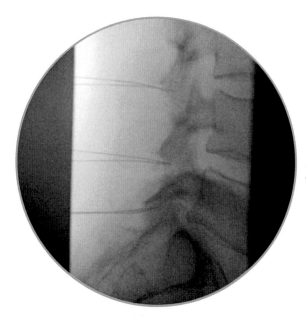

Figure 13-1S
Tilt: 0°
Oblique: 90° Right

Lateral View. Final needle positioning after placement within the bilateral L3-L4, L4-L5, and L5-S1 facet joints.

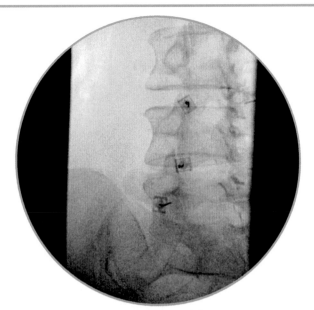

Figure 13-1T
Tilt: 0°
Oblique: 20° Left

Oblique View. Final needle positioning after placement with the left L3-L4, L4-L5, and L5-S1 facet joints – prior to administration of contrast.

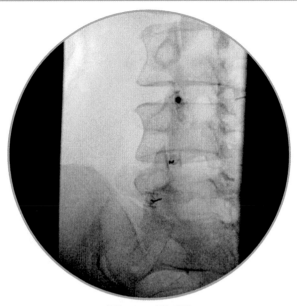

Figure 13-1U
Tilt: 0°
Oblique: 20° Left

Oblique View. After negative aspiration, contrast is administered with spread noted within the left L3-L4 facet joint.

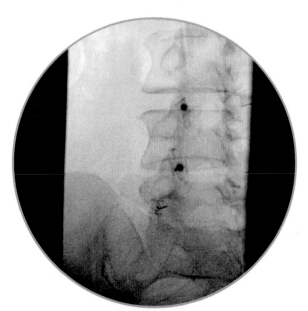

Figure 13-1V
Tilt: 0°
Oblique: 20° Left

Oblique View. After negative aspiration, contrast is administered with spread noted within the left L4-L5 facet joint.

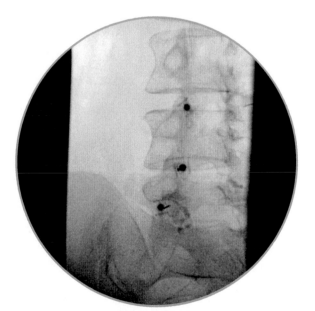

Figure 13-1W
Tilt: 0°
Oblique: 20° Left

Oblique View. After negative aspiration, contrast is administered with spread noted within the left L5-S1 facet joint.

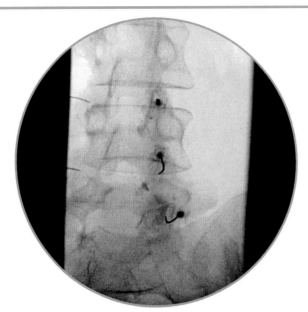

Figure 13-1X
Tilt: 0°
Oblique: 20° Right

Oblique View. Similar steps are followed for administration of contrast on the right side. Note the final intra-articular spread within the right L3-L4, L4-L5, and L5-S1 facet joints.

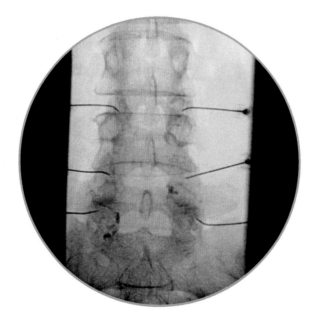

Figure 13-1Y
Tilt: 0°
Oblique: 0°

A/P View. Note the intra-articular spread of contrast in this view at the bilateral L3-L4, L4-L5, and L5-S1 facet joints.

See Page 282

Chapter 14
Cervical Facet Joint Injection

☐ Obtain an A/P view to locate the targeted levels, with the patient in the prone position. Consider taking a scout lateral view over the targeted facet joint to get an appreciation of the angle of the articular pillar. This helps with determining the caudal needle entry point (*see page 165 for an additional discussion regarding the superoinferior angle of the cervical articular pillar*). With the scout lateral view, a pointer can be placed over the lateral aspect of the patient's neck, and aligned to match the angle of the targeted joint (see Figure 14-1B). With this pointer angle maintained, approximate where the pointer crosses the posterior aspect of the patient's neck – this point can be used as an estimate for the caudal needle entry point that will create a trajectory to facilitate smooth entry into the targeted joint.

☐ Next, in the A/P view, the needle is placed at the previously estimated caudal needle entry point on the posterior neck, and over the midportion of the facet joints (see Figure 14-1C). The needle is advanced in a non-coaxial fashion towards the targeted cervical facet joint, making sure to keep it over the midportion of the facet joint in order to avoid inadvertent neural injury. The needle is advanced ideally until bony contact is made at the inferior portion of the facet joint. *Of note, as an alternative technique, a caudal tilt of the C-arm can be used to identify the targeted joint with placement of the needle in a coaxial fashion. However, tilting of the C-arm may cause distortion of targeted structures, making it more challenging to visuazlize the facet joint.*

☐ After contact with bone, a lateral view is obtained and the needle is adjusted in the cephalocaudad direction as needed until it is seen to be within the joint. The needle should not be advanced beyond the posterior half of the joint, as seen in the lateral view. *Of note, in the lower cervical segments, the needle tip may not be seen due to obstruction from the shoulders. In these instances, a contralateral oblique view should be used instead for placing the needle wthin the joint.*

☐ Next, after negative aspiration, contrast is administered in either the lateral or contralateral oblique view to ensure no vascular uptake with proper intra-articular spread.

☐ Finally, an A/P view is taken once again to ensure intraarticular spread and that the needle is near the mid-portion of the joint with respect to mediolateral positioning.

Right C3-C4, C4-C5, C5-C6
Facet Joint Injection

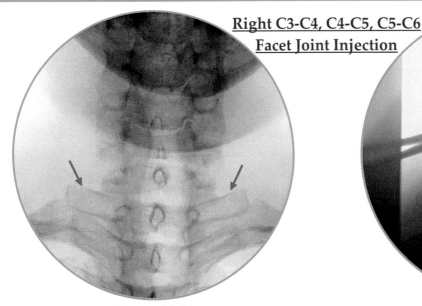

Figure 14-1A
Tilt: 10° Cephalad
Oblique: 0°

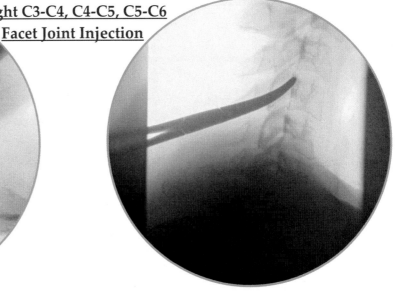

Figure 14-1B
Tilt: 10° Cephalad
Oblique: 90° Right

A/P View. Note the vertebral levels based off the T1 vertebra, which has large and exaggerated transverse processes (blue arrows). *In this case, a cephalad tilt better squares the endplates and removes the mandible from obstructing the mid to lower cervical segments.*

Lateral View. Pointer is placed over the lateral neck, at the C4 articular pillar and approximating the angle of the C3-C4 joint space. *With this angle of the pointer, estimate where the proximal end of the pointer crosses the posterior neck. This will be the caudal needle entry point for the C3-C4 facet joint.*

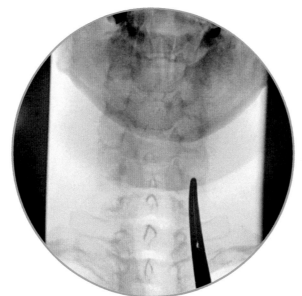

Figure 14-1C
Tilt: 10° Cephalad
Oblique: 0°

A/P View. Based off the pointer angle approximating the C3-C4 facet joint as discussed in Figure 14-1B, the proximal end of the pointer was noted to cross the posterior neck at the C6 level. *This needle entry point, over the middle of the facet joint, will allow entry into the C3-C4 joint.*

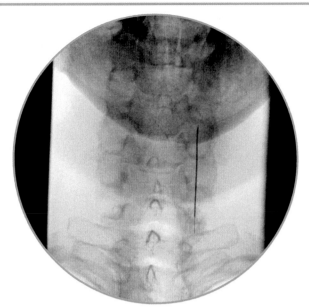

Figure 14-1D
Tilt: 10° Cephalad
Oblique: 0°

A/P View. The needle is advanced cephalad towards the targeted joint, making sure to stay over the mid-portion of the facet joint. Avoid going medially, to prevent inadvertent spinal cord injury. *Note that the needle is approaching C4 – advance until contact with bone.*

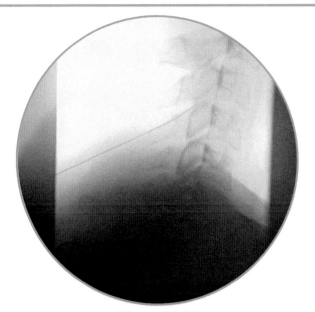

Figure 14-1E
Tilt: 10° Cephalad
Oblique: 90° Right

Lateral View. The needle is advanced into the C3-C4 facet joint. *Note that by first approximating the joint space angle using the scout lateral, the final needle trajectory is fairly parallel to the joint space.* The needle is kept in the posterior half of the joint to safely avoid vital neurovascular structures.

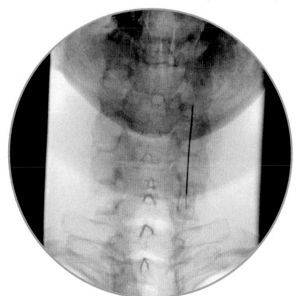

Figure 14-1F
Tilt: 10° Cephalad
Oblique: 0°

A/P View. Final needle position after entry into the right C3-C4 facet joint. Note that the needle tip is in the mid-portion of the facet joint, mediolaterally.

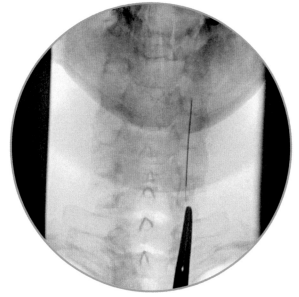

Figure 14-1G
Tilt: 10° Cephalad
Oblique: 0°

A/P View. As discussed previously, for the C3-C4 facet joint, the estimated needle entry point based off Figure 14-1B was noted to be at C6. Thus, using this same approximation, the pointer for needle entry into the C4-C5 facet joint is placed at C7.

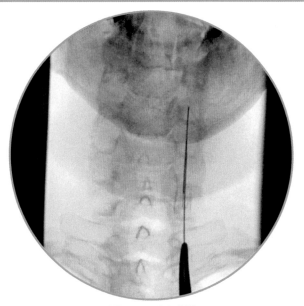

Figure 14-1H
Tilt: 10° Cephalad
Oblique: 0°

A/P View. The needle is advanced cephalad towards the targeted joint, staying over the mid-portion of the facet joint - *superimposed over the prior needle placed, and approaching C5*. Note that in a similar fashion, the pointer for needle entry into the C5-C6 joint is placed at T1.

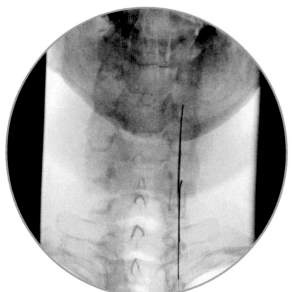

Figure 14-1I
Tilt: 10° Cephalad
Oblique: 0°

A/P View. The needle is advanced cephalad towards the targeted joint, making sure to stay over the mid-portion of the facet joint. Avoid going medially, in order to prevent spinal cord injury. *Note that the inferior most needle is approaching C6 – advance until contact with bone.*

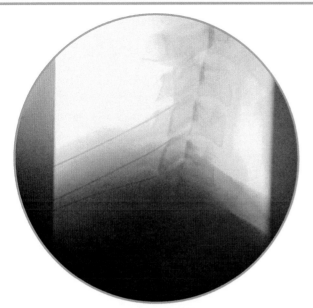

Figure 14-1J
Tilt: 10° Cephalad
Oblique: 90° Right

Lateral View. The inferior needles are advanced into the C4-C5 & C5-C6 facet joints, and placed in the posterior half of the joint to safely avoid vital neurovascular structures. *Note that a more caudal needle entry for the C5-C6 facet joint would have even better aligned with the joint space angle.*

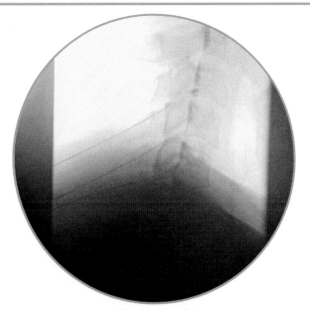

Figure 14-1K
Tilt: 10° Cephalad
Oblique: 90° Right

Lateral View. After negative aspiration, administration of contrast at the right C3-C4 facet joint shows proper intra-articular spread.

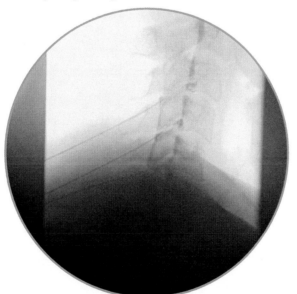

Figure 14-1L
Tilt: 10° Cephalad
Oblique: 90° Right

Lateral View. After negative aspiration, administration of contrast at the right C4-C5 facet joint shows proper intra-articular spread.

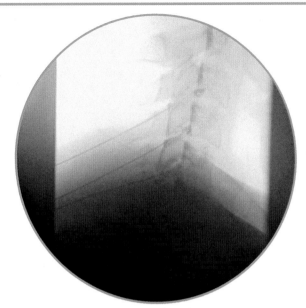

Figure 14-1M
Tilt: 10° Cephalad
Oblique: 90° Right

Lateral View. After negative aspiration, administration of contrast at the right C5-C6 facet joint shows proper intra-articular spread.

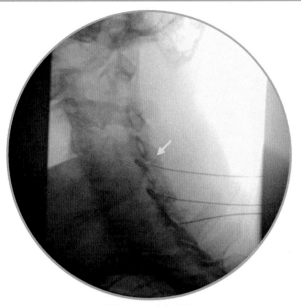

Figure 14-1N
Tilt: 10° Cephalad
Oblique: 45° Left

Contralateral Oblique View. In addition to a lateral view, or as an alternative, a CLO view can be obtained to confirm needle depth, placement within the facet joint, and placement posterior to the neural foramen. *Note the C3 articular pillar (yellow arrow) and C3-C4 foramen (blue star).*

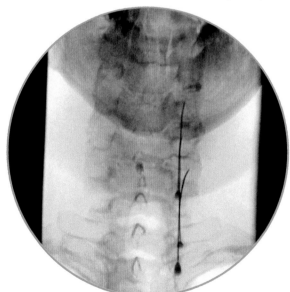

Figure 14-1O
Tilt: 10° Cephalad
Oblique: 0°

A/P view. Final needle position and contrast spread after intra-articular placement within the right C3-C4, C4-C5, and C5-C6 facet joints.

See Page 287

Chapter 15
Thoracic Facet Joint Injection

- Obtain an A/P view to locate the targeted levels. The thoracic facet joints are oriented in a near-coronal plane. As a result, this requires a significant caudal needle entry to place the needle within the joint. For entering a thoracic facet joint, needle entry should be at least one level below, at the inferior aspect of the pedicle (i.e., 6 o'clock position) – *see Figure 14-1A*.

- The needle is advanced from the caudal level towards the inferior pedicle of the targeted facet joint, making sure to keep the needle over the mid-portion of the facet joint at all times in order to avoid inadvertent neural injury. Once bone is contacted at the inferior pedicle of the targeted facet joint, a lateral view is obtained.

- In the lateral view, the needle is advanced using cephalocaudal adjustments as needed until the tip has entered the joint. The needle should not be advanced beyond the posterior half of the joint, as seen in the lateral view.

- In the lateral view, contrast is administered after negative aspiration to ensure proper intra-articular spread without vascular uptake.

- Finally, an A/P view is taken once again to ensure intraarticular spread and that the needle is near the mid-portion of the joint with respect to mediolateral positioning.

Right T8-T9, T9-T10, T10-T11
Facet Joint Injection

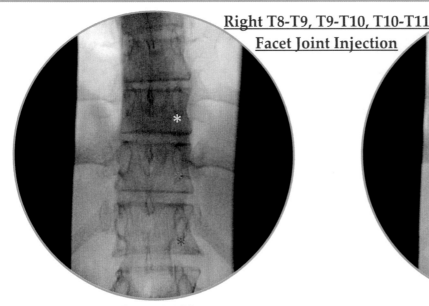

Figure 15-1A
Tilt: 0°
Oblique: 0°

A/P View. The steep angles of the thoracic facet joints require a caudal needle entry. *For the right T8-T9 facet joint, the needle entry point is as the inferior T10 pedicle (yellow star). Similarly, note the needle entry points for the right T9-T10 facet joint (blue star) and right T10-T11 facet joint (red star).*

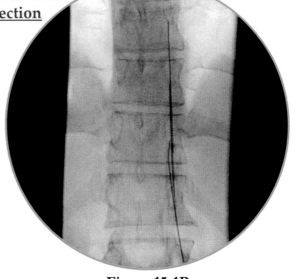

Figure 15-1B
Tilt: 0°
Oblique: 0°

A/P View. Each needle is placed at its entry point and advanced towards its respective facet joint. The needles are kept over the mid-portion of the facet joints and advanced to the inferior aspect of the pedicle at the targeted facet joint, until contact with bone.

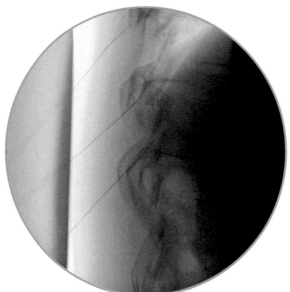

Figure 15-1C
Tilt: 0°
Oblique: 90° Right

Lateral View. The inferior most needle has been advanced into the right T10-T11 facet joint, ensuring that it stays in the posterior half of the joint to avoid vital neurovascular structures. *Note that the superior two needles have yet to be advanced into their respective joints.*

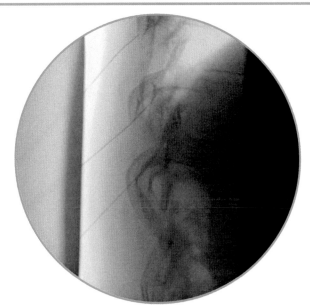

Figure 15-1D
Tilt: 0°
Oblique: 90° Right

Lateral View. After negative aspiration, administration of contrast shows intra-articular spread within the right T10-T11 facet joint.

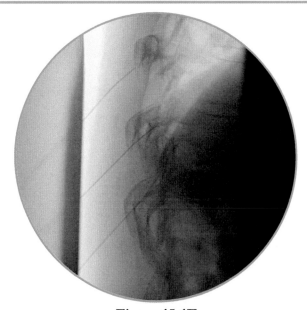

Figure 15-1E
Tilt: 0°
Oblique: 90° Right

Lateral View. The middle needle has been advanced into the right T9-T10 facet joint, ensuring that it stays in the posterior half of the joint to avoid vital neurovascular structures.

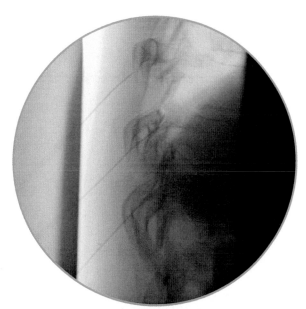

Figure 14-1F
Tilt: 0°
Oblique: 90° Right

Lateral View. After negative aspiration, administration of contrast shows intra-articular spread within the right T9-T10 facet joint.

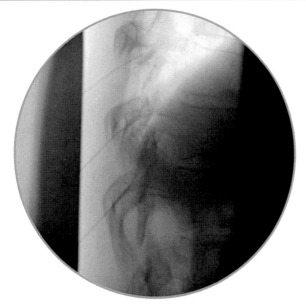

Figure 15-1G
Tilt: 0°
Oblique: 90° Right

Lateral View. The superior needle has been advanced into the right T8-T9 facet joint, ensuring that it stays in the posterior half of the joint to avoid vital neurovascular structures.

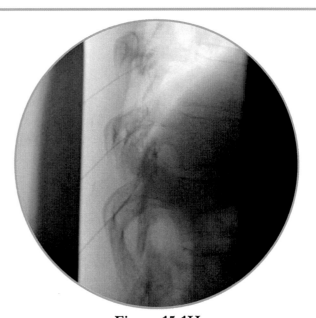

Figure 15-1H
Tilt: 0°
Oblique: 90° Right

Lateral View. After negative aspiration, administration of contrast shows intra-articular spread within the right T8-T9 facet joint.

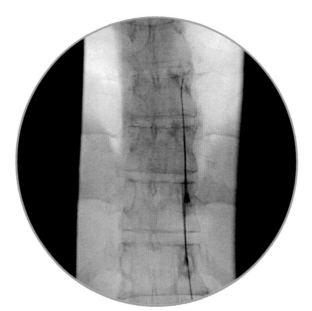

Figure 15-1I
Tilt: 0°
Oblique: 0°

A/P View. Final needle positioning after intra-articular placement within the right T8-T9, T9-T10, and T10-T11 facet joints. *Note that the needles are kept over the mid-portion of the facet joints — care should be taken to avoid medial needle placement to prevent inadvertent spinal cord injury.*

See Page 287

Chapter 16
Intercoccygeal Joint Injection

☐ Obtain a lateral view to locate the sacrococcygeal junction and targeted intercoccygeal joint. One may often be able to identify the coccygeal cornua in this view (see Figure 16-1B). The needle entry is in the midline of the patient's back and with a trajectory that matches the angle of the intercoccygeal joint. *Care should be taken to keep the needle near the midline by using intermittent A/P views as needed.*

☐ Once the needle is advanced within the joint, and after negative aspiration, contrast is administered to confirm proper intercoccygeal spread. *Of note, ensure that the needle is not advanced too far ventrally in order to avoid puncturing the bowels, which lie anterior to the sacrum.* Once appropriate spread is noted, an A/P view is obtained.

☐ In the A/P view, confirm that the needle tip remains near the midline with appropriate intercoccygeal contrast spread.

Intercoccygeal Joint Injection

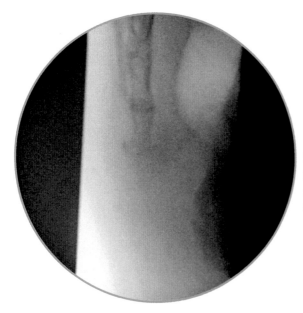

Figure 16-1A
Tilt: 0°
Oblique: 90° Right

Lateral View.   Collimation is used to focus on the sacrococcygeal junction and intercoccygeal joint. Note that the image can be made clearer by either adjusting the contrast settings or using further collimation.

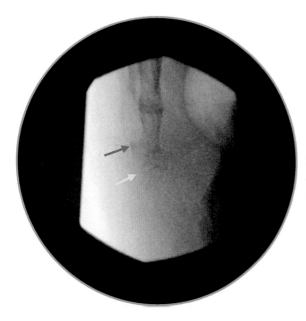

Figure 16-1B
Tilt: 0°
Oblique: 90° Right

Lateral View. Further collimation creates a clearer image – compare to Figure 16-1A. Note the coccygeal cornu (blue arrow) and intercoccygeal joint (yellow arrow).

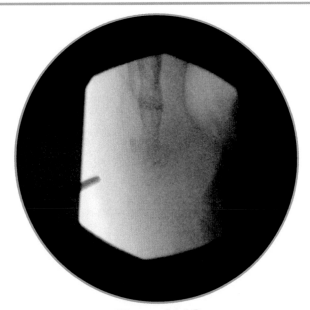

Figure 16-1C
Tilt: 0°
Oblique: 90° Right

Lateral View. Pointer showing the location of needle placement. Note how the pointer is slightly caudad to the joint space to create a needle trajectory that approximates the angle of the joint space, facilitating easier entry into the intercoccygeal joint.

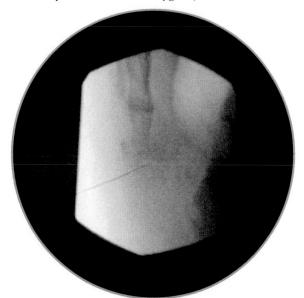

Figure 16-1D
Tilt: 0°
Oblique: 90° Right

Lateral View. Needle placement within the intercoccygeal joint. *Ensure that the needle is not advanced too far anteriorly, as the bowels lie ventral to the sacrum.*

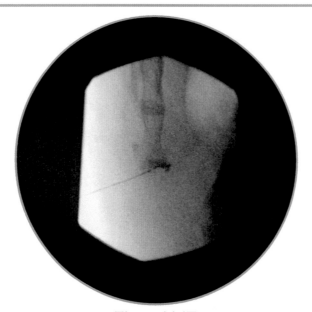

Figure 16-1E
Tilt: 0°
Oblique: 90° Right

Lateral View. After negative aspiration, administration of contrast shows spread within the intercoccygeal joint.

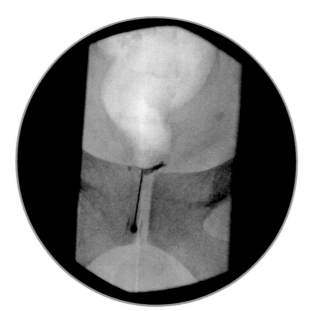

Figure 16-1F
Tilt: 0°
Oblique: 0°

A/P View. Note the spread of contrast outlining the intercoccygeal joint space in this view.

See Page 298

Chapter 17
Neuromodulation (Thoracolumbar)

- Obtain an A/P view to identify the targeted interspace to be entered. At this level, apply oblique rotation as needed to place the spinous process in the midline (i.e., "true" A/P), and cephalocaudal tilting as needed (typically caudal tilt) to square the endplates (see page 226 for further discussion). *Of note, if both endplates cannot be squared, preference should be given to squaring the SEP.* It is the author's preference to enter at the T12-L1 interspace, which has some key advantages such as a lack of significant lordosis in this region (allowing for easier needle placement & lead steering) and typically a lack of surgical hardware (which is often found at lower levels).

- For patients with average body habitus, the needle entry point should be at the medial border of the pedicle one level below the targeted interspace (i.e., 9 o'clock position for the right pedicle, 3 o'clock position for the left pedicle – *see page 224*). This will allow for a trajectory that has a needle angle of 45° or less to the skin, which is ideal for smooth lead placement and steering within the epidural space. *Patients with a thinner build will have a more superior needle entry, whereas more obese patients will have a more caudal needle entry (see pages 225 for further discussion).* It should be noted that if the needle angle is too steep, the patient may experience discomfort as the lead is subsequently passed and advanced through the needle due to more direct pressure from the lead on the dura.

- The needle is advanced from the entry point with the bevel facing down towards the midline of the targeted interspace (at an angle of 45° or less to the skin), until slight contact is made with the superior laminar edge at the targeted interspace. Next, after the needle has contacted bone, a lateral view is obtained where further needle advancement is carried out while concurrently assessing needle depth. *Of note, it is the author's preference to use a Coude needle, as this curved needle allows for additional control of mediolateral lead steerability in the subsequent steps.*

- In the lateral view, the needle is rotated 180° so the bevel is facing upward. Next, further advancement is carried out using the LOR technique. *Use the "V Technique" to ensure reliable and repeatable needle access of the epidural space without complication (see page 227 for further discussion).* Once LOR has been achieved, a lead is passed through the needle. Ensure that the lead is not advanced more than a few contacts out of the needle in the lateral view, since mediolateral lead positioning cannot be assessed in this view. Once there is confirmation that the lead has entered the posterior epidural space, an A/P view is obtained.

- In the A/P view, the lead is further steered to its final position, ensuring that it is kept in the midline, or slightly paramedian if targeting a specific side, to prevent inadvertent contact of the exiting nerve roots or placement in the anterior epidural space.

- Once the lead has been advanced to its final position in the A/P view, a lateral view is obtained once again to confirm that the entirety of the lead sits in the posterior epidural space. Impedances are checked and stimulation testing carried out as needed to ensure proper lead placement. *If needed, the leads may be adjusted to obtain adequate coverage of all typical painful areas.*

- The needles & guidewires are removed, and the leads are anchored to the skin (see page 229).

SCS
Thoracolumbar

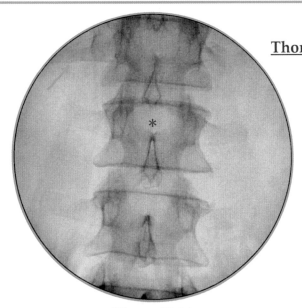

Figure 17-1A
Tilt: 0°
Oblique: 0°

A/P View. Note the targeted T12-L1 interspace (red star) and 12th rib (green arrow). The spinous process at the targeted interspace is fairly midline (i.e., "true" A/P) and the endplates squared. *Thus, no further fluoroscopic adjustments will be needed prior to needle placement.*

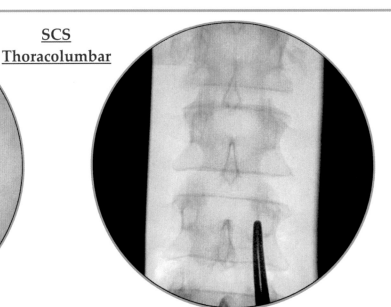

Figure 17-1B
Tilt: 0°
Oblique: 0°

A/P View. Pointer showing the location of percutaneous needle entry on the right, at the medial border of the pedicle (i.e., 9 o'clock position of the pedicle) one level below. *Note that this entry point is for an average-sized patient.*

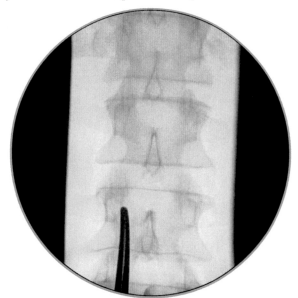

Figure 17-1C
Tilt: 0°
Oblique: 0°

A/P View. Pointer showing the location of percutaneous needle entry on the left, at the medial border of the pedicle (i.e., 3 o'clock position of the pedicle) one level below. *Note that this entry point is for an average-sized patient.*

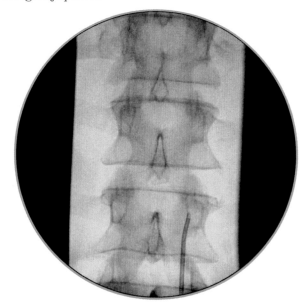

Figure 17-1D
Tilt: 0°
Oblique: 0°

A/P View. Needle entry on the right, with a planned trajectory towards the targeted T12-L1 interspace. *Note the curve of the Coude needle.*

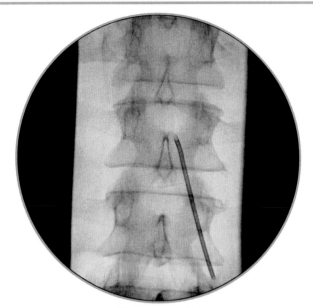

Figure 17-1E
Tilt: 0°
Oblique: 0°

A/P View. The needle is advanced until gentle contact is made with the right superior laminar edge at L1, near midline.

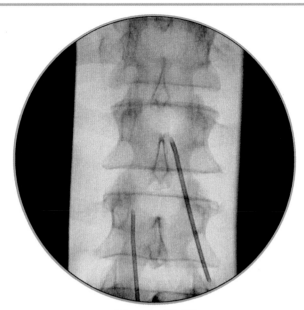

Figure 17-1F
Tilt: 0°
Oblique: 0°

A/P View. Needle entry on the left, with a planned trajectory towards the targeted T12-L1 interspace.

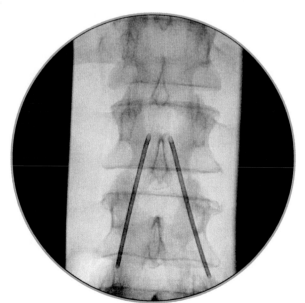

Figure 17-1G
Tilt: 0°
Oblique: 0°

A/P View. The needle is advanced until gentle contact is made with the left superior laminar edge at L1, near midline.

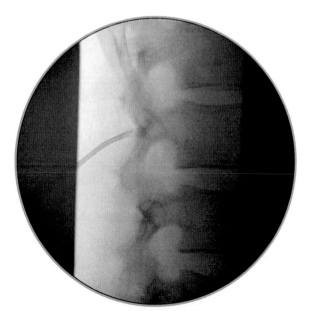

Figure 17-1H
Tilt: 0°
Oblique: 90° Right

Lateral View. Once each needle has contacted bone at the superior laminar edge in the prior view, a lateral view is obtained – *note the needle positioning in this view once the superior lamina has been contacted.* In this case, both needles are perfectly superimposed upon each other.

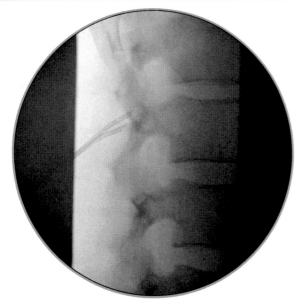

Figure 17-1I
Tilt: 0°
Oblique: 90° Right

Lateral View. The right needle is advanced just slightly, while angling the needle tip more cephalad to facilitate entry into the interspace. At this needle position, a LOR syringe is attached.

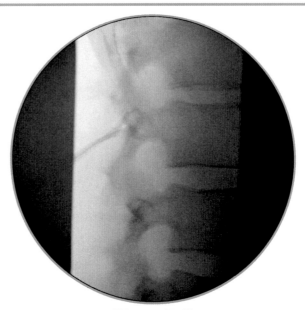

Figure 17-1J
Tilt: 0°
Oblique: 90° Right

Lateral View. The needle is rotated 180° so that the bevel is facing cephalad, allowing the lead to be steered in the cephalad direction. Next, needle advancement is carried out until LOR is achieved. Note the final position of the right needle once LOR has been attained.

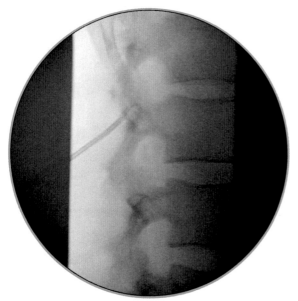

Figure 17-1K
Tilt: 0°
Oblique: 90° Right

Lateral View. Similar steps are carried out using the needle advancement technique previously described in Figures 17-1I & 17-1J. Note the final position of the needles after LOR has been attained – *in this case, the needles are perfectly superimposed upon each other.*

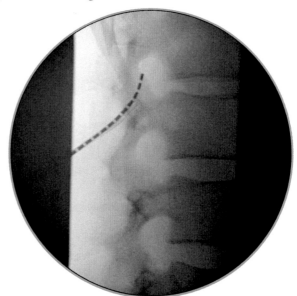

Figure 17-1L
Tilt: 0°
Oblique: 90° Right

Lateral View. A percutaneous lead is advanced through the right needle and into the posterior epidural space. Care should be taken not to advance the lead more than a few contacts into the epidural space, since mediolateral lead positioning cannot be assessed in this view.

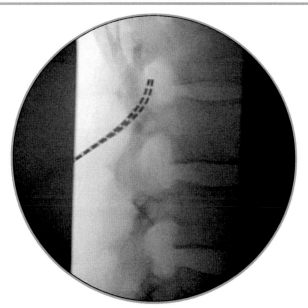

Figure 17-1M
Tilt: 0°
Oblique: 90° Right

Lateral View. A percutaneous lead is advanced through the left needle and into the posterior epidural space. Care should be taken not to advance the lead more than a few contacts into the epidural space, since mediolateral lead positioning cannot be assessed in this view.

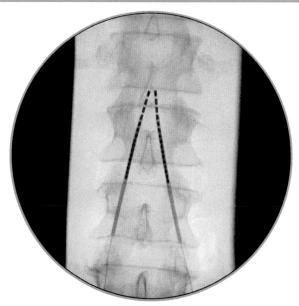

Figure 17-1N
Tilt: 0°
Oblique: 0°

A/P View. Further lead advancement is carried out in this view where mediolateral positioning can be assessed. Note how the left and right leads have entered the T12-L1 interspace and are heading towards the T12 vertebra.

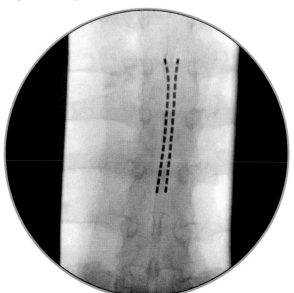

Figure 17-1O
Tilt: 0°
Oblique: 0°

A/P View. The leads are advanced towards the final position, lying in both a left and right paramedian position relative to the spinous processes. In this image, the leads have been advanced to a final position such that the tips lie at the top of T7.

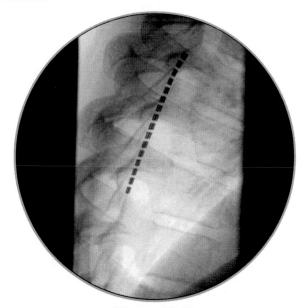

Figure 17-1P
Tilt: 0°
Oblique: 90° Right

Lateral View. Note the final position of the leads in the lateral view, with the tips at the top of T7 and the entirety of the lead lying in the posterior epidural space.

See Page 301

Additional Discussion:
Mediolateral Needle Entry – Why the Medial Border of the Pedicle?

From a mediolateral perspective, the percutaneous needle entry site is at the medial border of the pedicle one level below the targeted interspace. When the interspace is accessed near midline with this needle trajectory, the stimulator lead can be more easily steered to either a midline or paramedian position on the same side of needle placement (*see Figure 17-2A*). This entry point prevents unwanted veering of the lead towards the contralateral side, in the lateral gutter near the exiting nerve roots, or in the anterior epidural space.

If the needle is placed more medial than the medial border of the pedicle, it may encounter obstruction from the spinous process when attempting to access the targeted interspace (*see Figure 17-2B*).

If the needle is placed more lateral than the medial border of the pedicle, although the targeted interspace can be accessed near midline without obstruction, the needle trajectory created may cause subsequent lead placement to travel towards the contralateral side, or land in the gutter and subsequently the anterior epidural space (*See Figure 17-2B*).

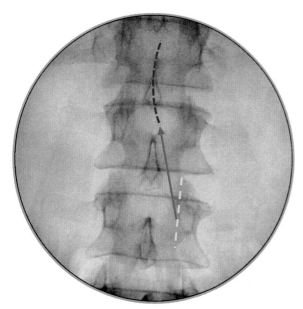

Figure 17-2A

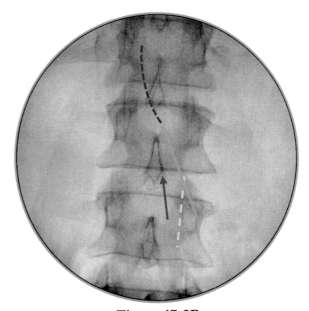

Figure 17-2B

A/P View. Note the line bisecting the medial border of the right L2 pedicle (yellow dashed line). Percutaneous needle entry at this mediolateral positioning allows the needle trajectory to access the interspace near midline and without obstruction (blue arrow). With this needle trajectory, the lead (purple dashed line) can be steered comfortably towards the midline or slightly paramedian and ipsilateral to needle placement. This prevents the lead from traveling too far laterally, avoiding the exiting nerve roots and the anterior epidural space.

A/P View. Percutaneous needle placement that is too far medial to the medial border of the pedicle (yellow dashed line) may create a needle trajectory (red arrow) that is unable to access the targeted interspace due to obstruction from the superior spinous process. Percutaneous needle placement that is too far lateral to the medial border of the pedicle may create a needle trajectory (green arrow) that causes the exiting lead (purple dashed line) to land on the contralateral side, despite multiple attempts at re-steering – this type of lead placement carries an increased risk of contacting an exiting nerve root or ending up in the anterior epidural

Additional Discussion:
Cephalocaudal Needle Entry – Why a Needle Angle of 45°?

Challenges with needle placement, interspace entry, and lead steering can be decreased significantly, if not completely avoided, with appropriate pre-procedural planning. Ideally, needle placement should be planned in such a way that it accesses the targeted interspace with a "needle to skin" angle of approximately 45° or less. This will allow easier lead steerability and less patient discomfort as the lead is placed through the needle and advanced to its final position. For patients with average body habitus, this desired angle is created with a percutaneous needle entry that is at the medial border of the pedicle <u>one vertebral level below the targeted interspace</u>. For example, if entering the T12-L1 interspace, percutaneous needle entry should be at approximately the medial border of the L2 pedicle. *Note that for patients with a larger body habitus, the desired angle is created by entering more caudal, since there will be more tissue to traverse before accessing the interspace. Similarly, for patients with a thinner body habitus, the desired angle is created by entering more cephalad, since there will be less tissue to traverse (see Figure 17-3).*

With experience, the proceduralist may become proficient at accurately estimating the percutaneous entry site by assessing patient body habitus or palpating over the spinous processes to approximate depth from skin to spinous process. However, it is the author's experience that with pre-procedural MRI analysis, challenges with needle entry, interspace access, and lead steerability, can be nearly completely eliminated. This is accomplished by reviewing the sagittal lumbar MRI and estimating the needle entry site needed to create the desired "needle to skin" angle of 45° or less – *see Figure 17-4 for an example of how to use an MRI to estimate the percutaneous needle entry site.*

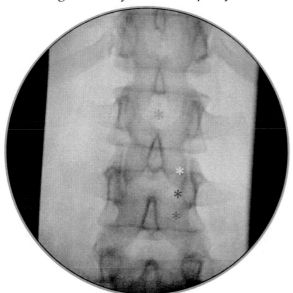

Figure 17-3
Tilt: 0°
Oblique: 0°

A/P View. Example of cephalocaudal percutaneous needle entry for accessing the T12-L1 interspace (green star) for average body habitus (red star), thinner body habitus (yellow star), and larger body habitus (blue star).

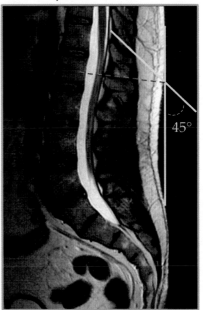

Figure 17-4
T2 Sagittal Lumbar MRI
Draw a line over the posterior skin. Next, draw a bisecting line from the T12-L1 epidural space which forms a 45° angle with the skin. Where the two lines intersect corresponds to the needle entry site, which in this case is approximately the medial border of the L2 pedicle (red dashed line) – as expected for average body habitus.

Additional Discussion:

How Fluoroscopic Tilting Affects the Needle Angle...

When setting up the fluoroscopic view for SCS needle placement, it is important to optimize visualization of the targeted interspace prior to needle placement.

1. Apply an oblique as needed to bring the spinous process at the desired interspace in the midline and equidistant between the pedicles. *For example, if targeting the T12-L1 interspace, the L1 spinous process should be brought to the midline using oblique adjustments as needed (compare Figure 17-5 to the fluoroscopically adjusted Figure 17-6 – left oblique applied).*

2. Apply cephalocaudal tilting as needed to square the endplates at the targeted interspace. *For example, if targeting the T12-L1 interspace, the L1 endplates should be squared since this will be the location of the visualized interspace. If only one endplate can be squared, preference should be given to squaring the SEP. In the lower thoracic and upper lumbar region, often a caudal tilt is needed to square the SEP given the natural curvature of the spine in this region (compare Figure 17-5 to the fluoroscopically adjusted Figure 17-6 – caudal tilt applied).*

If placing a needle *AFTER* applying a cephalocaudal tilt to square the endplates, the following principles should be understood:

☐ *First and Foremost...* for the average body habitus, placing the needle one level below the interspace *(at the medial border of the pedicle)* will create the desired angle (see page 225).

☐ If the needle is placed at the same location (i.e., one level below and at the medial border of the pedicle) <u>AFTER applying a caudal tilt</u> to square the endplates, the needle angle created will be less than 45°. *In patients with a thinner body habitus, if the angle becomes too shallow, one may not be able to access the epidural space. In such a scenario, the caudal fluoroscopic tilting needed to square the endplates will necessitate a more cephalad needle entry.*

☐ If the needle is placed at the same location (i.e., one level below at the medial border of the pedicle) <u>AFTER applying a cephalad tilt</u> to square the endplates, the needle angle created will be more than 45°. *Thus, cephalad tilting may necessitate a more caudad needle entry.*

Figure 17-5 **Figure 17-6**

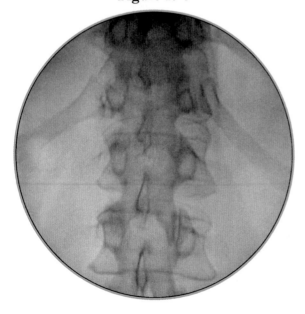
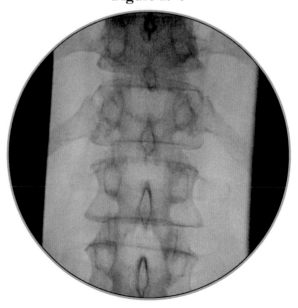

Additional Discussion:
Dr. Singh's "V Technique" for Reliable & Safe Epidural Access

It is important that the proceduralist has an understanding of the expected location of the needle tip when loss of resistance (LOR) is to be achieved. This understanding allows the proceduralist to avoid unsafe needle advancement that may lead to a dural puncture or neural compromise. By using the described "V technique" (see Figures 17-7A & 17-7B), needle tip location for epidural access can be predicted and achieved safely, in a reliable and repeatable manner...

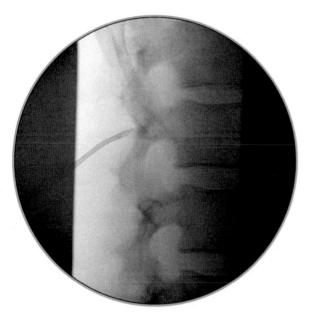

Figure 17-7A
Tilt: 0°
Oblique: 90° Right

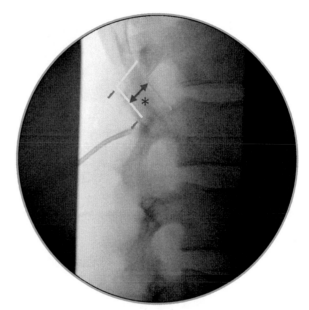

Figure 17-7B
Tilt: 0°
Oblique: 90° Right

Lateral View. The needle is seen to be touching the superior laminar edge of L1.

Note that just superior to the needle tip, the T12 IAP and L1 SAP form a sideways "V" *(see Figure 17-7B for further explanation).*

Lateral View. Figure 17-7A reproduced. Note the sideways "V" formed by the IAP and SAP superior to the needle tip, both anteriorly (green lines) and posteriorly (yellow lines).

The needle trajectory for accessing the epidural space should be in between the blue hash marks – preferably exactly in the middle.

LOR can be expected somewhere in between the inferior legs of the anterior and posterior "V" *(red double arrow).* In patients without significant LF hypertrophy, LOR will be attained near the middle of this region *(purple star)* – See Figure 17-8.

Of note, during needle advancement, if the needle tip reaches the inferior leg of the anterior "V" and LOR has still not been obtained, do NOT advance any further to avoid a dural puncture. Instead, obtain an A/P view to assess the mediolateral positioning of the needle, and ensure sure that the needle has not veered too far lateral.

Additional Discussion:
Dr. Singh's "V Technique" Continued...

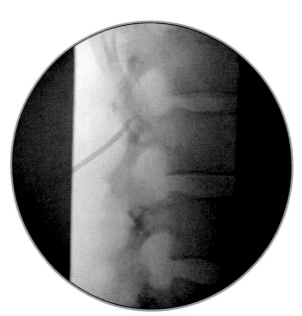

Figure 17-8
Tilt: 0°
Oblique: 90° Right

Lateral View. In this image, LOR has been achieved.

Note the needle trajectory relative to the inferior leg of the posterior "V" (compare to the points discussed in Figure 17-7B).

Also note the location of the needle tip when LOR has been achieved relative to the inferior leg of both the posterior and anterior "V" (compare to the points discussed in Figure 17-7B).

The needle tip should never be advanced beyond the inferior leg of the anterior "V".

Additional Discussion:
Anchoring SCS Trial Leads Without Sutures

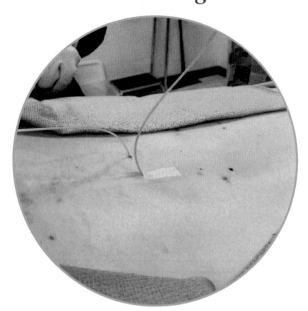

Figure 17-9A

Steri-Strips™ 1/8" x 3" are cut in half so that they are 1/8" by 1.5". Next, one cut Steri-Strip™ is placed such that half is on the skin (superior to the lead) and the other half is on the lead itself – *the lead should be in the middle of the Steri-Strip™ width-wise for a secure attachment.*

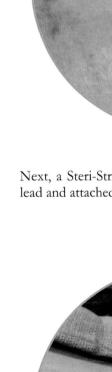

Figure 17-9B

Next, a Steri-Strip™ is similarly placed inferior to the lead and attached to the previously placed Steri-Strip.

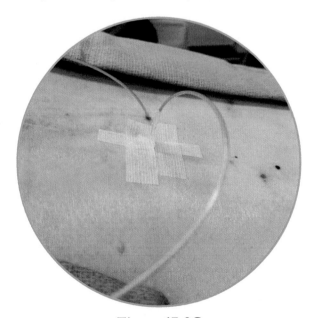

Figure 17-9C

Steri-Strips™ are placed horizontally over the skin and on top of the previously placed Steri-Strips™, both above and below the lead. *Note that the Steri-Strips™ should be hugging against the lead for a secure attachment.*

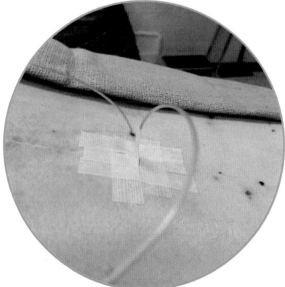

Figure 17-9D

Finally, two more Steri-Strips™ are placed vertically over the skin on top of the previously placed horizontal Steri-Strips™. This creates a crisscross type pattern that secures the lead to the skin without the need for sutures.

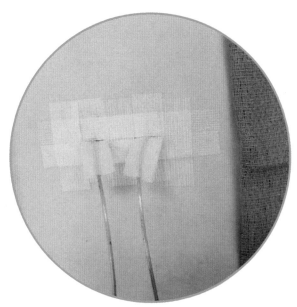

Figure 17-9E

Note the appearance after all Steri-Strips™ have been placed over each lead using the previously outlined steps.

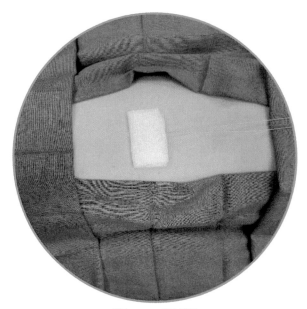

Figure 17-9F

After securing each lead with the Steri-Strips™, a 4"x4" Gauze is folded in half and placed over the Steri-Strips™.

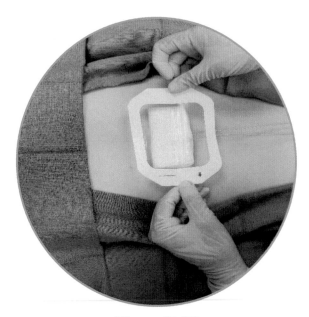

Figure 17-9G

A Tegaderm (4" x 4.75") is placed over the Gauze.

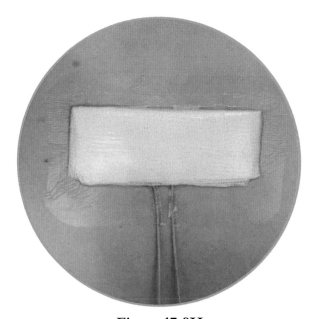

Figure 17-9H

Note the final appearance after anchoring and securing the leads to the skin using the previously described steps.

Chapter 18
Neuromodulation (Cervicothoracic)

- Obtain an A/P view to identify the targeted interspace to be entered, which often is C7-T1 or T1-T2 for cervical lead placement. Apply oblique rotation as needed to keep the spinous process at the targeted interspace in the midline (i.e., "true" A/P). Apply cephalocaudal tilting as needed to square the endplates. *If both endplates cannot be squared, preference should be given to squaring the SEP.*

- For patients with average body habitus, the needle entry point should be at the medial border of the pedicle one level below (i.e., 9 o'clock position for the right pedicle, 3 o'clock position for the left pedicle). This will allow for a needle trajectory that has an angle of 45° or less to the skin, which is ideal for smooth lead placement and steering within the epidural space. It should be noted that if the needle angle is too steep, the patient may experience discomfort with lead placement due to more direct pressure on the dura as the lead passes through the needle and is advanced. *Patients with a thinner build will have a more superior needle entry, whereas more obese patients will have a more caudal needle entry (see pages 225-226 for further discussion)*

- The needle is advanced from the entry point with the bevel facing down towards the midline of the targeted interspace (at an angle of 45° or less to the skin), until slight contact is made with the superior laminar edge at the targeted interspace. *It is the author's preference to use a Coude needle, as this curved needle allows for additional control of mediolateral lead steerability. However, some may find that the use of a straight needle is easier for entering the epidural space due to a smaller interspace in the cervicothoracic region compared to the thoracolumbar region.* After contact with bone, a contralateral oblique (CLO) view is obtained where further needle advancement is carried out while assessing needle depth. *A CLO view is preferred to a lateral view, given the potential for the shoulders obstructing clear visualization of the needle tip in the lower cervical region.*

- In the CLO view, the needle is rotated 180° so the bevel is facing upward. Next, further advancement is carried out using the LOR technique (see Chapter 6 for procedural tips on cervical interspace entry using the CLO view and the VILL). Once LOR has been achieved, a lead is passed through the needle. Ensure that the lead is not advanced more than a few contacts out of the needle, as mediolateral lead positioning cannot be assessed in this view. Once there is confirmation that the lead is entering the posterior epidural space, an A/P view is obtained.

- In the A/P view, the lead is steered to its final position, ensuring that the lead is kept in the midline, or paramedian, to prevent inadvertent contact of the exiting nerve roots or placement in the anterior epidural space.

- Once the lead has been advanced to its final position in the A/P view, a final lateral and/or CLO view is also obtained to confirm that the entirety of the lead sits in the posterior epidural space. Impedances are checked and stimulation testing carried out as needed to ensure proper lead placement. *If needed, the leads may be adjusted to obtain adequate coverage of all painful areas.*

- The needles and guidewires are removed, and the leads are anchored to the skin (see pages 229-230).

<u>SCS</u>
<u>Cervicothoracic</u>

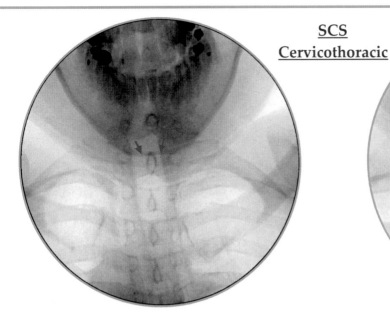

Figure 18-1A
Tilt: 10° Cephalad
Oblique: 0°

A/P View. For a planned C7-T1 interspace entry, a cephalad tilt is applied to better square the T1 SEP (red arrows).

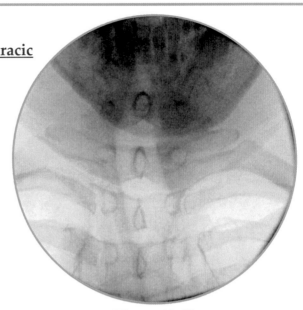

Figure 18-1B
Tilt: 10° Cephalad
Oblique: 3° Right

A/P View. A very slight right oblique is applied to bring the T1 spinous process more midline and equidistant between the pedicles ('true" A/P). *Compare the T1 spinous process position in this view to Figure 18-1A.*

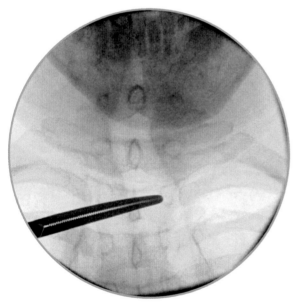

Figure 18-1C
Tilt: 10° Cephalad
Oblique: 3° Right

A/P View.   Pointer showing the location of percutaneous needle entry one level below the targeted interspace and at the medial border of the right T2 pedicle (9 o'clock position).

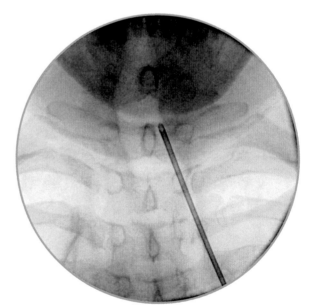

Figure 18-1D
Tilt: 10° Cephalad
Oblique: 3° Right

A/P View.   Needle placement with the trajectory towards the C7-T1 interspace, and near midline. The needle tip is advanced no further than the T1 laminar edge, and until gentle contact with bone.

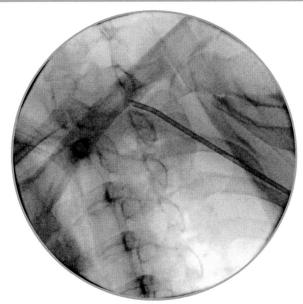

Figure 18-1E
Tilt: 10° Cephalad
Oblique: 50° Left

Contralateral Oblique View. After gentle contact with bone, the needle is advanced just slightly, while angling the needle tip more cephalad to facilitate entry into the interspace. At this needle position (dorsal to the VILL – *see Chapter 6 for further discussion*), attach a LOR syringe.

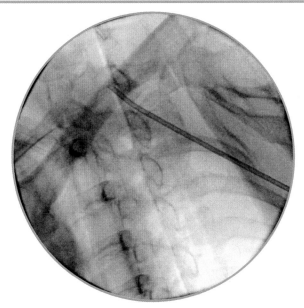

Figure 18-1F
Tilt: 10° Cephalad
Oblique: 50° Left

Contralateral Oblique View. The needle is rotated 180° so that the bevel is facing cephalad, allowing the lead to be steered in the cephalad direction. Next, needle advancement is carried out until LOR is achieved – just anterior to the VILL.

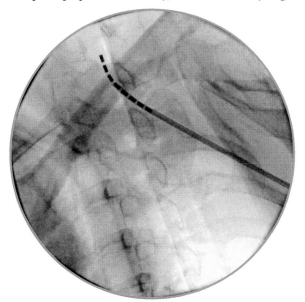

Figure 18-1G
Tilt: 10° Cephalad
Oblique: 50° Left

Contralateral Oblique View. A lead is placed through the needle and advanced into the epidural space. Note that the lead is not advanced beyond a few contacts out of the needle, since mediolateral positioning cannot be assessed in this view. Next, an A/P view is obtained.

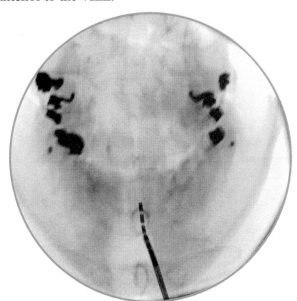

Figure 18-1H
Tilt: 10° Cephalad
Oblique: 0°

A/P View. The lead is seen to be just a few contacts out of the needle tip. The lead should be steered to its final position in this view, where mediolateral positioning can be seen. *Care should be taken to keep the lead near the midline, in order to maintain it in the posterior epidural space.*

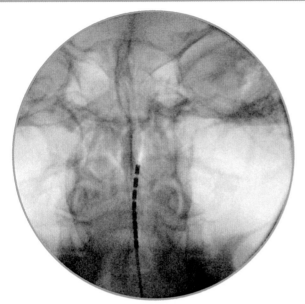

Figure 18-1I
Tilt: 10° Cephalad
Oblique: 0°

A/P View. The lead is steered to the top of C2. Note that the lead is placed in a right paramedian position, to target the patient's symptomatic side.

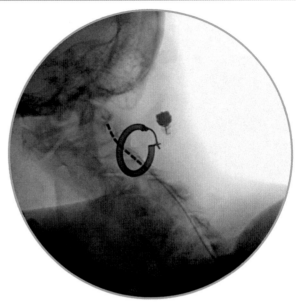

Figure 18-1J
Tilt: 10° Cephalad
Oblique: 50° Left

Contralateral Oblique View. Note the final positioning of the lead at the top of C2 in this view. Also, note the patient's earring overlying the lead. *One should consider removing all jewelry prior to beginning the procedure to provide fluoroscopic views free of visual obstruction.*

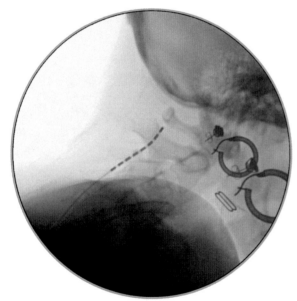

Figure 18-1K
Tilt: 0°
Oblique: 90° Right

Lateral View. Note the final positioning of the lead at the top of C2 in this view.

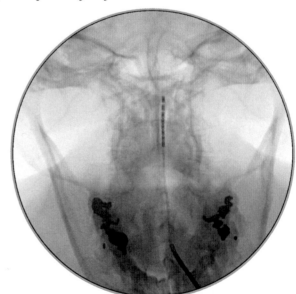

Figure 18-1L
Tilt: 0°
Oblique: 0°

A/P View. After removing the collimation, note the final positioning of the lead at the top of C2.

See Page 300

Additional Discussion:
Cervical Lead Placement with Thoracolumbar Entry

Placement of a cervical lead can also be accomplished by entering in the thoracolumbar interspace and steering cephalad, similar to the placement techniques discussed in Chapter 17. If entering in the thoracolumbar region for cervical lead placement, a longer lead (e.g., 70 cm) will be required.

Below is an example of using the thoracolumbar percutaneous entry approach for placement of one thoracic (50 cm) and two cervical (70 cm) leads.

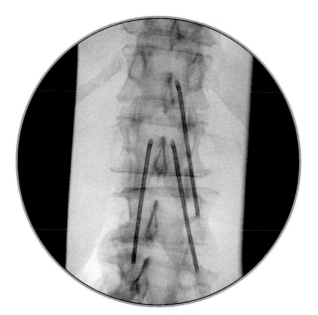

Figure 18-2A
Tilt: 0°
Oblique: 0°

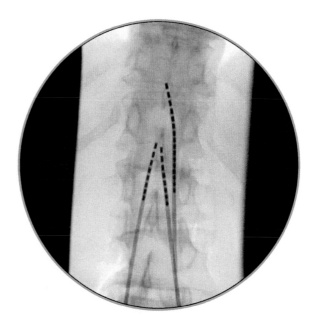

Figure 18-2B
Tilt: 0°
Oblique: 0°

A/P View. Using the steps previously described in Chapter 17, the needles are placed at the medial border of the pedicle one level below the targeted interspace. In this case, the superior needle will be used for placement of the thoracic lead (T11-T12 interspace entry), and the inferior needles will be used for placement of the two cervical leads (T12-L1 interspace entry).

A/P View. Each lead has been placed into the epidural space. The two inferior 8 contact leads will be steered into the upper cervical spine, and the superior 16 contact lead will be steered into the mid thoracic spine.

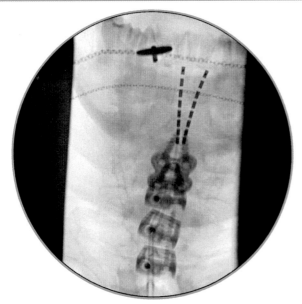

Figure 18-2C
Tilt: 0°
Oblique: 0°

A/P View. Note the final positioning of the cervical leads, lying in a paramedian position on each side.

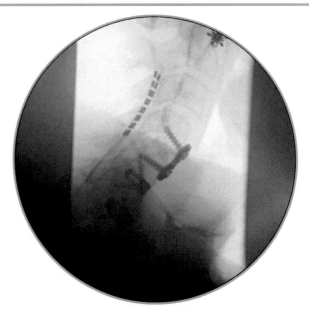

Figure 18-2D
Tilt: 0°
Oblique: 90° Right

Lateral View. Note the final positioning of the cervical leads in the posterior epidural space, with the tips at the C2-C3 intervertebral level.

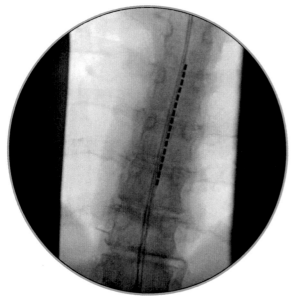

Figure 18-2E
Tilt: 0°
Oblique: 0°

A/P View. Note the final positioning of the thoracic lead at the top of T7, lying a in a midline to slightly right paramedian position.

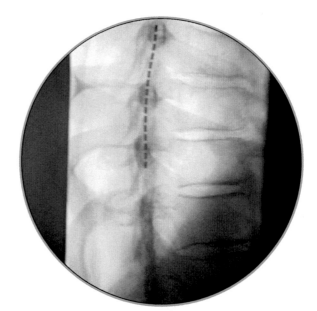

Figure 18-2F
Tilt: 0°
Oblique: 90° Right

Lateral View. Note the final positioning of the thoracic lead in the posterior epidural space.

See Page 302

Chapter 19
Glenohumeral Intra-Articular Joint Injection

- With the patient in the supine position, and with the palm of the hand facing up, obtain a P/A view to identify the glenohumeral joint. For the left shoulder, the needle is placed coaxially anywhere from the 10 o'clock to 12 o'clock position over the humeral head. For the right shoulder, the needle is placed coaxially anywhere from the 12 o'clock to 2 o'clock position over the humeral head. By using this approach, and not entering the actual articulating surface, one may avoid potential damage to the joint cartilage.

- The needle is advanced until contact is made with the humeral head. After contact with bone, it is helpful to "wiggle" a bent needle tip to ensure that it is firmly under the capsule.

- Next, after negative aspiration, contrast is administered to ensure subcapsular spread and along the joint line.

Left Shoulder Joint Injection

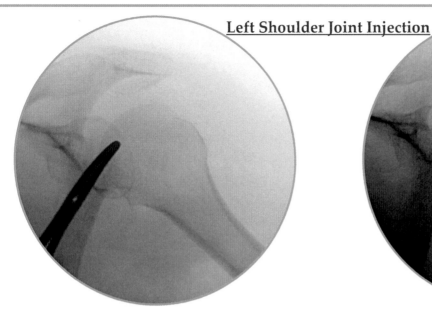

Figure 19-1A
Tilt: 0°
Oblique: 0°

P/A View.   Pointer showing the location of needle placement over the 12 o'clock position of the left humeral head.

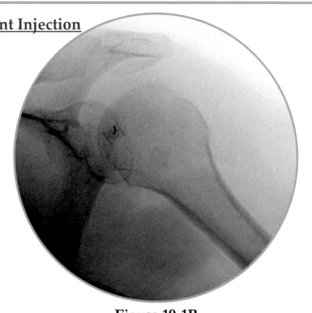

Figure 19-1B
Tilt: 0°
Oblique: 0°

P/A View.   Coaxial needle placement near the 12 o'clock position of the humeral head. After contact with bone, the needle is rotated and "wiggled" to get the tip firmly under the capsule of the joint.

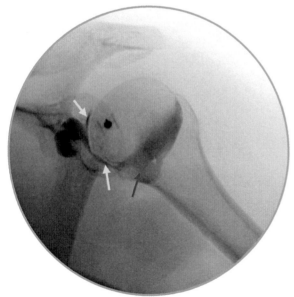

Figure 19-1C
Tilt: 0°
Oblique: 0°

P/A View.   After negative aspiration, contrast is administered showing subcapsular spread (red arrow) and spread along the joint line (yellow arrows).

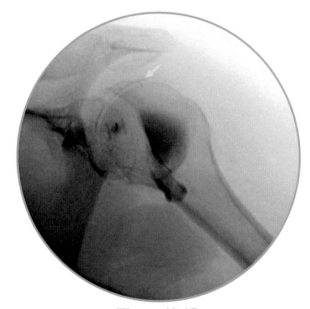

Figure 19-1D
Tilt: 0°
Oblique: 0°

P/A View. After injection of the medication solution, note the further spread of contrast under the joint capsule and more diffusely along the joint line (yellow arrow) – confirming intra-articular spread.

See Page 304

Chapter 20
Acromioclavicular Intra-Articular Joint Injection

☐ With the patient in the supine position, obtain a P/A view to identify the acromioclavicular (AC) joint. *A slight ipsilateral oblique may be used to further open the joint.*

☐ The needle is advanced coaxially until it is seated within the joint. Of note, often a subtle increase in resistance can be felt as the needle enters the joint.

☐ Next, after negative aspiration, contrast is administered to ensure proper intra-articular spread.

Right AC Joint Injection

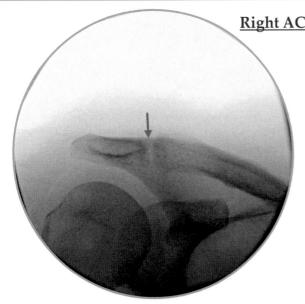

Figure 20-1A
Tilt: 0°
Oblique: 0°

P/A View. Note the right AC joint (blue arrow).

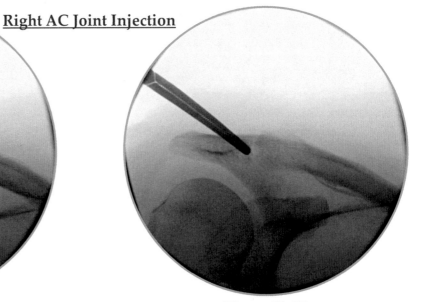

Figure 20-1B
Tilt: 5° Left
Oblique: 0°

P/A View. Applying a slight ipsilateral oblique can assist in further opening the joint. Pointer at the location of the right AC joint.

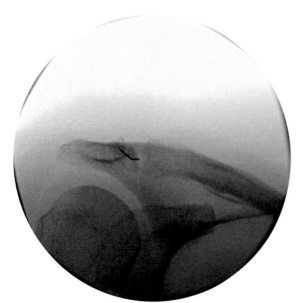

Figure 20-1C
Tilt: 5° Left
Oblique: 0°

P/A View. Coaxial needle placement within the right AC joint. *Often a subtle increase in resistance can be felt once the needle enters the joint.*

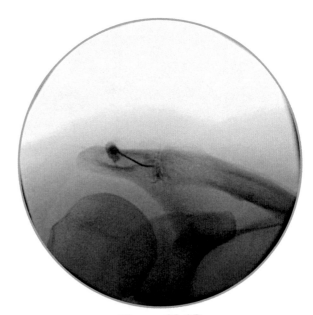

Figure 20-1D
Tilt: 0°
Oblique: 0°

P/A View. After negative aspiration, contrast agent is administerd, showing proper intra-articular spread.

See Page 306

Chapter 21
Greater Trochanteric Bursa Injection

Method 1 *(author's preferred method)*:

☐ With the patient in the prone position, obtain an A/P view to identify the targeted greater trochanter.

☐ Next, apply an ipsilateral oblique of approximately 45°. The needle is advanced in a coaxial view towards the lateral aspect and middle portion of the greater trochanter, until contact with bone.

☐ Next, an A/P view is taken to ensure that the needle is at the lateral edge of the middle portion of the greater trochanter. If needed, small mediolateral adjustments can be made to get the needle tip at the lateral edge of the greater trochanter.

☐ After negative aspiration, contrast is administered to ensure proper spread about the greater trochanteric bursa.

Method 2:

☐ With the patient in the prone position, obtain an A/P view to identify the targeted greater trochanter. In this view, the greater trochanter is palpated and needle entry is performed from a lateral approach. The needle is advanced in a non-coaxial fashion until contact is made with bone.

> *Of note, this approach is more easily performed in thinner patients, since the greater trochanter may be difficult to palpate in those with a larger body habitus, which is one of the reasons why this is not the author's preferred approach.*

☐ After negative aspiration, contrast is administered to ensure proper spread about the greater trochanteric bursa.

Left GTB Injection
Method 1

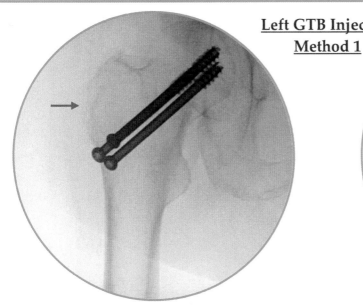

Figure 21-1A
Tilt: 0°
Oblique: 0°

A/P View. Note the left greater trochanter (blue arrow), and internal fixation hardware consisting of cannulated compression screws placed for a left femoral neck fracture.

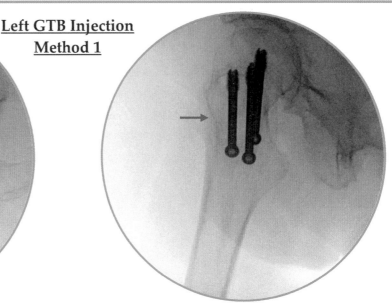

Figure 21-1B
Tilt: 0°
Oblique: 45° Left

Oblique View. An ipsilateral oblique is applied to create a needle trajectory that allows placement at the trochanteric bursa. Note the lateral edge of the greater trochanter in this view (blue arrow).

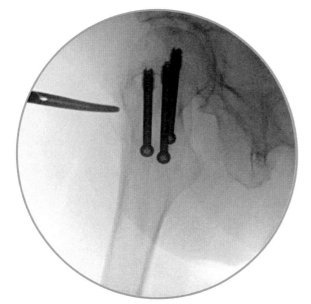

Figure 21-1C
Tilt: 0°
Oblique: 45° Left

Oblique View. Pointer showing the location of needle placement at the lateral edge of the greater trochanter.

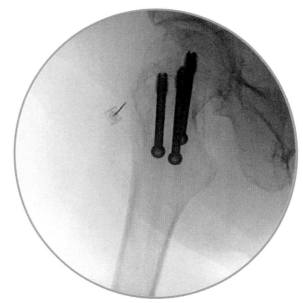

Figure 21-1D
Tilt: 0°
Oblique: 45° Left

Oblique View. Coaxial needle placement at the lateral margin of the greater trochanter. The needle is advanced until contact with bone. Next, an A/P view is obtained.

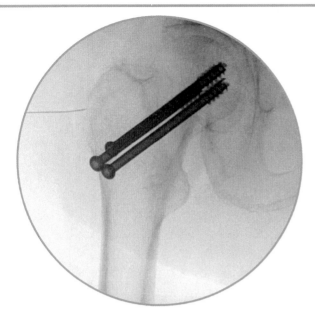

Figure 21-1E
Tilt: 0°
Oblique: 0°

A/P View. Note that in this view the needle is seen to be at the lateral margin of the left greater trochanter. *If this is not seen, the needle is adjusted mediolaterally as needed until the tip is at the lateral edge of the greater trochanter.*

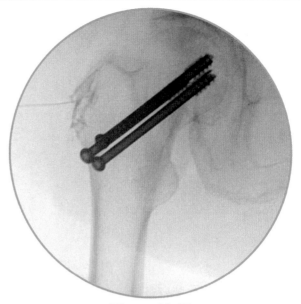

Figure 21-1F
Tilt: 0°
Oblique: 0°

A/P View. After negative aspiration, contrast is administered showing spread at the left greater trochanteric bursa.

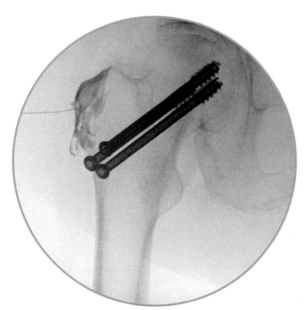

Figure 21-1G
Tilt: 0°
Oblique: 0°

A/P View. Further administration of contrast confirms spread outlining the left greater trochanteric bursa.

See Page 304

Left GTB Injection
Method 2

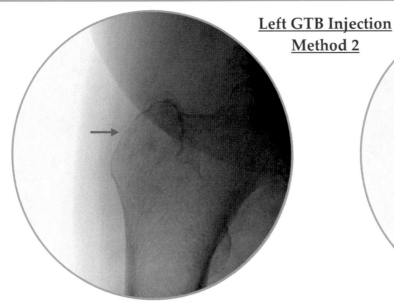

Figure 21-2A
Tilt: 0°
Oblique: 0°

A/P View. Note the left greater trochanter (blue arrow).

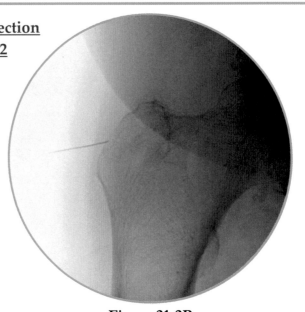

Figure 21-2B
Tilt: 0°
Oblique: 0°

A/P View. The greater trochanter is identified through direct palpation laterally. Once felt, the needle is placed at this location and advanced in a non-coaxial fashion using fluoroscopic guidance, until contact with the lateral margin of the greater trochanter.

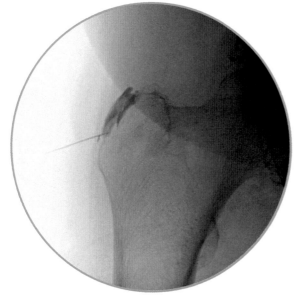

Figure 21-2C
Tilt: 0°
Oblique: 0°

A/P View. After negative aspiration, contrast is administered showing spread at the left greater trochanteric bursa.

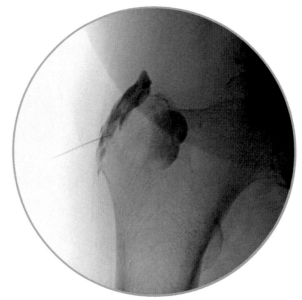

Figure 21-2D
Tilt: 0°
Oblique: 0°

A/P View. Further administration of contrast confirms spread outlining the left greater trochanteric bursa.

Chapter 22
Hip Intra-Articular Joint Injection

☐ With the patient in the supine position, a P/A view is taken to identify the targeted femoral head and neck. The needle is advanced in a coaxial view towards the lateral aspect of the femoral neck, until contact is made with bone. By using this approach, and not entering the actual articulating surface, one may avoid potential damage to the joint cartilage.

☐ After contact with bone, it is helpful to "wiggle" a bent needle tip to ensure that it is firmly under the hip joint capsule.

☐ Next, after negative aspiration, contrast is administered to ensure subcapsular spread and along the joint line.

   The proceduralist can often see a "halo" as the contrast encircles the femoral head/neck junction (see Figure 22-1C).

Left Hip Joint Injection

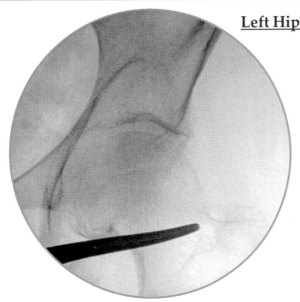

Figure 22-1A
Tilt: 0°
Oblique: 0°

P/A View. Pointer showing the location of needle placement over the lateral aspect of the femoral neck.

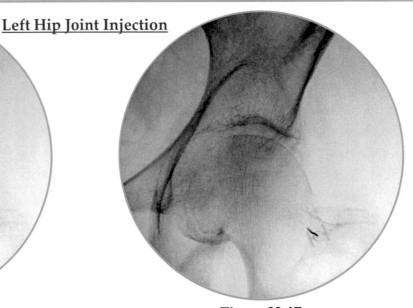

Figure 22-1B
Tilt: 0°
Oblique: 0°

P/A View. Coaxial needle placement at the lateral aspect of the femoral neck, until contact with bone.

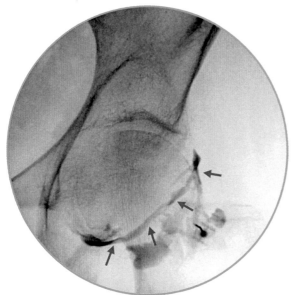

Figure 22-1C
Tilt: 0°
Oblique: 0°

P/A View. After negative aspiration, contrast is administered. Note the subcapsular spread and "halo sign" around the femoral head/neck junction (red arrows).

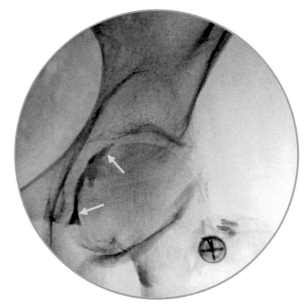

Figure 22-1D
Tilt: 0°
Oblique: 0°

P/A View. After administration of the medication solution, note the diffuse spread of contrast outlining the joint line (yellow arrows) – confirming intra-articular spread.

See Page 304

Chapter 23
Ischial Bursa Injection

- With the patient in the prone position, an A/P view is taken to identify the ischial tuberosity of the targeted ischium.

- The needle is advanced coaxially towards the bony prominence of the ischium at the location of the ischial bursa, until contact with bone.

- Next, after negative aspiration, contrast is administered to ensure spread at the ischial bursa.

Left Ischial Bursa Injection

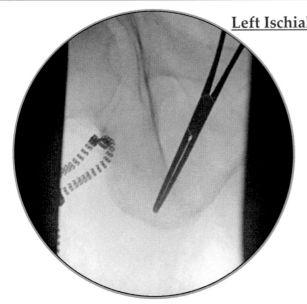

Figure 23-1A
Tilt: 0°
Oblique: 0°

A/P View. Pointer over the left ischial tuberosity.

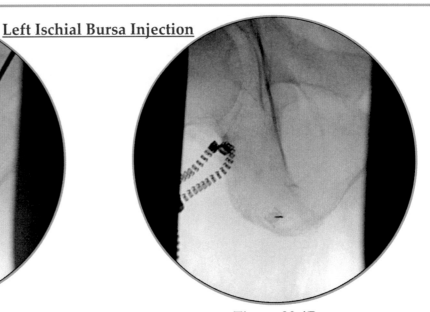

Figure 23-1B
Tilt: 0°
Oblique: 0°

A/P View. Coaxial needle placement at the left ischium, until contact with bone.

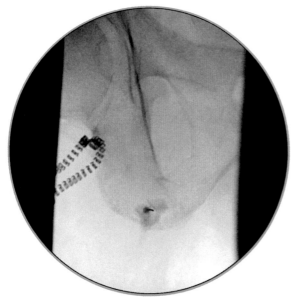

Figure 23-1C
Tilt: 0°
Oblique: 0°

A/P View. After negative aspiration, contrast is administered showing spread at the left ischial bursa.

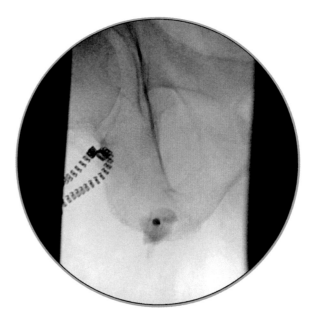

Figure 23-1D
Tilt: 0°
Oblique: 0°

A/P View. Further administration of contrast confirms spread at the left ischial bursa.

See Page 304

Chapter 24
Knee Intra-Articular Joint Injection

☐ With the patient in the supine position, a P/A view is taken to identify the targeted knee joint. The needle is advanced in the lateral aspect of the joint space, and directed towards the midline. Often, the proceduralist may feel a distinct loss of resistance once the needle is intra-articular. Alternatively, once the needle is firmly seeded in the subcutaneous tissue, the proceduralist may choose to attach a syringe with local anesthetic and inject gently as the needle is advanced towards its final destination, observing for a distinct loss of resistance.

> *The medial joint space can be entered using a similar technique as described above. However, in many cases, the medial joint space shows more degenerative change than the lateral joint space, making intra-articular needle entry more challenging from the medial approach.*

☐ After intra-articular needle placement and negative aspiration, contrast agent is administered to confirm proper intra-articular spread. This is noted with the classic "Mustache Sign," as contrast spread is seen to outline the medial and lateral joint spaces *(see Figure 24-1D)*.

Left Knee

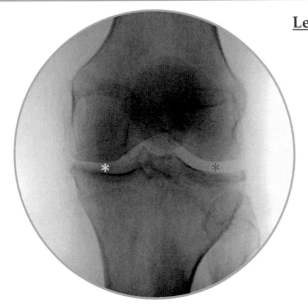

Figure 24-1A
Tilt: 0°
Oblique: 0°

P/A View. Note the lateral (blue star) and medial (yellow star) joint spaces.

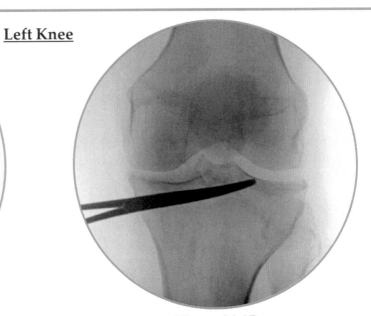

Figure 24-1B
Tilt: 0°
Oblique: 0°

P/A View. Pointer showing the location of needle placement just inferior to the lateral joint space.

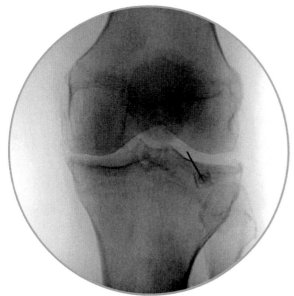

Figure 24-1C
Tilt: 0°
Oblique: 0°

P/A View. Needle placement into the lateral joint space of the left knee. The needle is advanced until a loss of resistance is felt.

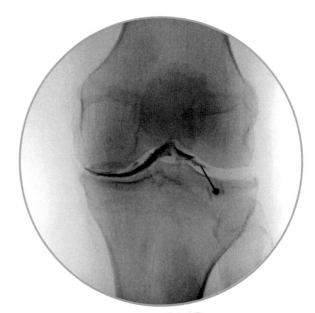

Figure 24-1D
Tilt: 0°
Oblique: 0°

P/A View. After negative aspiration, contrast is administered. Note the intra-articular spread and classic "mustache sign" spreading into the medial joint space.

See Page 304

**Bilateral Knee
Severe Osteoarthritis**

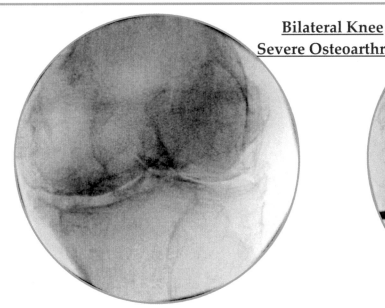

Figure 24-2A
Tilt: 0°
Oblique: 0°

P/A View. Note the severe osteoarthritis of the left knee, which is nearly bone on bone both medially and laterally.

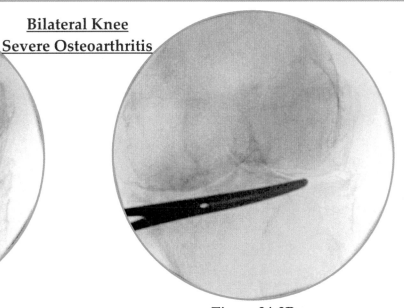

Figure 24-2B
Tilt: 0°
Oblique: 0°

P/A View. Pointer showing the location of needle placement at the lateral joint space.

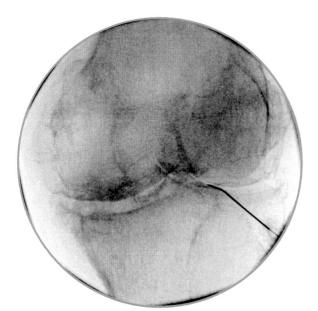

Figure 24-2C
Tilt: 0°
Oblique: 0°

P/A View. Needle placement into the lateral joint space of the left knee. The needle is advanced until a loss of resistance is felt.

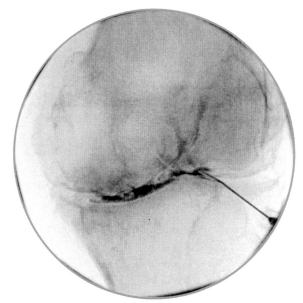

Figure 24-2D
Tilt: 0°
Oblique: 0°

P/A View. After negative aspiration, contrast is administered. Note the intra-articular spread and classic "mustache sign" spreading into the medial joint space.

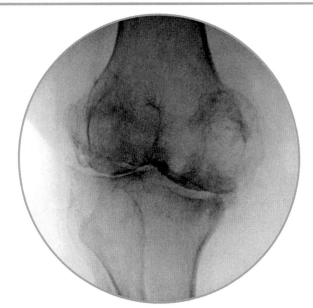

Figure 24-2E
Tilt: 0°
Oblique: 0°

P/A View. Note the severe osteoarthritis of the right knee, which is nearly bone on bone both medially and laterally.

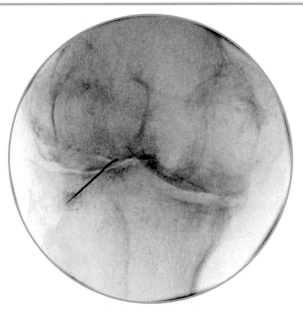

Figure 24-2F
Tilt: 0°
Oblique: 0°

P/A View. Needle placement into the lateral joint space of the right knee. The needle is advanced until a loss of resistance is felt.

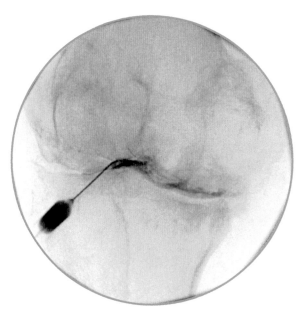

Figure 24-2G
Tilt: 0°
Oblique: 0°

P/A View.   After negative aspiration, contrast is administered. Note the intra-articular spread and classic "mustache sign" spreading into the medial joint space.

See Page 305

Chapter 25
Ganglion of Impar Injection

☐ Obtain a lateral view to locate the sacrococcygeal junction and intercoccygeal joint, as the needle can be advanced through either location for this procedure. The needle entry is in the midline of the patient's back and with a trajectory that matches the angle of the either the sacrococcygeal junction or intercoccygeal joint. *Care should be taken to keep the needle near the midline throughout advancement, and the use of intermittent A/P views should be used as needed to ensure such.*

☐ The needle is advanced until the tip is seen to be just ventral to the anterior sacrum. Care should be taken to NOT advance the needle much further than just beyond the anterior sacrum, in order to avoid puncture of the bowel contents (which lie further anterior).

☐ Next, after negative aspiration, contrast agent is administered to confirm spread anterior to the sacrum and posterior to the bowels.

☐ Finally, an A/P view is taken to confirm that the needle tip is near the midline with appropriate contrast spread.

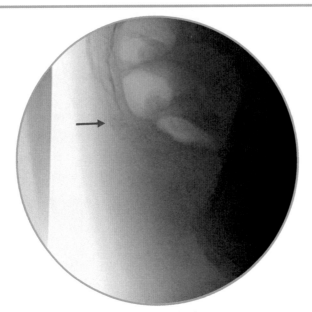

Figure 25-1A
Tilt: 0°
Oblique: 90° Right

Lateral View. Collimation is used to provide a clearer view of the sacrum and coccyx. Note the sacrococcygeal junction (red arrow).

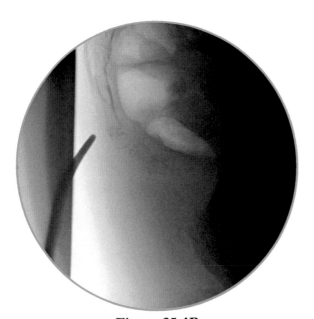

Figure 25-1B
Tilt: 0°
Oblique: 90° Right

Lateral View. Pointer showing the location of needle placement at the level of the sacrococcygeal junction.

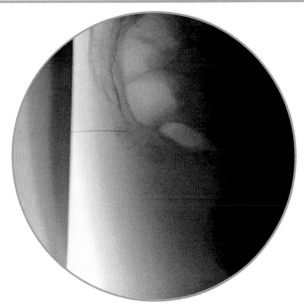

Figure 25-1C
Tilt: 0°
Oblique: 90° Right

Lateral View. Needle placement within the sacrococcygeal junction. Note that the needle still needs to be further advanced to get just anterior to the sacrum, in order to target the Ganglion of Impar – *see Figure 25-1D.*

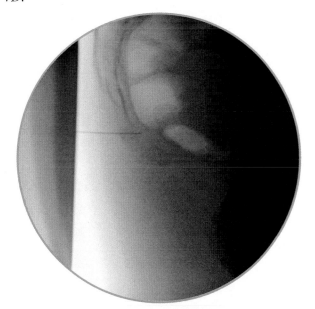

Figure 25-1D
Tilt: 0°
Oblique: 90° Right

Lateral View. Note that the needle has been advanced just ventral to the sacrum, but posterior to the bowel contents.

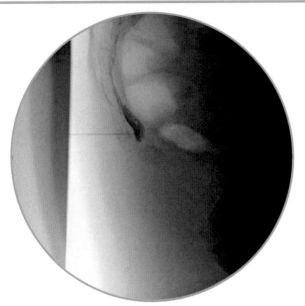

Figure 25-1E
Tilt: 0°
Oblique: 90° Right

Lateral View. After negative aspiration, contrast is administered. Note the spread anterior to the sacrum, but posterior to the bowel gas pattern – confirming spread at the Ganglion of Impar.

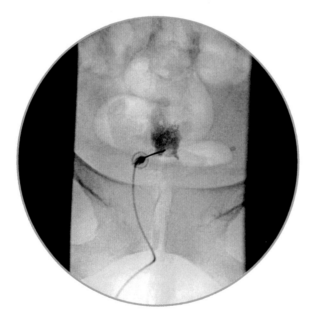

Figure 25-1F
Tilt: 0°
Oblique: 0°

A/P View. Note the midline spread of contrast in this view, outlining the location of the Ganglion of Impar.

See Page 308

Chapter 26
Piriformis Muscle Injection

☐ Obtain an A/P view to identify the location of the targeted piriformis muscle, which can be accomplished by using anatomical landmarks. The piriformis muscle is located lateral to the sacrum at approximately the S3 level and just inferior to the ipsilateral sacroiliac joint (see Figure 26-1C).

☐ The needle is placed coaxially at the location of the targeted piriformis muscle, inferior to the ipsilateral sacroiliac joint and lateral to the sacrum at approximately the S3 level. Often, a subtle increase in resistance may be felt once the needle enters the muscle. *If there is any question regarding needle depth during advancement, intermittent lateral views should be taken to assess depth.* Once the needle approaches the piriformis muscle, a lateral view is obtained.

☐ In the lateral view, the needle is further advanced until the tip is just anterior to the sacrum.

☐ After negative aspiration, contrast agent is administered to confirm spread about the piriformis muscle.

☐ Finally, an A/P view is obtained once again to confirm appropriate spread outlining the targeted piriformis muscle.

Left Piriformis

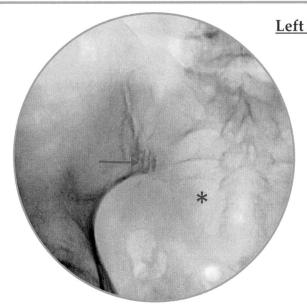

Figure 26-1A
Tilt: 0°
Oblique: 0°

A/P View. Note the left SI joint (blue arrow) and sacrum (red star). The piriformis muscle is just inferior to the SI joint and lateral to the sacrum at approximately the S3 level.

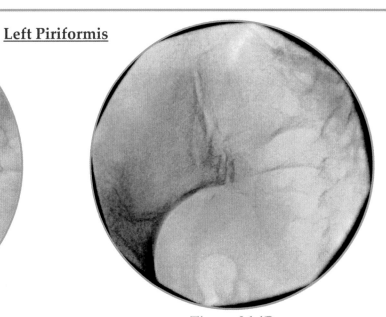

Figure 26-1B
Tilt: 0°
Oblique: 0°

A/P View. The use of collimation not only provides less radiation exposure to both the proceduralist and patient, but also allows one to focus on the targeted region.

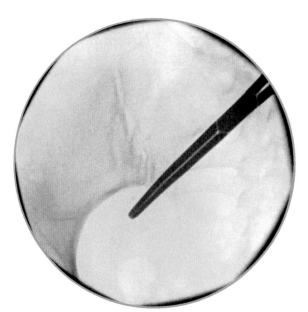

Figure 26-1C
Tilt: 0°
Oblique: 0°

A/P View. Pointer at the location of needle placement over the left piriformis muscle – just inferior to the SI joint and lateral to the sacrum at approximately the S3 level.

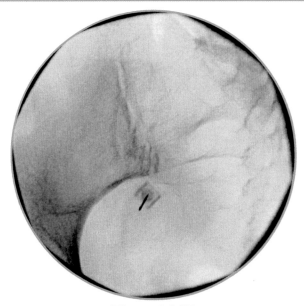

Figure 26-1D
Tilt: 0°
Oblique: 0°

A/P View. Coaxial needle placement at the left piriformis muscle. Often, when the needle enters the piriformis muscle, a subtle increase in resistance can be felt. *If there is any question as to the needle depth, intermittent lateral views should be checked.*

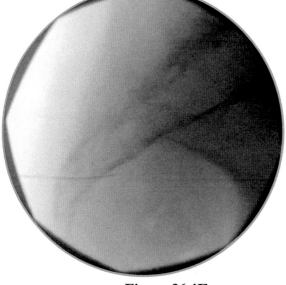

Figure 26-1E
Tilt: 0°
Oblique: 90° Right

Lateral View. The needle is advanced until the tip is just ventral to the anterior sacrum.

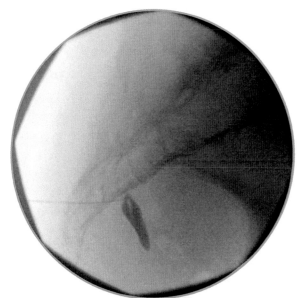

Figure 26-1F
Tilt: 0°
Oblique: 90° Right

Lateral View. After negative aspiration, contrast is administered showing spread about the piriformis muscle.

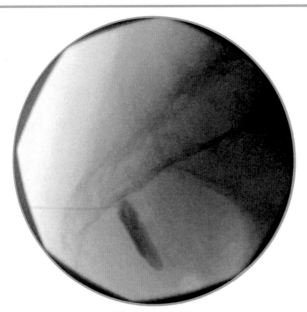

Figure 26-1G
Tilt: 0°
Oblique: 90° Right

Lateral View. Further administration of contrast confirms spread along the piriformis muscle.

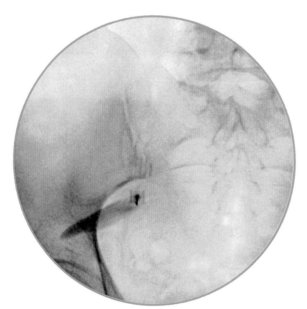

Figure 26-1H
Tilt: 0°
Oblique: 0°

A/P View. Note the contrast spread about the left piriformis muscle in this view.

See Page 310

Left Piriformis
Deconditioned Muscle

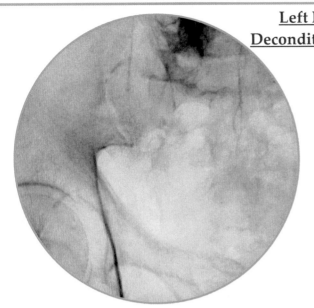

Figure 26-2A
Tilt: 0°
Oblique: 0°

A/P View. Note the left SI joint and sacrum. The piriformis muscle is located just inferior to the SI joint and lateral to the sacrum at approximately the S3 level.

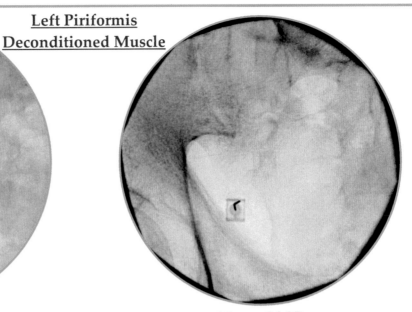

Figure 26-2B
Tilt: 0°
Oblique: 0°

A/P View. Coaxial needle placement at the left piriformis muscle. Often, when the needle enters the piriformis muscle, a subtle increase in resistance can be felt. *If there is any question as to the needle depth, intermittent lateral views should be checked.*

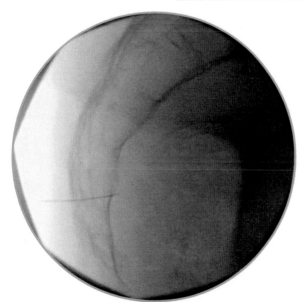

Figure 26-2C
Tilt: 0°
Oblique: 90° Right

Lateral View. The needle is advanced until the tip is just ventral to the anterior sacrum.

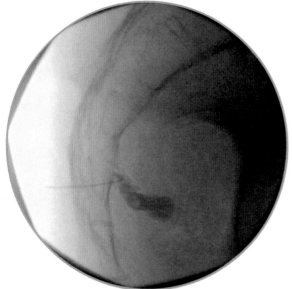

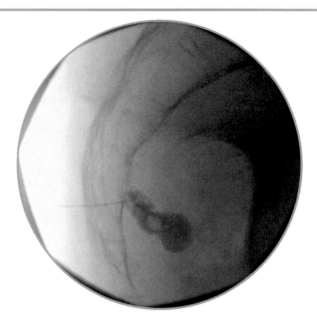

Figure 26-2D
Tilt: 0°
Oblique: 90° Right

Figure 26-2E
Tilt: 0°
Oblique: 90° Right

Lateral View. After negative aspiration, contrast is administered, showing spread about the piriformis muscle. *This is a deconditioned piriformis muscle in a fairly elderly patient.*

Lateral View. Further administration of contrast confirms spread along the piriformis muscle.

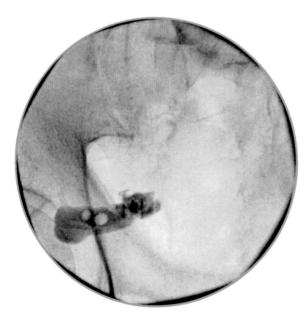

Figure 26-2F
Tilt: 0°
Oblique: 0°

A/P View. Note the contrast spread about the left piriformis muscle in this view.

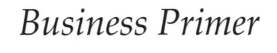

Business Primer

Chapter 27
Business Primer Introduction

"A business absolutely devoted to service will have one worry about profits. They will be embarrassingly large."

-Henry Ford

The majority of this text is focused on improving pain, function, and quality of life, by presenting best procedural practices as it relates to a myriad of interventional pain procedures – *because above all else is service to the patient*. At the core of every proceduralist should be the patient's best interest and how to hone one's procedural skills to best fulfill this interest.

Yet, in order for a practice to be successful and endure the ever changing world of healthcare, it must be run with healthy business principles in place. Unfortunately, more often than not, formal medical training does not provide the proceduralist with the necessary knowledge or business acumen needed to run a medical practice. The purpose of the subsequent chapters is not to transform the proceduralist into a business expert, but rather to provide answers to some of the fundamental questions of running a private interventional pain practice.

For example…
-How much is a vial of Methylprednisolone vs. Dexamethasone vs. Triamcinolone?
-For a given procedure, how much does it actually cost per mL to use local anesthetic?
-What is the price difference between a 3.5" vs. 5" Quincke spinal needle?
-For a given procedure, does a bilateral or two level ipsilateral approach have a higher profit margin?
-What is the actual profit margin for a given procedure when the cost of goods is accounted for?

In the following chapters, the reader will find answers to all of the above questions. In addition, for <u>every procedure described in part 1</u> of this textbook, the reader will find the corresponding current procedural terminology (CPT) code(s) needed for correct billing (with appropriate modifiers – *see Appendix B on page 312-313 for a comprehensive list*), and the exact expense & revenue analysis. For each procedure, this analysis includes:
- A breakdown of each supply used with the corresponding cost.
- A breakdown of all reimbursements (e.g., procedural, drug used, drug wasted, etc.).
- A quick snapshot summary of the total supply cost, total reimbursement, and the overall profit (see page 266 for further discussion).

***It should be noted that the supply costs presented are based off negotiated 2020 rates from various vendors (see Appendix A on page 311 for a comprehensive list of supply costs). The reimbursement presented is based off the Medicare Q4 2020 fee schedule.

The profit presented in each subsequent chapter is in the form of "Gross Profit Margin":

$$Gross\ Profit\ Margin = \frac{Revenue - Cost\ of\ Goods}{Revenue} x\ 100$$

The reasoning behind presenting *gross* profit margin is due to the fact that the variables "revenue" and "cost of goods" can be more easily compared across multiple practices. In contrast, presenting a comparison of *net* profit margin across varying practices would be much more challenging, given the higher variability of an individual practice's operating expenses (e.g., renting vs. owning equipment, renting vs. owning real estate, interest, taxes, cost of staff/employees, cost of EMR, etc.). Thus, by looking at the gross profit margin, the reader can more easily compare the revenue of a given procedure (i.e., Medicare fee schedule for a specified CPT code) and the cost of goods (i.e., cost of a specific supply) to his or her own practice.

The reimbursement and cost of goods will undoubtedly vary based off region. In addition, with respect to the cost of goods, in certain instances more favorable pricing will be seen with group purchasing organizations (GPO). Nonetheless, the data presented herein will allow the reader to use the presented information as a reference to determine both efficiencies and inefficiencies within his or her own practice. For example, there may be instances where one finds that they are overpaying significantly on a supply compared to what is presented. This can be an opportunity to reach out to a given vendor(s) to discuss efficiencies in pricing. There may be other instances where the reader finds that he or she is obtaining comparable, or perhaps even more favorable, pricing compared to what is presented, which can provide reassurance on how the practice is running.

Lastly, it is certainly understood that many readers of this text may not actually be in a private practice setting. Nonetheless, the information presented still holds significant value in enhancing the proceduralist's understanding of gross profitability for a variety of interventional pain procedures. This information may also serve to assist the proceduralist with negotiating salaries & bonuses, hiring of additional staff, or justifying additional practice expenditures.

In summary, there are two ways to increase the "Gross Profit Margin" of any given procedure – increase the revenue (which the proceduralist has little to no control over) OR decrease the cost of goods. It is the author's goal that by presenting "real world" expense and revenue analysis from a busy and efficient interventional pain practice, the reader will be able to compare, and where needed improve, the efficiency of his or her own practice.

Chapter 28

Expense & Revenue Analysis
Lumbar & Sacral
Transforaminal Epidural Steroid Injection

<u>**TFESI**</u>
<u>**Single Level (Right or Left) – Lumbar or Sacral**</u>

Expenses

	Cost:
Supplies:	
☐ Pain Pack (1)	$5.04
☐ Gloves Sterile size 7.5	$0.73
☐ Earloop Mask	$0.06
☐ Quincke (Spinal Needle) 22 Gauge 3.5" (1)	$1.08
☐ Extension Tubing (1)	$0.84
Medications:	
☐ Dexamethasone 10 mg/mL – 1 mL SDV (1)	$1.79
☐ Bupivacaine 0.25% – 10 mL SDV (1)	$1.04
☐ Omnipaque 240 mg/mL – 50 mL SDV (1)	$3.99
☐ Lidocaine 1% 50 mL MDV (5 mL)	$0.16
Total	$14.73

Medicare Reimbursement

CPT Code	Units	Modifier	Reimbursement:
64483	1	RT or LT	$230.05
J1100	10		$1.02
Q9966	1		$0.33
Q9966	49	JW	$16.17
		Total	$247.57

Total Reimbursement	**Total Supply Cost**	**Profit**
$247.57	**$14.73**	**$232.84**

Gross Profit Margin

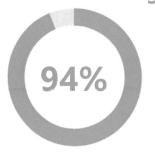

94%

<u>**TFESI**</u>
<u>**Two Level Ipsilateral (Left) – Lumbar or Sacral**</u>

Expenses

	Cost:
Supplies:	
☐ Pain Pack (1)	$5.04
☐ Gloves Sterile size 7.5	$0.73
☐ Earloop Mask	$0.06
☐ Quincke (Spinal Needle) 22 Gauge 3.5" (2)	$2.16
☐ Extension Tubing (1)	$0.84
Medications:	
☐ Dexamethasone 10 mg/mL – 1 mL SDV (2)	$3.58
☐ Bupivacaine 0.25% – 10 mL SDV (1)	$1.04
☐ Omnipaque 240 mg/mL – 50 mL SDV (1)	$3.99
☐ Lidocaine 1% 50 mL MDV (7 mL)	$0.22
Total	$17.66

Medicare Reimbursement

CPT Code	Units	Modifier	Reimbursement:
64483	1	LT	$230.05
64484	1	LT	$101.79
J1100	20		$2.05
Q9966	2		$0.66
Q9966	48	JW	$15.79
		Total	$350.34

Total Reimbursement	Total Supply Cost	Profit
$350.34	**$17.66**	**$332.68**

Gross Profit Margin

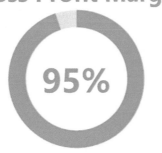

95%

<u>TFESI</u>
<u>Single Level (Bilateral) – Lumbar or Sacral</u>

Expenses

	Cost:
Supplies:	
☐ Pain Pack (1)	$5.04
☐ Gloves Sterile size 7.5	$0.73
☐ Earloop Mask	$0.06
☐ Towels Disposable 4/pack (1)	$1.86
☐ Quincke (Spinal Needle) 22 Gauge 3.5" (2)	$2.16
☐ Extension Tubing (1)	$0.84
Medications:	
☐ Dexamethasone 10 mg/mL – 1 mL SDV (2)	$3.58
☐ Bupivacaine 0.25% – 10 mL SDV (1)	$1.04
☐ Omnipaque 240 mg/mL – 50 mL SDV (1)	$3.99
☐ Lidocaine 1% 50 mL MDV (7 mL)	$0.22
Total	$19.52

Medicare Reimbursement

CPT Code	Units	Modifier		Reimbursement:
64483	1	50		$345.08
J1100	20			$2.05
Q9966	2			$0.66
Q9966	48	JW		$15.79
			Total	$363.58

Total Reimbursement	**Total Supply Cost**	**Profit**
$363.58	$19.52	$344.06

Gross Profit Margin

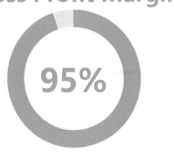

95%

<u>**TFESI**</u>
<u>**Three Level Ipsilateral (Right or Left) – Lumbar or Sacral**</u>

Expenses

		Cost:
Supplies:		
☐	Pain Pack (1)	$5.04
☐	Gloves Sterile size 7.5	$0.73
☐	Earloop Mask	$0.06
☐	Towels Disposable 4/pack (1)	$1.86
☐	Quincke (Spinal Needle) 22 Gauge 3.5" (3)	$3.24
☐	Extension Tubing (1)	$0.84
Medications:		
☐	Dexamethasone 10 mg/mL – 1 mL SDV (2)	$3.58
☐	Bupivacaine 0.25% – 10 mL SDV (1)	$1.04
☐	Omnipaque 240 mg/mL – 50 mL SDV (1)	$3.99
☐	Lidocaine 1% 50 mL MDV (7 mL)	$0.22
	Total	$20.60

Medicare Reimbursement

CPT Code	Units	Modifier		Reimbursement:
64483	1	RT or LT		$230.05
64484	2	RT or LT		$203.58
J1100	20			$2.05
Q9966	3			$0.99
Q9966	47	JW		$15.56
			Total	$452.23

Total Reimbursement	Total Supply Cost	Profit
$452.23	**$20.60**	**$431.63**

Gross Profit Margin

95%

TFESI
Two Level (Bilateral + Right) – Lumbar or Sacral

Expenses

	Cost:
Supplies:	
☐ Pain Pack (1)	$5.04
☐ Gloves Sterile size 7.5	$0.73
☐ Earloop Mask	$0.06
☐ Towels Disposable 4/pack (1)	$1.86
☐ Quincke (Spinal Needle) 22 Gauge 3.5" (3)	$3.24
☐ Extension Tubing (1)	$0.84
Medications:	
☐ Dexamethasone 10 mg/mL – 1 mL SDV (2)	$3.58
☐ Bupivacaine 0.25% – 10 mL SDV (1)	$1.04
☐ Omnipaque 240 mg/mL – 50 mL SDV (1)	$3.99
☐ Lidocaine 1% 50 mL MDV (7 mL)	$0.22
Total	$20.60

Medicare Reimbursement

CPT Code	Units	Modifier	Reimbursement:
64483	1	50	$345.08
64484	1	RT	$101.79
J1100	20		$2.05
Q9966	3		$0.99
Q9966	47	JW	$15.56
		Total	$465.47

Total Reimbursement	Total Supply Cost	Profit
$465.47	**$20.60**	**$444.87**

Gross Profit Margin

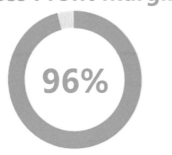

96%

Chapter 29

Expense & Revenue Analysis
Caudal & Lumbar Interlaminar Epidural Steroid Injection

<u>Caudal Epidural</u>

Expenses

		Cost:
Supplies:		
☐	Pain Pack (1)	$5.04
☐	Gloves Sterile size 7.5	$0.73
☐	Earloop Mask	$0.06
☐	Quincke (Spinal Needle) 22 Gauge 3.5" (1)	$1.08
☐	Extension Tubing (1)	$0.84
Medications:		
☐	Methylprednisolone 80 mg/mL – 1 mL SDV (1)	$13.93
☐	Preservative Free Normal Saline NaCl 0.9% – 10 mL SDV (1)	$0.55
☐	Bupivacaine 0.25% – 10 mL SDV (1)	$1.04
☐	Omnipaque 240 mg/mL – 50 mL SDV (1)	$3.99
☐	Lidocaine 1% 50 mL MDV (5 mL)	$0.16
	Total	$27.42

Medicare Reimbursement

CPT Code	Units	Modifier	Reimbursement:
62323	1		$248.26
J1040	1		$11.19
Q9966	2		$0.66
Q9966	48	JW	$15.79
		Total	$275.90

Total Reimbursement	Total Supply Cost	Profit
$275.90	**$27.42**	**$248.48**

Gross Profit Margin

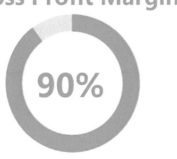

90%

Interlaminar ESI – Lumbar

Expenses

		Cost:
Supplies:		
☐	Pain Pack (1)	$5.04
☐	Gloves Sterile size 7.5	$0.73
☐	Earloop Mask	$0.06
☐	Tuohy 18 Gauge 3.5" Needle (1)	$2.74
☐	Loss of Resistance 10 mL Syringe	$1.60
☐	Extension Tubing (1)	$0.84
Medications:		
☐	Methylprednisolone 80 mg/mL – 1 mL SDV (1)	$13.93
☐	Preservative Free Normal Saline NaCl 0.9% – 10 mL SDV (1)	$0.55
☐	Omnipaque 240 mg/mL – 50 mL SDV (1)	$3.99
☐	Lidocaine 1% 50 mL MDV (5 mL)	$0.16
	Total	$29.64

Medicare Reimbursement

CPT Code	Units	Modifier	Reimbursement:
62323	1		$248.26
J1040	1		$11.19
Q9966	2		$0.66
Q9966	48	JW	$15.79
		Total	$275.90

Total Reimbursement	Total Supply Cost	Profit
$275.90	**$29.64**	**$246.26**

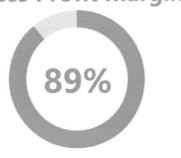

Gross Profit Margin

89%

Chapter 30

Expense & Revenue Analysis
Cervical & Thoracic
Interlaminar Epidural Steroid Injection

Interlaminar ESI – Cervical or Thoracic

Expenses

		Cost:
Supplies:		
☐	Pain Pack (1)	$5.04
☐	Gloves Sterile size 7.5	$0.73
☐	Earloop Mask	$0.06
☐	Tuohy 18 Gauge 3.5" Needle (1)	$2.74
☐	Loss of Resistance 10 mL Syringe	$1.60
☐	Extension Tubing (1)	$0.84
Medications:		
☐	Methylprednisolone 80 mg/mL – 1 mL SDV (1)	$13.93
☐	Preservative Free Normal Saline NaCl 0.9% – 10 mL SDV (1)	$0.55
☐	Omnipaque 240 mg/mL – 50 mL SDV (1)	$3.99
☐	Lidocaine 1% 50 mL MDV (5 mL)	$0.16
	Total	$29.64

Medicare Reimbursement

CPT Code	Units	Modifier		Reimbursement:
62321	1			$251.36
J1040	1			$11.19
Q9966	2			$0.66
Q9966	48	JW		$15.79
			Total	$279.00

Total Reimbursement	Total Supply Cost	Profit
$279.00	**$29.64**	**$249.36**

Gross Profit Margin

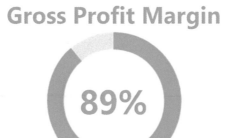

89%

Chapter 31

Expense & Revenue Analysis
Lumbar & Sacral
Facet Joint Injection/Medial Branch Block

MBB
Three Level Ipsilateral (Right) – Lumbar or Sacral

Expenses

	Cost:
Supplies:	
☐ Pain Pack (1)	$5.04
☐ Gloves Sterile size 7.5	$0.73
☐ Earloop Mask	$0.06
☐ Towels Disposable 4/pack (1)	$1.86
☐ Quincke (Spinal Needle) 22 Gauge 3.5" (4)	$4.32
☐ Extension Tubing (1)	$0.84
Medications:	
☐ Bupivacaine 0.25% – 50 mL MDV (2 mL)	$0.10
☐ Omnipaque 240 mg/mL – 50 mL SDV (1)	$3.99
☐ Lidocaine 1% 50 mL MDV (7 mL)	$0.22
Total	$17.16

Medicare Reimbursement

CPT Code	Units	Modifier		Reimbursement:
64493	1	RT		$168.89
64494	1	RT		$87.57
64495	1	RT		$87.57
Q9966	1			$0.33
			Total	$344.36

Total Reimbursement	**Total Supply Cost**	**Profit**
$344.36	$17.16	$327.20

Gross Profit Margin

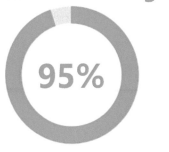

95%

MBB
Three Level (Bilateral) – Lumbar or Sacral

Expenses

	Cost:

Supplies:

	Cost:
☐ Pain Pack (1)	$5.04
☐ Gloves Sterile size 7.5	$0.73
☐ Earloop Mask	$0.06
☐ Towels Disposable 4/pack (1)	$1.86
☐ Quincke (Spinal Needle) 22 Gauge 3.5" (8)	$8.64
☐ Extension Tubing (1)	$0.84

Medications:

	Cost:
☐ Bupivacaine 0.25% – 50 mL MDV (4 mL)	$0.19
☐ Omnipaque 240 mg/mL – 50 mL SDV (1)	$3.99
☐ Lidocaine 1% 50 mL MDV (10 mL)	$0.32
Total	$21.67

Medicare Reimbursement

CPT Code	Units	Modifier		Reimbursement:
64493	1	50		$253.34
64494	1	50		$131.36
64495	1	50		$131.36
Q9966	2			$0.66
			Total	$516.72

Total Reimbursement	Total Supply Cost	Profit
$516.72	**$21.67**	**$495.05**

Gross Profit Margin

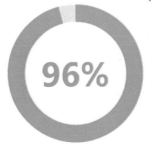

96%

<u>Facet Joint</u>
<u>Three Level (Bilateral) – Lumbar or Sacral</u>

Expenses

		Cost:
Supplies:		
☐	Pain Pack (1)	$5.04
☐	Gloves Sterile size 7.5	$0.73
☐	Earloop Mask	$0.06
☐	Towels Disposable 4/pack (1)	$1.86
☐	Quincke (Spinal Needle) 22 Gauge 3.5" (6)	$6.48
☐	Extension Tubing (1)	$0.84
Medications:		
☐	Triamcinolone 400 mg/10 mL MDV (2 mL)	$4.83
☐	Bupivacaine 0.25% – 50 mL MDV (4 mL)	$0.19
☐	Omnipaque 240 mg/mL – 50 mL SDV (1)	$3.99
☐	Lidocaine 1% 50 mL MDV (8 mL)	$0.25
	Total	$24.27

Medicare Reimbursement

CPT Code	Units	Modifier		Reimbursement:
64493	1	50		$253.34
64494	1	50		$131.36
64495	1	50		$131.36
J3301	8			$10.64
Q9966	2			$0.66
			Total	$527.36

Total Reimbursement	**Total Supply Cost**	**Profit**
$527.36	$24.27	$503.09

Gross Profit Margin

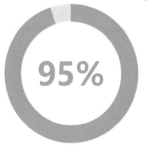

95%

Chapter 32

Expense & Revenue Analysis
Lumbar & Sacral
Radiofrequency Nerve Ablation

RFNA
Three Level Ipsilateral (Right or Left) – Lumbar or Sacral

Expenses

	Cost:
Supplies:	
☐ Pain Pack (1)	$5.04
☐ Gloves Sterile size 7.5	$0.73
☐ Earloop Mask	$0.06
☐ Radiofrequency Needle 18 Gauge 100 mm with 10 mm active tip (4)	$48.00
☐ Grounding Pad (1)	$8.00
☐ Towels Disposable 4/pack (2)	$3.73
☐ Tegaderm 4 x 4.75 (1)	$0.61
Medications:	
☐ Lidocaine 1% 50 mL MDV (10 mL)	$0.32
Total	$66.49

Medicare Reimbursement

CPT Code	Units	Modifier		Reimbursement:
64635	1	RT or LT		$405.40
64636	2	RT or LT		$331.24
			Total	$736.64

Total Reimbursement	**Total Supply Cost**	**Profit**
$736.64	$66.49	$670.15

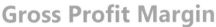

Gross Profit Margin

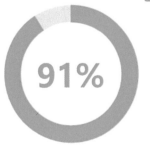

91%

¹*The cost of non-disposable RF electrodes are not included under "Expenses" since this is a one time non-recurring expense.*

Chapter 33

Expense & Revenue Analysis
Cervical & Thoracic
Facet Joint Injection/Medial Branch Block

MBB
Three Level Ipsilateral (Left) – Cervical or Thoracic

Expenses

		Cost:
Supplies:		
☐	Pain Pack (1)	$5.04
☐	Gloves Sterile size 7.5	$0.73
☐	Earloop Mask	$0.06
☐	Towels Disposable 4/pack (1)	$1.86
☐	Quincke (Spinal Needle) 22 Gauge 3.5" (4)	$4.32
☐	Extension Tubing (1)	$0.84
Medications:		
☐	Bupivacaine 0.25% – 50 mL MDV (2 mL)	$0.10
☐	Omnipaque 240 mg/mL – 50 mL SDV (1)	$3.99
☐	Lidocaine 1% 50 mL MDV (7 mL)	$0.22
	Total	$17.16

Medicare Reimbursement

CPT Code	Units	Modifier		Reimbursement:
64490	1	LT		$186.50
64491	1	LT		$94.54
64492	1	LT		$95.20
Q9966	1			$0.33
			Total	$375.05

Total Reimbursement	Total Supply Cost	Profit
$376.57	**$17.16**	**$359.41**

Gross Profit Margin

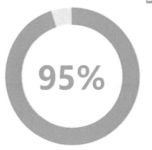

95%

Facet Joint
Three Level Ipsilateral (Right) – Cervical or Thoracic

Expenses	Cost:
Supplies:	
☐ Pain Pack (1)	$5.04
☐ Gloves Sterile size 7.5	$0.73
☐ Earloop Mask	$0.06
☐ Towels Disposable 4/pack (1)	$1.86
☐ Quincke (Spinal Needle) 22 Gauge 3.5" (3)	$3.24
☐ Extension Tubing (1)	$0.84
Medications:	
☐ Triamcinolone 400 mg/10 mL MDV (1 mL)	$2.41
☐ Bupivacaine 0.25% – 50 mL MDV (2 mL)	$0.10
☐ Omnipaque 240 mg/mL – 50 mL SDV (1)	$3.99
☐ Lidocaine 1% 50 mL MDV (7 mL)	$0.22
Total	$18.49

Medicare Reimbursement

CPT Code	Units	Modifier	Reimbursement:
64490	1	RT	$186.50
64491	1	RT	$94.54
64492	1	RT	$95.20
J3301	4		$5.32
Q9966	1		$0.33
		Total	$381.89

Total Reimbursement	Total Supply Cost	Profit
$381.89	**$18.49**	**$363.40**

Gross Profit Margin

95%

Chapter 34

Expense & Revenue Analysis
Cervical & Thoracic
Radiofrequency Nerve Ablation

RFNA
Three Level Ipsilateral (Left) – Cervical or Thoracic

Expenses

		Cost:
Supplies:		
☐	Pain Pack (1)	$5.04
☐	Gloves Sterile size 7.5	$0.73
☐	Earloop Mask	$0.06
☐	Radiofrequency Needle 18 Gauge 100 mm with 10 mm active tip (4)	$48.00
☐	Grounding Pad (1)	$8.00
☐	Towels Disposable 4/pack (2)	$3.73
☐	Tegaderm 4 x 4.75 (1)	$0.61
Medications:		
☐	Dexamethasone 10 mg/mL – 1 mL SDV (1)	$1.79
☐	Lidocaine 1% 50 mL MDV (10 mL)	$0.32
	Total	$68.28

Medicare Reimbursement

CPT Code	Units	Modifier		Reimbursement:
64633	1	LT		$410.08
64634	2	LT		$363.48
J1100	10			$1.02
			Total	$774.58

Total Reimbursement	**Total Supply Cost**	**Profit**
$774.58	**$68.28**	**$706.30**

Gross Profit Margin

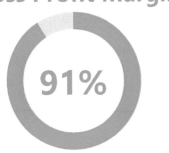

91%

¹*The cost of non-disposable RF electrodes are not included under "Expenses" since this is a one time non-recurring expense.*

Chapter 35

Expense & Revenue Analysis
Sacroiliac Joint Radiofrequency Nerve Ablation

RFNA
Sacroiliac Joint (Right)

Expenses

		Cost:
Supplies:		
☐	Pain Pack (1)	$5.04
☐	Gloves Sterile size 7.5	$0.73
☐	Earloop Mask	$0.06
☐	Radiofrequency Needle 18 Gauge 100 mm with 10 mm active tip (6)	$72.00
☐	Palisade Guide Block	$85.00
☐	Towels Disposable 4/pack (2)	$3.73
☐	Tegaderm 4 x 4.75 (1)	$0.61
Medications:		
☐	Lidocaine 1% 50 mL MDV (10 mL)	$0.32
	Total	$167.49

Medicare Reimbursement

CPT Code	Units	Modifier		Reimbursement:
64625	1	RT		$485.35
			Total	$485.35

Total Reimbursement	Total Supply Cost	Profit
$485.35	**$167.49**	**$317.86**

Gross Profit Margin

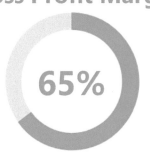

65%

¹*The cost of non-disposable RF electrodes are not included under "Expenses" since this is a one time non-recurring expense.*

Chapter 36

Expense & Revenue Analysis
Sacroiliac Joint Injection

<u>SI Joint</u>
<u>(Right or Left)</u>

Expenses

Supplies:	Cost:
☐ Pain Pack (1)	$5.04
☐ Gloves Sterile size 7.5	$0.73
☐ Earloop Mask	$0.06
☐ Quincke (Spinal Needle) 22 Gauge 3.5" (1)	$1.08
☐ Extension Tubing (1)	$0.84

Medications:	
☐ Triamcinolone 400 mg/10 mL MDV (1 mL)	$2.41
☐ Bupivacaine 0.25% – 50 mL MDV (1 mL)	$0.05
☐ Omnipaque 240 mg/mL – 50 mL SDV (1)	$3.99
☐ Lidocaine 1% 50 mL MDV (5 mL)	$0.16
Total	$14.36

Medicare Reimbursement

CPT Code	Units	Modifier	Reimbursement:
27096	1	RT or LT	$158.19
J3301	4		$5.32
Q9966	1		$0.33
		Total	$163.84

Total Reimbursement	Total Supply Cost	Profit
$163.84	**$14.36**	**$149.48**

Gross Profit Margin

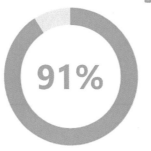

91%

SI Joint
(Bilateral)

Expenses

		Cost:
Supplies:		
☐	Pain Pack (1)	$5.04
☐	Gloves Sterile size 7.5	$0.73
☐	Earloop Mask	$0.06
☐	Quincke (Spinal Needle) 22 Gauge 3.5" (2)	$2.16
☐	Extension Tubing (1)	$0.84
Medications:		
☐	Triamcinolone 400 mg/10 mL MDV (2 mL)	$4.83
☐	Bupivacaine 0.25% – 50 mL MDV (2 mL)	$0.10
☐	Omnipaque 240 mg/mL – 50 mL SDV (1)	$3.99
☐	Lidocaine 1% 50 mL MDV (5 mL)	$0.16
	Total	$17.91

Medicare Reimbursement

CPT Code	Units	Modifier		Reimbursement:
27096	1	50		$237.29
J3301	8			$10.64
Q9966	1			$0.33
			Total	$248.26

Total Reimbursement	**Total Supply Cost**	**Profit**
$248.26	$17.91	$230.35

Gross Profit Margin

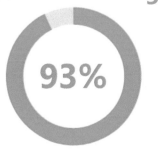

93%

Chapter 37

Expense & Revenue Analysis
Intercoccygeal Joint Injection

Intercoccygeal Joint

Expenses

		Cost:
Supplies:		
☐	Pain Pack (1)	$5.04
☐	Gloves Sterile size 7.5	$0.73
☐	Earloop Mask	$0.06
☐	Quincke (Spinal Needle) 22 Gauge 3.5" (1)	$1.08
☐	Extension Tubing (1)	$0.84
Medications:		
☐	Triamcinolone 400 mg/10 mL MDV (1 mL)	$2.41
☐	Bupivacaine 0.25% – 50 mL MDV (1 mL)	$0.05
☐	Omnipaque 240 mg/mL – 50 mL SDV (1)	$3.99
☐	Lidocaine 1% 50 mL MDV (3 mL)	$0.10
	Total	$14.30

Medicare Reimbursement

CPT Code	Units	Modifier		Reimbursement:
20605	1			$52.22
77003	1			$96.44
J3301	4			$5.32
Q9966	1			$0.33
			Total	$154.31

Total Reimbursement	**Total Supply Cost**	**Profit**
$154.31	$14.30	$140.01

Gross Profit Margin

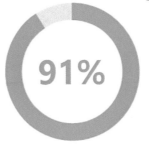

91%

Chapter 38

Expense & Revenue Analysis
Spinal Cord Stimulation (Neuromodulation)

<u>SCS</u>
<u>Single Lead</u>

Expenses

		Cost:
Supplies:		
☐	Pain Pack (1)	$5.04
☐	Gloves Sterile size 7.5	$0.73
☐	Earloop Mask	$0.06
☐	Towels Disposable 4/pack (2)	$3.73
☐	Trial Lead Kit 50 cm (1)	$150.00
☐	OR Cable and Extension (1)	$1.00
☐	Patient Trial Kit (1)	$1.00
☐	Coude Epidural Needle 14 Gauge 4" (1)	$1.00
☐	Loss of Resistance 10 mL Syringe	$1.60
☐	Steri-strips 1/8" x 3" (1)	$0.82
☐	Tegaderm 4 x 4.75 (1)	$0.61
Medications:		
☐	Lidocaine 1% 50 mL MDV (10 mL)	$0.32
	Total	$165.91

Medicare Reimbursement

CPT Code	Units	Modifier		Reimbursement:
63650	1			$1,820.51
95972	1	59		$56.89
			Total	$1,877.4

Total Reimbursement	Total Supply Cost	Profit
$1,877.40	**$165.91**	**$1,711.49**

Gross Profit Margin

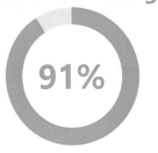

91%

<u>SCS</u>
<u>Two Leads</u>

Expenses

Supplies:	Cost:
☐ Pain Pack (1)	$5.04
☐ Gloves Sterile size 7.5	$0.73
☐ Earloop Mask	$0.06
☐ Towels Disposable 4/pack (2)	$3.73
☐ Trial Lead Kit 50 cm (2)	$300.00
☐ OR Cable and Extension (2)	$2.00
☐ Patient Trial Kit (1)	$1.00
☐ Coude Epidural Needle 14 Gauge 4" (2)	$2.00
☐ Loss of Resistance 10 mL Syringe	$1.60
☐ Steri-strips 1/8" x 3" (1)	$0.82
☐ Tegaderm 4 x 4.75 (1)	$0.61

Medications:	
☐ Lidocaine 1% 50 mL MDV (10 mL)	$0.32
Total	$317.91

Medicare Reimbursement

CPT Code	Units	Modifier	Reimbursement:
63650	2		$2,730.77
95972	1	59	$56.89
		Total	$2787.66

Total Reimbursement	Total Supply Cost	Profit
$2,787.66	**$317.91**	**$2,469.75**

Gross Profit Margin

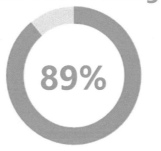

89%

<u>SCS</u>
<u>Three Leads</u>

Expenses

	Cost:
<u>Supplies:</u>	
☐ Pain Pack (1)	$5.04
☐ Gloves Sterile size 7.5	$0.73
☐ Earloop Mask	$0.06
☐ Towels Disposable 4/pack (2)	$3.73
☐ Trial Lead Kit 50 cm (1)	$150.00
☐ Trial Lead Kit 70 cm (2)	$300.00
☐ OR Cable and Extension (3)	$3.00
☐ Patient Trial Kit (1)	$1.00
☐ Coude Epidural Needle 14 Gauge 4" (3)	$3.00
☐ Loss of Resistance 10 mL Syringe	$1.60
☐ Steri-strips 1/8" x 3" (2)	$1.65
☐ Tegaderm 4 x 4.75 (2)	$1.22
<u>Medications:</u>	
☐ Lidocaine 1% 50 mL MDV (10 mL)	$0.32
Total	$471.35

Medicare Reimbursement

CPT Code	Units	Modifier		Reimbursement:
63650	3			$3,641.02
95972	1	59		$56.89
			Total	$3,697.91

Total Reimbursement	Total Supply Cost	Profit
$3,697.91	**$471.35**	**$3,226.68**

Gross Profit Margin

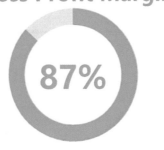

87%

Chapter 39

Expense & Revenue Analysis
Large & Intermediate Joint/Bursa Injection

Large Joint/Bursa
(Left)

Expenses

		Cost:
Supplies:		
☐	Pain Pack (1)	$5.04
☐	Gloves Sterile size 7.5	$0.73
☐	Earloop Mask	$0.06
☐	Quincke (Spinal Needle) 22 Gauge 3.5" (1)	$1.08
☐	Extension Tubing (1)	$0.84
Medications:		
☐	Triamcinolone 400 mg/10 mL MDV (1 mL)	$2.41
☐	Bupivacaine 0.25% – 50 mL MDV (4 mL)	$0.19
☐	Omnipaque 240 mg/mL – 50 mL SDV (1)	$3.99
☐	Lidocaine 1% 50 mL MDV (3 mL)	$0.10
	Total	$14.44

Medicare Reimbursement

CPT Code	Units	Modifier	Reimbursement:
20610	1	LT	$62.12
77002	1		$102.87
J3301	4		$5.32
Q9966	1		$0.33
		Total	$170.64

Total Reimbursement	**Total Supply Cost**	**Profit**
$170.64	$14.44	$156.20

Gross Profit Margin

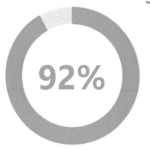

92%

Large Joint/Bursa
(Bilateral)

Expenses	
	Cost:
Supplies:	
☐ Pain Pack (1)	$5.04
☐ Gloves Sterile size 7.5	$0.73
☐ Earloop Mask	$0.06
☐ Quincke (Spinal Needle) 22 Gauge 3.5" (2)	$2.16
☐ Extension Tubing (1)	$0.84
Medications:	
☐ Triamcinolone 400 mg/10 mL MDV (2 mL)	$4.83
☐ Bupivacaine 0.25% – 50 mL MDV (8 mL)	$0.39
☐ Omnipaque 240 mg/mL – 50 mL SDV (1)	$3.99
☐ Lidocaine 1% 50 mL MDV (5 mL)	$0.16
Total	$18.20

Medicare Reimbursement				
				Reimbursement:
CPT Code	**Units**	**Modifier**		
20610	1	50		$93.18
77002	1			$102.87
J3301	8			$10.64
Q9966	2			$0.66
			Total	$207.35

Total Reimbursement	**Total Supply Cost**	**Profit**
$207.35	$18.20	$189.15

Gross Profit Margin

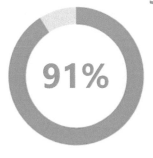

91%

Intermediate Joint/Bursa
(Right)

Expenses

	Cost:
Supplies:	
☐ Pain Pack (1)	$5.04
☐ Gloves Sterile size 7.5	$0.73
☐ Earloop Mask	$0.06
☐ Quincke (Spinal Needle) 22 Gauge 3.5" (1)	$1.08
☐ Extension Tubing (1)	$0.84
Medications:	
☐ Triamcinolone 400 mg/10 mL MDV (0.5 mL)	$1.21
☐ Bupivacaine 0.25% – 50 mL MDV (0.5 mL)	$0.02
☐ Omnipaque 240 mg/mL – 50 mL SDV (1)	$3.99
☐ Lidocaine 1% 50 mL MDV (1 mL)	$0.03
Total	$13.00

Medicare Reimbursement

CPT Code	Units	Modifier	Reimbursement:
20605	1	RT	$52.22
77002	1		$102.87
J3301	2		$2.66
Q9966	1		$0.33
		Total	$158.08

Total Reimbursement	**Total Supply Cost**	**Profit**
$158.08	$13.00	$145.08

Gross Profit Margin

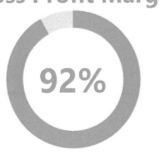

92%

Chapter 40

Expense & Revenue Analysis
Ganglion of Impar Injection

Ganglion of Impar

Expenses

	Cost:
Supplies:	
☐ Pain Pack (1)	$5.04
☐ Gloves Sterile size 7.5	$0.73
☐ Earloop Mask	$0.06
☐ Quincke (Spinal Needle) 22 Gauge 3.5" (1)	$1.08
☐ Extension Tubing (1)	$0.84
Medications:	
☐ Methylprednisolone 80 mg/mL – 1 mL SDV (1)	$13.93
☐ Bupivacaine 0.25% – 50 mL MDV (7 mL)	$0.34
☐ Omnipaque 240 mg/mL – 50 mL SDV (1)	$3.99
☐ Lidocaine 1% 50 mL MDV (3 mL)	$0.10
Total	$26.11

Medicare Reimbursement

CPT Code	Units	Modifier	Reimbursement:
64520	1		$222.81
J1040	1		$11.19
Q9966	2		$0.66
		Total	$234.66

Total Reimbursement	**Total Supply Cost**	**Profit**
$234.66	$26.11	$208.55

Gross Profit Margin

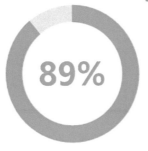

89%

Chapter 41

Expense & Revenue Analysis
Piriformis Muscle Injection

Piriformis Muscle
(Left)

Expenses

	Cost:
Supplies:	
☐ Pain Pack (1)	$5.04
☐ Gloves Sterile size 7.5	$0.73
☐ Earloop Mask	$0.06
☐ Quincke (Spinal Needle) 22 Gauge 3.5" (1)	$1.08
☐ Extension Tubing (1)	$0.84
Medications:	
☐ Triamcinolone 400 mg/10 mL MDV (1 mL)	$2.41
☐ Bupivacaine 0.25% – 50 mL MDV (4 mL)	$0.19
☐ Omnipaque 240 mg/mL – 50 mL SDV (1)	$3.99
☐ Lidocaine 1% 50 mL MDV (3 mL)	$0.10
Total	$14.44

Medicare Reimbursement

CPT Code	Units	Modifier	Reimbursement:
20552	1	LT	$53.47
77002	1		$102.87
J3301	4		$5.32
Q9966	1		$0.33
		Total	$161.99

Total Reimbursement	Total Supply Cost	Profit
$161.99	**$14.44**	**$147.55**

Gross Profit Margin

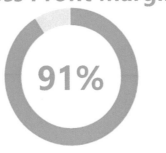

91%

Appendix A

Procedural Supply Costs

22G x 3.5" Spinal Needle	$107.52/#100
22G x 5" Spinal Needle	$63.76/#25
22G x 7" Spinal Needle (Reli)	$65.80/#25
18G x 3.5" Tuohy Needle	$68.42/#25
18G x 5" Tuohy Needle	$112.09/#25
ᵗPain Pack	$161.23/#32
LOR Syringe 10 cc	$80.09/#50
Extension Tubing 8"	$42.00/#50
Tegaderm 4x4.75	$30.48/#50
ChloraPrep 3 mL	$26.26/#25
Towels 17x27 4/pk	$37.25/#80
Gloves Latex 7.5 - Encore	$36.70/#50
Gloves Latex Free 7.5 - Gammex	$59.76/#50
18G x 15 cm RF Needle	$12.00/#1
18G x 10 cm RF Needle	$12.00 #1
Grounding Pad	$40/#5

SCS Supply Costs

Trial Lead Kit 50 cm	$150.00/#1
Trial Lead Kit 70 cm	$150.00/#1
OR Cable and Extension	$1.00/#1
Patient Trial Kit	$1.00/#1
Epimed Coude Needle	$1.00/#1

Medication Costs

Dexamethasone 10 mg/mL	$1.79/(1 mL vial)
Methylprednisolone 80 mg/mL	$13.93/(1 mL vial)
Triamcinolone 400 mg/10 mL	$24.13/(10 mL vial)
ᵗOmnipaque 240 mg/ml - 50 mL	$3.99/(50 mL vial)
NaCl 0.9% Preservative Free - 10 mL	$0.55/(10 mL vial)
Lidocaine 1% MDV - 50 mL	$1.59/(50 mL vial)
Bupivacaine 0.25% SDV - 10 mL	$1.04/(10 mL vial)
Bupivacaine 0.25% MDV - 30 mL	$1.19/(30 mL vial)
Bupivacaine 0.25% MDV - 50 mL	$2.41/(50 mL vial)

ᵗ Contents include Syringe 5 ml (1), Syringe 10 mL (1), Syringe 3 mL (1), Gauze (4), Needle counter (1), Drape (1), Needle 27Gx1.5" (1), Needle 18Gx1.5" (3), Chlorhexidine applicator (2)

ᴴ In some instances, higher volume vials have a lesser cost than smaller volume vials. In such scenarios, the most cost effective vial is presented.

Appendix B

Modifiers

11	Reduced Fee Amount 11
16	Reduced Fee Amount 16
17	Reduced Fee Amount 17
22	Unusual procedural services
23	Unusual anesthesia
24	Unrelated evaluation and management service by the same physician during a postoperative period
25	Significant, separately identifiable evaluation and management service by the same physician on the same day of the procedure or other service
26	Professional component
27	Multiple outpatient hospital e/m encounters on the same date
32	Mandated services
33	Preventive service when the Primary purpose of the service is the delivery of an evidence bases service
47	Anesthesia by surgeon
50	Bilateral procedure
51	Multiple procedures
52	Reduced services
53	Discontinued procedure
54	Surgical care only
55	Postoperative management only
56	Preoperative management only
57	Decision for surgery
58	Staged or related procedure or service by the same physician during the postoperative period
59	Distinct procedural service
62	Two surgeons
63	Procedure performed on infants less than 4 kg
66	Surgical team
73	Discontinued out-patient hospital/ambulatory surgery center (asc) procedure prior to the administration of anesthesia
74	Discontinued out-patient hospital/ambulatory surgery center (asc) procedure after administration of anesthesia
76	Repeat procedure by same physician
77	Repeat procedure by another physician
78	Return to the operating room for a related procedure during the postoperative period
79	Unrelated procedure or service by the same physician during the postoperative period
80	Assistant surgeon

81	Minimum assistant surgeon
82	Assistant surgeon (when qualified resident surgeon not available)
90	Reference (outside) laboratory
91	Repeat clinical diagnostic laboratory test
95	Synchronous Telemed Service Via Real-Time Interactive Audio and Video Telecom System
96	Habilitative Services
97	Rehabilitative Services
99	Multiple modifiers
JW	Drug/Biological amount discarded/not administered
LT	Left side
RT	Right side

Index

V

Made in the USA
Las Vegas, NV
11 January 2022

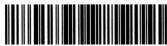

40934640R00202